RESPITE CARE

RESPITE CARE
SUPPORT FOR PERSONS WITH DEVELOPMENTAL DISABILITIES AND THEIR FAMILIES

Edited by

Christine L. Salisbury, Ph.D.
Assistant Professor
Division of Professional Education
University Center at Binghamton
State University of New York

and

James Intagliata, Ph.D.
Formerly, Director of Research
University Affiliated Facility
University of Missouri-Kansas City

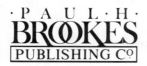

·P A U L·H·
BROOKES
PUBLISHING Cº

Baltimore • London

Paul H. Brookes Publishing Co.
Post Office Box 10624
Baltimore, Maryland 21285-0624

Typeset by The Composing Room, Grand Rapids, Michigan.
Manufactured in the United States of America by
The Maple Press Company, York, Pennsylvania.

Library of Congress Cataloging-in-Publication Data
Main entry under title:

Respite care.

    Includes bibliographies and index.
    1. Developmentally disabled children—Respite care—Addresses,
essays, lectures.   2. Respite care—Addresses, essays, lectures.
    3. Developmentally disabled children—Family relationships—Addresses,
essays, lectures.   I. Salisbury, Christine L., 1951–   II.
Intagliata, James. [DNLM: 1. Child Development Disorders.
2. Family.   3. Respite Care. WS 350.6 R434]
HV891.R47   1986   362.4′048′088054   85-29076
ISBN 0-933716-60-5 (pbk.)

CONTENTS

CONTRIBUTORS

Jan Blacher, Ph.D.
Associate Professor
School of Education
University of California
Riverside, CA 92521

Harriet Horowitz Bongiorno
3010 Yale Street
Endwell, NY 13760

Paul J. Castellani, Ph.D.
Director of Program Research
New York State Office of Mental
   Retardation/Developmental
   Disabilities
44 Holland Avenue
Albany, NY 12229

Paul D. Cotten, Ph.D.
Director
Boswell Retardation Center
P.O. Box 128
Sanatorium, MS 39112

Noreen Quinn Curran
Advocacy Associates
33-A Harvard Street, Suite 201
Brookline Village, MA 02146

Barbara Coyne Cutler, M.Ed.
APT Project
Autism Services Association
99 School Street
Weston, MA 02193

Andrew L. Egel, Ph.D.
Department of Special Education
University of Maryland
College Park, MD 20742

Janet T. Ferguson, M.S.W.
Lindsay/Ferguson Associates
2324 West Main Street
Kalamazoo, MI 49007

Darald Hanusa, M.S.W.
Harry A. Waisman Center on Mental
   Retardation
University of Wisconsin
Madison, WI 53706

James Intagliata, Ph.D.
Management Consultant
1160 South Clinton Avenue
Oak Park, IL 60304

Matthew P. Janicki, Ph.D.
Director of Planning
New York State Office of Mental
   Retardation/Developmental
   Disabilities
44 Holland Avenue
Albany, NY 12229

Marty Wyngaarden Krauss, Ph.D.
Director
Social Science Research
Eunice Kennedy Shriver Center
Waltham, MA 02254

Joel M. Levy, CSW, F.A.A.M.D.
Executive Director
Young Adult Institute and Workshop,
   Inc.
460 West 34th Street
New York, NY 10001

Philip H. Levy, Ph.D.
Associate Executive Director
Young Adult Institute and Workshop,
  Inc.
460 West 34th Street
New York, NY 10001

Sally A. Lindsay, M.A.
Lindsay/Ferguson Associates
2324 West Main Street
Kalamazoo, MI 49007

Nancy A. Neef, Ph.D.
Assistant Professor
Division of Education
The Johns Hopkins University
Baltimore, MD 21212

Peggy Ogle, Ph.D.
Department of Special Education
University of Maryland
College Park, MD 20742

J. Macon Parrish, Ph.D.
Director of Training and Outpatient
  Services
Department of Behavioral Psychology
The John F. Kennedy Institute
and
Assistant Professor
Department of Psychiatry
The Johns Hopkins University School
  of Medicine
707 North Broadway
Baltimore, MD 21205

Thomas H. Powell, Ed.D.
Connecticut's University Affiliated
  Program
School of Education
The University of Connecticut
Storrs, CT 06268

Phyllis Prado, M.S.
Formerly, Coordinator
UCLA Project on Severely Impaired
  Young Children and Their Families
Mental Retardation Research Center,
  NDI
University of California
Los Angeles, CA 90024

Christine L. Salisbury, Ph.D.
Assistant Professor
Division of Professional Education
University Center at Binghamton
State University of New York
Binghamton, NY 13901

Marsha Mailick Seltzer, Ph.D.
Associate Chairperson and
  Professor/Research Sequence
Boston University
School of Social Work
264 Bay State Road
Boston, MA 02215

Mary A. Slater, Ph.D.
Assistant Professor of Pediatrics
Texas Tech University Health Sciences
  Center
Amarillo, TX 79106-1797

Judy Stoycheff, R.N.
Harry A. Waisman Center on Mental
  Retardation
University of Wisconsin
Madison, WI 53706

Lynn McDonald Wikler, ACSW, Ph.D.
Assistant Professor
School of Social Work
and
Waisman Center on Mental Retardation
  and Human Development
425 Henry Mall
University of Wisconsin
Madison, WI 53706

FOREWORD

This book is about providing respite care to families who have a member with a disability. Respite care refers to services provided to families to enable them to take a break from the responsibility of caring for a member with a disability. That member may be a child, middle-age adult, or an elderly person. Respite care can best be understood from the perspective of the families who need it. The following excerpt from the *Lawrence Journal World* (a newspaper in Lawrence, Kansas) describes a community-based respite care program and, in particular, a child and family who benefited from it:

> Carol Schaub, Trinity board member and mother of client Becky Schaub, confirms the difficulty of finding specially trained people like the Trinity volunteer who stays with her 13-year-old handicapped daughter.
>
> Becky does not walk or talk, so the person who stays with her must be able to anticipate her needs and wants, Mrs. Schaub says.
>
> Becky was born with a severe lack of muscle tone and since January has been struggling with respiratory failure. An oxygen unit stands ready near her bed, and a nurse from the Douglas County Visiting Nurses Association keeps the vigil every night while she sleeps. Anyone caring for Becky must know how to connect oxygen to her tracheostomy.
>
> Becky's respite caregiver is her primary teacher at Cordley School, Tami Connor. Like many Trinity volunteers, Ms. Connor brings to this work specialized professional background in service to persons with handicaps.
>
> Mrs. Schaub explains, "We've worked with Tami very extensively in the school system and for a while, we were doing home training in physical therapy as well.
>
> Tami is very willing to take on a very big responsibility. Not many people are.
>
> For the first time since Becky was hospitalized last winter, Mrs. Schaub and her husband, Sherry, were planning a "respite" weekend to take their 19-year-old daughter to her summer job.
>
> Becky was to be cared for during the daytime by Ms. Connor and during the night by the visiting nurse. The Schaub's 14-year-old daughter, also well versed in Becky's care, would be home too.
>
> "We're going to try it again," Mrs. Schaub says.

The prospect makes her nervous but, she explains, since Becky got sick it's been very difficult to balance her needs which can be critical, with the needs of their two other daughters.

We can extract major points and principles from this "window" into family life. Some of these include:

- Parents experience difficulty in locating people who are competent in responding to the needs of their child.
- Many people are unwilling to assume the responsibility of respite care.
- Parents place great value on developing trust and confidence in the care provider.
- Parents of children with disabilities often go for extended periods of time without a break from their caregiving responsibilities.
- Leaving a child with a careprovider can create anxiety for parents.
- Families need assistance in balancing the needs of all family members.

Facts like these have led to respite care becoming a cornerstone of family support services.

Are you a family member or professional interested in enhancing family well-being by exploring the benefits that can be derived from respite care? If so, we want to highlight for you why we think this book can be a helpful resource. We believe it can provide you with answers to the most important questions about respite care. Some of the questions addressed in this book for which you will be able to find answers include:

- Why do families with a member having a disability need additional support beyond that available through personal and social support networks?
- What are the financial disincentives for families when they keep members with a disability at home as contrasted to placing them in institutional settings?
- What models are available for individualizing respite care according to the unique needs of a family?
- How can respite care serve as a preventive measure to buffer stress in a family?
- What are the relevant issues in providing respite care to persons at various points of the lifespan?
- Does respite care accomplish what it purports to accomplish?
- What research is available on the impact of respite care?

The editors of this book, Chris Salisbury and Jim Intagliata, have distinguished themselves nationally as leading experts on the topics of respite services and family adjustment. They are eminently qualified to synthesize the literature in this important area. Furthermore, they have selected an outstanding cast of authors who have the credentials and expertise to address their topics. The result of this synergistic effort is a book whose "whole is greater than the sum of its parts." This book represents state-of-the-art knowledge on respite care and surpasses any other source as a comprehensive, substantive, and relevant compilation.

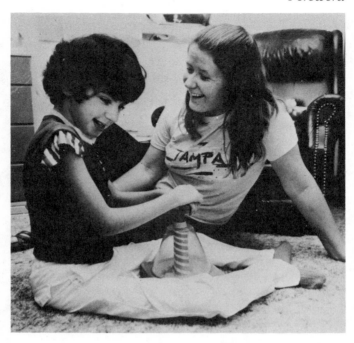

We have benefited greatly from reading this book, and we believe that you will, too. The ultimate beneficiaries of this book, however, should be families like the Schaubs in Lawrence, Kansas, and in every other town across the nation. We must be ever mindful that respite care is a *means* rather than an *end* in itself. It is a means to enhancing quality of life for families and persons with disabilities. The extent to which respite services actually enhance quality of life will probably depend as much on the relationship that is established between the careprovider and the family as anything else. The models, research, training programs, staffing patterns, and other important aspects of respite care are critically important and must be solidly investigated and developed; however, the ultimate key is likely to be in the affective realm of relationship. We urge you, as you participate in respite experiences with families and persons with disabilities, to strive first and foremost to establish a human and supportive relationship, which is what enhanced quality of life is all about. Becky Schaub and Tami Connor experienced the magic of relationship. Look at their photograph above and see for yourself.

Ann P. Turnbull, Ed.D.
Holly Anne Benson, M.Ed.
Bureau of Child Research
and
Department of Special Education
University of Kansas
Lawrence

PREFACE

The need of families for support in general and for respite care in particular has emerged as one of the most important issues to be addressed in the 1980s by policymakers, service providers, and researchers in the field of developmental disabilities. Although families of persons with developmental disabilities have always been in need of support, the salience of this need has emerged more and more dramatically as the system of care has gradually shifted to a community-based orientation. A major tenet of this community-based service system is the value and importance of being able to maintain individuals with developmental disabilities in the homes of their natural families. As a result of deinstitutionalization efforts, more families than ever before are now attempting to meet the needs of children with more severe disabilities in their own homes. These facts, along with a more general societal concern about the stability of the family, have resulted in the issue of family support services occupying a high-priority on the policy agenda at the federal, state, and local levels.

This book represents an effort to respond to the growing need for information on respite care and family support services by providing readers with a perspective on the rationale for and design and evaluation of respite care programs. It is intended to enable readers to understand more clearly the specific needs that these services are attempting to address, the variety of program models that are available, and the key factors that need to be considered not only when developing and implementing respite care programs, but also when assessing their value and impact. In an effort to present the broadest and most useful perspective on respite care, the editors purposefully solicited a collection of authors who represent a wide variety of relevant viewpoints on respite services. Included are those of policymakers, program developers and implementers, researchers, and also parents of individuals with developmental disabilities. By sharing these multiple perspectives, the editors hope that readers will not only broaden their understanding, but improve their ability to make a more significant contribution to the development of services that support families most effectively.

This volume has been organized into three major sections: 1) rationale and need for respite services, 2) issues and models for delivering respite services, and 3) evaluating respite services.

PART I: RATIONALE AND NEED

In Chapter 1, Salisbury provides a broader context within which to understand the significance of respite services for persons with developmental disabilities. She does this by reviewing the literature on the impact of the birth of any child on a family unit, giving special attention to the research on family stress and the role that social support and networks play in helping families to cope and adjust. She highlights the special stresses and demands placed on families of children with developmental disabilities and concludes by describing the importance of respite services as an essential type of support needed by these families.

In Chapter 2, Powell and Ogle provide an in-depth look at the impact that a child with developmental disabilities has on other siblings in the family, and the various factors that influence the nature and magnitude of this impact. They point out the special needs of, and types of adjustments required by, siblings of a person with developmental disabilities. They close by highlighting not only the critical functions that respite services can serve for siblings but also the special role that siblings can play in serving as a lifelong support to their brother or sister with developmental disabilities.

In Chapter 3, Janicki, Krauss, Cotten, and Seltzer discuss the special respite care needs of the growing population of older adults with developmental disabilities. They point out that program planners must begin to give far greater attention to developing the particular types of respite care and other kinds of support services needed by this older population. They suggest that such services will play a crucial role in helping to maintain these individuals in their present natural-family and age-integrated community residential settings.

In Chapter 4, Slater offers a view of the national perspective on respite care for families with children with developmental disabilities. She presents and reviews the results of a number of statewide respite care surveys as well as national surveys of respite care programs and of broader-ranging family support programs in which respite care is but a part. She discusses the major findings of these surveys and highlights the need for developing not only a wide array of formal supportive services for families but also family support programs that give family members greater control in determining their primary needs as well as opportunities to meet these needs in as normalized a fashion as possible.

In Chapter 5, Curran and Bongiorno bring Part I to a conclusion by providing their individual perspectives on the need for and value of respite care based on their own experience as parents of children with developmental disabilities.

PART II: ISSUES AND MODELS

In Chapter 6, Levy and Levy present an overview of the range of respite care models that are currently in use both for in-house and out-of-house respite. They also briefly discuss some fiscal issues and considerations regarding respite care. They conclude by describing their experience with the development of a community respite care program in the New York metropolitan area and emphasize a number of specific issues that must be faced by anyone who is developing or delivering respite care services.

In Chapter 7, Parrish, Egel, and Neef provide a model for respite care provider training that utilizes a competency-based approach. They make the important point that the quality of training provided to respite care workers is a crucial element in the success of any respite care program. The key to the competency-based approach that they describe is its emphasis on participants acquiring and maintaining behavioral skills in contrast to a focus on the provision of general information designed to improve attitude or increase knowledge.

In Chapter 8, Ferguson and Lindsay provide a detailed description of the Respite Care Co-op Program that was begun in Kalamazoo, Michigan. This unique approach enables parents of children with developmental disabilities to join together to develop their own cooperative respite care service and support group as they need and want it. This program model is strongly parent directed with professionals playing a more supportive and facilitating role. The authors discuss what it takes to make the program work, its potential problems and pitfalls, and its unique benefits for participating parents and families.

In Chapter 9, Cutler describes another specific approach to providing respite services—a community-based respite residence program. She offers this model as an important respite alternative, especially for meeting the needs of families with children, adolescents, or adults who have severe behavioral or medical problems. She points out that unless respite alternatives such as the respite community residence are developed to meet the specific special needs of the most severely disabled and underserved population, there is a high risk that such individuals may be institutionalized when their natural family support system can no longer cope.

In Chapter 10, Salisbury develops the premise that integrated, generic community services, while not specifically designed to provide respite care, offer an important untapped source of respite for families of individuals with developmental disabilities. She discusses the need for and value of integrating persons with developmental disabilities into generic community service programs. She concludes by identifying the major factors that presently impede such integration and by discussing how these barriers might be overcome.

In Chapter 11, Blacher and Prado provide a comprehensive look at the role that public schooling plays in providing respite for all families, with or without a handicapped child. They discuss how PL 94-142, the Education for All Handicapped Children Act, has resulted in parents of handicapped children (even those with severe disabilities) being freed from the burden of care for a significant portion of each weekday. In addition, these parents are also now able to interact with school or day care teachers who became important informational and personal supportive resources on whom they can rely.

In Chapter 12, Curran and Bongiorno conclude Part II of this volume by once again sharing their personal perspectives as parents of individuals with developmental disabilities. In their comments, they identify what characteristics of respite care programs they feel are most influential in affecting parents' use of and comfort with respite care. They pay particular attention to ease of access, cost, and the selection and training of the individuals who serve as respite care workers.

PART III: EVALUATING RESPITE SERVICES

In Chapter 13, Wikler, Hanusa, and Stoycheff present process evaluation as a method for better understanding the ways in which respite care may function to alleviate the stresses of families with developmentally disabled children. Two examples of process evaluation are described, one focusing on monitoring changes in the behavior problems of the child and the other on the stress levels of each family. In closing, they emphasize not only the need to offer respite care services that are uniquely tailored to the circumstances of particular families, but also the need to incorporate a process focus into evaluations so that the individual nuances of each family's personal experiences can be more carefully observed and understood.

In Chapter 14, Intagliata presents a comprehensive review of outcome evaluation studies of respite services. In order to systematize the review and to guide the development and design of future outcome studies, he introduces a conceptual framework that identifies key independent, intervening, and outcome variables that must be considered in respite care research. After evaluating the degree to which currently available evaluation data substantiates the beneficial impacts of respite care, he closes the chapter by presenting a number of significant issues and problems that remain to be addressed by those engaged in the design, administration, and evaluation of respite care programs.

In Chapter 15, Castellani presents an analysis of the central issues that must be addressed in developing policies to guide the provision of respite services. He discusses the fact that respite care services expand the thrust of services to include not only the individual with developmental disabilities but also the family and the resulting difficulties that this presents for policymakers and legislators. He also addresses the issues regarding how such services can be funded and how explicit, equitable mechanisms need to be developed for making choices among those demanding what are likely to be limited respite services.

In Chapter 16, Curran and Bongiorno close the book by sharing their personal perspective on the individual and family impact of respite services. Both parents emphasize the important role that respite has or might have played in their lives and strongly encourage other parents to make active use of such a supportive resource in order to alleviate stress and prevent "burnout."

This book departs from previous texts on respite care (McGee, Smith, & Kenney, 1982; Raub, 1982; Warren & Dickman, 1981) in that it places the design, development, and evaluation of respite services within the broader context of the theory and research on family stress, adaptation, and coping. Although respite services are being expanded on a national level to include the frail elderly, chronically ill, and mentally ill populations, the editors have chosen to restrict the content to respite services for children with developmental disabilities and their families. There are generic features of the processes and information contained in this volume that transcend populations. Consequently, individuals working with groups other than persons with developmental disabilities may well find this a useful text. The chapters that follow provide a broad base of information from the personal and professional vantage points of each of the contributors.

REFERENCES

McGee, J.J., Smith, P.M., & Kenney, M. (1982). *Giving families a break: Strategies for respite care*. Omaha, NE: Media Resource Center, Meyer Children's Rehabilitation Institute.

Raub, M.J. (1982). *How to start a respite program*. Sacramento: State of California Council on Developmental Disabilities.

Warren, R., & Dickman, I.R. (1981). *For this respite, much thanks*. New York: United Cerebral Palsy Association, Inc.

To the memory of my Dad—
who by his example taught me great lessons
in compassion and optimism. And,
For Chuck, Melissa, Brett, Mom, Jan, and Tony—
whose love and support has helped me to
understand what "family" is all about.

CS

To Shari—
for her constancy of love and support.

JI

Part I

RATIONALE AND NEED FOR RESPITE SERVICES

Chapter 1

PARENTHOOD AND THE NEED FOR RESPITE

Christine L. Salisbury

Entry into parenthood creates structural and functional changes in the family unit (Hill, 1949; Hobbs, 1965; Jacoby, 1969; LeMasters, 1957; Rollins & Galligan, 1978). Behavioral changes in the dynamics of the family are generally considered to be stressful, particularly for families with younger, rather than older, children (Boss, 1980; Hoffman & Manis, 1978; Howard, 1978; Lamb, 1978; Neugarten, 1976). Parents typically rely on their own coping responses, intrafamilial assistance, and extrafamilial social supports to mitigate the effects of parenting stressors (McCubbin, Joy, Cauble, Comeau, Patterson, & Needles, 1980; Miller & Sollie, 1980). However, as Rollins and Galligan (1978) point out, questions remain regarding the factors that influence the magnitude of the stresses of becoming a parent.

To set the proper normative context for studying the stress experienced by families who have a child with developmental disabilities, it is important to understand the birth of any child as a stressor that produces some level of disorganization within the family unit. If we can understand the patterns of stress and coping found within any family that must adapt to the birth of a new child, we can better understand the dynamics of those families with an atypical child. This information has implications for the development of both generic and specialized supportive services for these families.

This book addresses the concept of respite for families with children who have developmental disabilities. Despite its relatively recent emergence as a special topic in the literature, respite care is being increasingly recognized for its potential as a crucial resource and special type of social support to families with dependent members. By delineating the relationships between respite services and the literature dealing with parenting stress and social support, this chapter lays the framework for understanding the significance of respite services.

SOCIAL SUPPORT AND SOCIAL NETWORKS

The quality of support received from social support networks plays a key role in mitigating the effects of stress; examining this support shifts the emphasis from why families fail to how families succeed (McCubbin & Boss, 1980). Social networks consist of relationships with neighbors, family and kin, co-workers, and other acquaintances who interact with the individual or family (McCubbin et al., 1980; Unger & Powell, 1980). Research findings support the inclination of individuals to draw on informal support resources in a time of need. This pattern prevails even when formal resources are available and are specifically designed to address the individual's presenting problem (Unger & Powell, 1980). Consequently, it cannot be assumed that individuals will be knowledgeable about or choose to use community resources in meeting family problems.

Social networks provide instrumental, emotional, and referral and information functions to individuals and families (Cobb, 1976; McCubbin et al., 1980; Unger & Powell, 1980). To understand better the relationship of atypical children, stress, and supportive resources to family functioning, it is useful to review the impact of and adaptation to the birth and development of the nonhandicapped child.

PARENTING THE NONHANDICAPPED CHILD

Impact of the Child

Family Structure and Roles Family interactions occur within the context of the family's structure and the roles that individual members assume in meeting the regulatory needs of the family unit (Boss, 1980; Minuchin, 1974). The established patterns of interactions and role delineation, as well as the overall balance in family functioning, are generally upset by the transition into parenthood and the arrival of a new family member. Roles and relationships must be adjusted to compensate for the added responsibilities associated with the birth of the child. Research on parenthood suggests that stress results from lack of role clarity, variability in expectations between husband and wife, and role overload (Aldous, 1978; Burr, 1970). A recurring theme in the literature on typical families is the normalcy of stress in parenthood and the concomitant buffering of its effects through various adaptive responses.

Several researchers have described a relationship between family size and parental stress (Bossard & Boll, 1956; Knox & Wilson, 1978). In these studies, as family size grew, there were increases in family tensions, demands on parents' finite time and energies, and physical exhaustion, and reductions in the amount of time spent on housework and community participation. These effects appear to be less pronounced with the addition of later children and with movement along the life cycle of the family (Hoffman & Manis, 1978).

Greater levels of stress are generally reported by single parents. Research on the relationship between marital status and parenting reveals that single parents are more socially isolated, receive less emotional and familial support, have less stable social networks, and are at greater risk for economic hardship (McLanahan, 1983; Weintraub & Wolf, 1983; Wikler, Haack, & Intagliata, 1984). Families headed by a female are more likely to be in a lower-income bracket than families headed by a male. Women more frequently lack the job skills, child care, and community support necessary to surmount the economic obstacles to self-sufficiency. The "emotional overload" that accrues from the social, economic, and psychological hardships of single parenthood often results in increased stress and depression (Burden, 1980).

The parent's relation to the child appears to influence perceptions of the parenting experience. Research by Miller and Sollie (1980) revealed that new mothers report higher stress than new fathers, and wives are more likely than husbands to view their marriages as changing in a negative way. This report and others indicate that mothers assume more responsibility for child rearing, perceive themselves as having less social support, and view the parenting experience with more mixed feelings, particularly in the early years (Hoffman & Manis, 1978; Rollins & Galligan, 1978).

Ragozin, Basham, Crnic, Greenberg, and Robinson (1982) provide a different view of the parenting experience. Their investigation found that parenting roles were significantly related both to maternal age and role satisfaction. Increased maternal age was related to greater satisfaction with parenting, increases in caregiving roles, and decreased time away from the child. Taken together with previous research, this study indicates that mothers appear to make an adjustment over time to the roles and responsibilities of parenthood.

Quality of Life   Several researchers have investigated the impact of children on the quality of the marital relationship and overall family functioning. Marital satisfaction appears to decrease markedly with the birth of the first child and is less affected by the arrival of later children (Hoffman & Manis, 1978; Rollins & Galligan, 1978). Although research has not convincingly supported the description of early parenthood as a "crisis" situation, considerable data are available to substantiate the increase in tensions, anxiety, and marital strain occurring at that time (LeMasters, 1957; Miller & Sollie, 1980; Spanier, Lewis, & Cole, 1975).

Hoffman and Manis (1978) conducted a well-controlled national study of the effects of children on the marital relationship. Loss of freedom was the most frequently cited disadvantage stated by parents of young, nonhandicapped children. However, some of the parents conceptualized this loss as movement toward maturation and adulthood, whereas others perceived it as a burden. Financial disadvantages and concerns about the child's health and safety were also frequently mentioned by parents. These concerns were perceived as having less impact as the child grew older.

Despite the preponderance of negative statements by young parents, their evaluation of parenthood was primarily positive. Parents tended to view the children as strengthening the marriage, providing a symbol of unity, and affording them opportunities for shared joy. Parents of older children similarly evaluated the experience as a predominantly positive one, involving periods of adjustment and increasing marital harmony. Research by Russell (1974) and others on reactions to parenthood support the findings of Hoffman & Manis's study.

Child Characteristics Age of the child can influence the relative amount of stress experienced by parents. Theoretical and empirical studies suggest a relationship between stress and the development of the child over time: Stress occurs in young families when significant adaptation is required on both functional and structural levels within the family due to the arrival of the new child (Boss, 1980; Duvall, 1972; Hoffman & Manis, 1978; Rapoport, 1963; Rollins & Galligan, 1978). As the child matures, the family system faces structural and functional changes brought on by such events as school entry, adolescence, graduation, and marriage. Each family development stage creates stress as a result of changes in family membership, relationships, and roles. Transition into life cycle stages is also presumed to produce stress (cf. Boss, 1980), although data on such processes are limited. Burr's (1970) research suggested that adolescence was a time in the life cycle when marital satisfaction, financial management, sex, and allocation of household tasks were at their lowest points.

The association among family change, child rearing, and stress has not been disputed in the literature. However, the variables associated with the production of stress are increasingly being seen from a multivariate, rather than univariate, perspective. Consequently, adjustment to parenthood must be viewed as an interaction among personal, family, and community variables (Korn, Chess, & Fernandez, 1978; Lerner & Spanier, 1978). The following section provides a brief summary of the coping and adaptation responses employed by parents of normally developing children.

Adaptation to the Nonhandicapped Child

Coping and adaptation in families with nonhandicapped children are accomplished through the use of resources both internal and external to the family. The internal stresses of the family, although controllable to some degree by family size and spacing of children, are also linked to the life stage and the family's configuration (Bell, Johnson, McGillicuddy-Delisi, & Sigel, 1980). McCubbin, Boss, and Wilson (cited in Miller & Sollie, 1980, p. 32) noted that successful adaptation to stress involves resources internal to the family (i.e., integration and adaptability) and the use of coping strategies to strengthen organization and functioning, including the utilization of community and social supports.

Social networks are most often analyzed in terms of their size, boundary density, and network density. Network size is predictive of more positive adjustment when individuals are the target of study (Wilcox, 1981). In general, the larger the social network, the greater the likelihood of successful coping and adaptation. Network density refers to the extent to which members of an individual's social network know each other, independent of the target person. Density provides a measure of the interrelatedness of the network. High-density networks may foster a close, supportive environment, or when high degrees of consensus exist among the network members, they may stifle independent action. Large, less dense networks are generally associated with positive adjustment (Caplan, 1982; Hirsch, 1980; Wilcox, 1981). Boundary density is a measure of the membership overlap between two or more individuals. Moderate levels of shared network members are associated with positive adjustment (Bott, 1971), whereas tightly linked (i.e., high density) networks can contribute to poor postdivorce adjustments (Wilcox, 1981). The extended family can incite stress and stimulate family conflict (Ackerman, 1963). Divergent expectations for social participation can also create marital conflict, as can the demands for reciprocity inherent in informal aid-giving arrangements (Garigue, 1956; Unger & Powell, 1980).

Research reviewed by Dunst, Trivette, and Cross (1986) indicates that married mothers who are involved in "tightly knitted" social networks expressed satisfaction with their domestic and maternal roles (Abernathy, 1973; Bott, 1971). Investigations of unmarried mothers suggest that support from social networks is generally unrelated to maternal role satisfaction. Dunst and colleagues concluded that "the extent to which increased role responsibility resulting from nonpresence of a spouse is lessened by extra-family support appears minimal" (p. 6). Such information may have significant bearing on the focus of intervention services with single parents.

Recent research by Ventura and Boss (1983) conducted with parents of new babies revealed three principal coping factors or patterns among the parents: 1) seeking social support and self-development, 2) maintaining family integrity, and 3) being religious, thankful, and content. Mothers reported using more of the 28 component coping strategies than did fathers. Fathers reported engaging in social activities to be more helpful in reducing parenthood stress than did mothers. Coping patterns of seeking social support and maintaining family integrity were found to be affected by sex of the respondent in a replication of Ventura and Boss's procedures with an additional 100 families. Differences were found for sex of child, with parents of boys reporting greater use of the coping behaviors for maintaining family integrity. Comparisons between families in which the newborn was the first child and in which it was a later-born child revealed no significant differences in the use of coping patterns. This study indicates that active strategies are employed by both parents in reducing the normative stressors associated with parenthood.

Education and attempts at increasing individual preparedness for parenthood can influence the prospective parent's self-confidence. Parents in Miller and Sollie's (1980) study indicated that learning to be more flexible, learning to be better organized, continuing some activities that were engaged in before the birth of the child, and sharing caregiving responsibilities were important strategies for adapting to parenthood stress. In addition, many respondents utilized neighbors and friends as social supports for advice, information, and caregiving of the child. These parents emphasized the importance for both the husband and the wife of taking time away from the baby. One of the most stressful aspects of parenthood, particularly for the wife, was the problem of balancing motherhood and a career. This finding is supported by research into dual-career families (Skinner, 1980) and the integrative writings of Lamb (1978).

Social networks within the community can also be used to enhance family adaptation and coping. Geismar (1971) links family well-being to community resources. Community support provides two types of aid: 1) primary provisions for survival and maintenance of a minimal level of social functioning and 2) secondary provisions to facilitate social participation, social control, mobility, social and political expression, and adequate living arrangements (cited in McCubbin et al., 1980, p. 864). Consequently, the quality of the community's resources plays a key role in supporting families at both the primary and secondary levels. Insufficient services can be expected to produce hardships for families attempting to meet potentially stressful life events.

There appears to be a prescriptive relationship between when and how networks are used by families under stress. Research suggests that high-contact neighborhood networks tend to be utilized for short-term emergencies, whereas kin groups are used for long-term commitments (Litwak & Szelenyi, 1969). Network density and frequency of contact appear to be positively related to extent of help received and the effectiveness of the network. These relationships are characterized as supplementary in that they augment the resources available within the family system. Informal networks are also used by families and individuals to provide advice and information that can eventually link them to formalized community resources (Freidson, 1960). However, the use and diversity of social networks can also be influenced by the cultural values, peer groups, ethnicity, and religious affiliation of user groups (Unger & Powell, 1980). Consequently, although patterns have been identified in the literature, providers of support services must assess the family's network on an *a priori* basis and throughout the intervention process to ensure that anticipated outcomes are indeed realized.

Considerable research indicates that social support has positive mediational effects on personal and familial well-being (Bott, 1971; McCubbin et al., 1980; Mitchell & Trickett, 1980), and can influence attitudes toward parenting (Ragozin et al., 1982), parent-child interaction patterns (Embry, 1980; Hetherington, Cox, & Cox, 1978; Weintraub & Wolf, 1983) and child development outcomes (Crockenberg, 1981; Ragozin et al., 1982). The broad potential influence of social support on the milieu of the family makes it particularly attractive as a target for intervention.

Despite the existence and use of need-meeting resources, there are times when families appear to lack recuperative power. As McCubbin et al. (1980) point out, problems will likely surface when the family is facing other life changes, and there is a "pile up" or cumulative effect of life stressors. In this case, typical resources are insufficient to enable the family to cope with additional changes. Families have been characterized as vulnerable when significant acute (e.g., short-term emergencies, such as death of spouse) and chronic (e.g., long term commitments, such as caring for a dependent family member) events drain the resources of the family unit, producing high levels of unresolved stress (McCubbin et al., 1980). In these situations, social support and social network resources can mediate the effects of stress and can promote the family's recovery from crisis (Geismar, 1971; McCubbin et al., 1980; Unger & Powell, 1980).

PARENTING THE HANDICAPPED CHILD

Recent research has begun to examine the complex interactive relationship of child, family, and social network variables as contributors to and mediators of stress (Beckman, 1983; Blacher, 1984; Howard, 1978; Korn et al., 1978; Salisbury, 1984; Turnbull, Summers, & Brotherson, 1983; Wright, Granger, & Sameroff, 1984). By placing the birth and development of the handicapped child within the theoretical and empirical framework of normative child-rearing stresses, the role of child, family, and community characteristics can be further examined in an attempt to understand better the family's adjustment to the handicapped child.

Impact of the Child

Family Structure and Roles   Throughout the literature, amount of care-giving demands and the concomitant disruption of family routines appear as recurring factors associated with increased stress in families with handicapped members (Beckman-Bell, 1981; Blacher, 1984; Bristol, 1979; Bristol &

Schopler, 1984; Cummings, 1976; Dunlap & Hollingsworth, 1979; Gallagher, Cross, & Scharfman, 1981; Gath, 1973; Korn et al., 1978; McAndrew, 1976; Salisbury, 1985; Seltzer & Krauss, 1984; Tausig, 1985; Wikler, 1981). The prolonged dependency of chronically ill and developmentally disabled children requires parents to do more for them for longer periods of time than is required for parents of nonhandicapped children. Disruption of family routines can occur because of intensive time demands posed by the handicapped infant (Gabel, McDowell, & Cerreto, 1983). The duration of basic care, coupled with the diverse medical, physical, and behavioral needs of the child, creates increased stress in these families.

Stress is reported to be even higher in single-parent families with handicapped children (Beckman, 1983; Dunst et al., 1986, Holroyd, 1974; Salisbury, 1985; Wikler et al., 1984), and with mothers than with fathers (Price-Bonham & Addison, 1978). The relationship between single parenthood and child-rearing stress is a complex one, clouded by the interplay of reduced economic and social support resources. Although significant differences between mothers and fathers have been reported on measures of stress (Bradshaw & Lawton, 1978; Burden, 1980; Holroyd, 1974; Salisbury, 1985), research also suggests elevated anxiety levels among fathers (Cummings, 1976). Clearly, additional research is needed before statements about the psychosocial health and dysfunction of parents of these children can be made.

Siblings of handicapped children, particularly sisters, are often depicted as being at greater risk for adjustment problems (Cairns, Clark, Smith, & Lansky, 1978; Gath, 1978; Tew & Lawrence, 1973). However, many of these reports obtained data from parents of the siblings, rather than from the siblings themselves. A more optimistic view of family functioning and sibling relationships is presented by other researchers (Caldwell & Guze, 1960; Cleveland & Miller, 1977; Lavigne & Ryan, 1979). As with the mother-father data, additional research is needed before definitive trends can be discerned.

Quality of Life   The presence of a handicapped child has historically been regarded as a source of stress and impairment to family functioning (Beckman-Bell, 1981; Farber, 1959, 1960; Fotheringham & Creal, 1974; Fowle, 1968; Gath, 1977; Holroyd, 1974; McAndrew, 1976; Satterwhite, 1978; Schonell & Watts, 1956; Wikler, 1981). These studies suggest that the presence of the child is related to financial problems, social isolation, marital discord, sibling adjustment problems, restrictions on family activities, health problems, household disorganization, and disruptions of relationships with family and friends. Investigations have focused on the global impact of the child on family functioning. This proliferation of studies on global impact has unfortunately typecast families with handicapped children as "doomed to dysfunction." Such a position fails to account for those families who are coping and adjusting to life with a handicapped member, as well as for the myriad of factors that contribute to stress and coping in individual families.

It has long been assumed that the presence of a handicapped child has a deleterious effect on marital integration. Although data have been reported on higher-than-normal divorce rates (Love, 1973; Tew, Lawrence, Payne, & Rawnsley, 1977) and increased marital discord (Featherstone, 1980; Gath, 1977), several investigations refute the presumption of negative impact (Dorner, 1975; Farber, 1959; Fotheringham, Skelton, & Hoddinott, 1972; Fowle, 1968; Korn et al., 1978; Starr, 1981; Vance, Fazan, Satterwhite, & Pless, 1980; Waisbren, 1980). These studies indicate that parental discord, divorce rates, and impaired marital integration are no greater than in the general population. Consequently, the overestimation of negative impact common among professionals (Blackard & Barsch, 1982) perpetuates a myth founded more on emotional perception and clinical impressions than on empirical evidence.

Comparative research, such as the examples provided below, provides preliminary evidence to substantiate the presence of increased levels of stress in families with handicapped children. However, the limited data base precludes our ability to judge the effectiveness of coping and adaptation among these families. Consequently, where these families fall relative to the general population of parents coping with same age children is not clear. Additional comparative research is desperately needed in order to understand better the continuum of adaptation among families and the parallels that exist with parents of normally developing children.

Satterwhite (1978) studied families with chronically ill children and found reported increases in financial worries, marital friction, concern about child health, and interruptions in family travel plans. However, when a sample of families with chronically ill children was compared with a sample of matched controls with healthy children, no significant differences were found (Vance et al., 1980).

Ruhe (1984) compared the distribution and amount of time spent by mothers of young nonhandicapped, mildly handicapped, and severely handicapped children in leisure, home care and child care activities during school and vacation times. Measures of stress, coping, and perceived quality of life were administered in conjunction with structured interviews. Mothers of severely handicapped children spent significantly more time in child care and expended more time with that child relative to the amount of time spent with other children in the family. Amount of time spent in child care was positively related to higher stress and negatively related to scores on the coping measure. Despite these findings, there were no significant differences between the three groups on perceived quality of life or on time spent on leisure or home care activities. Mothers of severely handicapped children in this sample were apparently adjusting to a life-style of higher stress and reduced coping resources. However, they did not perceive themselves as socially constrained or as having a poorer quality of life. Small sample size and broad domain definitions were acknowledged limitations in this study that may have obscured group differences on the questionnaire measures.

Friedrich and Friedrich (1981) surveyed 34 mothers of handicapped and nonhandicapped children ranging in age from 2 to 16 years of age, using a variety of measures. The handicapped children were rated as functioning in the mild and moderate ranges of retardation. Mothers of handicapped children reported less marital satisfaction, less social support, less religiosity, and poorer psychological well-being than their counterparts. The authors highlighted the fact that the mothers of handicapped children "not only appear to report more stress . . . but also fewer psychosocial assets to help ameliorate the continual impact of this stress" (p. 553). The authors emphasized the need for community social support resources to mitigate the effects of child-rearing stresses in families with handicapped children.

Salisbury (1985) investigated the nature of stress in a sample of families with young (ages 2 months to 4 years) handicapped and nonhandicapped children drawn from regular and special education preschools in four metropolitan-rural communities. Mothers and fathers completed the adapted version (Salisbury, 1986) of the Questionnaire on Resources and Stress-Short Form (Holroyd, 1982). Results revealed significantly greater levels of stress for parents of handicapped children. These differences were attributable to stresses regarding the long-term care, physical limitations, and cognitive development of their child. Single parents of handicapped children reported more stress when the child's physical caregiving needs were high. Single parents in both groups reported more stress than did their married counterparts. Parents of handicapped children were no more likely than those with nonhandicapped children to report problems in marital integration or personal well-being. Thus, although young handicapped children pose significant concerns for their parents, the spillover effects of these worries to other aspects of family life appear minimal.

Child Characteristics Researchers have examined the handicapped child's characteristics in an attempt to determine more clearly potential sources of stress. Parents of handicapped children report increased stress when the child is older (Bristol & Schopler, 1984; Farber, 1959; Suelze & Keenan, 1981; Wikler, Wasow, & Hatfield, 1981); more severely handicapped (Beckman, 1983; Saenger, 1965; Vickers, 1968); and male (Saenger, 1965). These studies suggest that inherent, unalterable child characteristics play a significant role in the production of stress for some families. Yet, the absence of comparative research and description of adaptive responses by families who appear to be coping restricts our ability to draw conclusions about the populations of families with dependent children.

The link between the child's level of functioning and the multiplicity of caregiving demands is a logical and empirically supported one (cf. Beckman-Bell, 1981; Bristol & Schopler, 1984). Yet, the stresses within these families are not necessarily correlated with the severity of the child's condition (Bradshaw & Lawton, 1978; Burden, 1980), nor is there evidence that there will be concomitant dysfunction in the marital relationship (Longo & Bond, 1984). As Korn et al. (1978) observed in their sample of rubella children, "marital discord specifically due or related to the handicapped child is relatively infrequent among the parents in our . . . sample" (p. 324). Rather, Korn and colleagues linked family disruption to the excessive care demands of the children.

The chronicity of the child's handicapping condition, coupled with the often higher level of caregiving demands, is viewed as placing long-term, extraordinary stress on the family unit. This chronic recurring need to adapt and confront the permanence of the child's handicap has been addressed by other authors (cf. Olshansky, 1962; Turnbull et al., 1983; Wikler, 1981). However, the role of social networks in reducing the burden of care in these families has not been adequately examined. Consequently, there are few data on the mediating effects of social support for families with high-demand children. However, the needs expressed by these families are known. Respite from caregiving demands, time to engage in personal and social activities, and time to spend with spouse and other children are ranked high on the list of critical needs expressed by these parents (Blacher, 1984; Bristol & Schopler, 1984; Ruhe, 1984; Salisbury, 1984; Seltzer & Krauss, 1984).

The relationship of age of the handicapped child to stress in families with handicapped children has only recently been addressed. Salisbury (1984) examined stress in 189 families with handicapped children in broad pre-school, school-age, and postschool-age groupings. Significant differences in parent stress were found between age groups on matters related to life-span care, cognitive impairment, pessimism, and financial stress. Pessimism and concern over care of their aging disabled son or daughter were greatest in parents of postschool-age children. Consistent with previous literature, the school-age years were a time when financial hardships were felt most. Concern over the developmental prognoses of their child was greatest in families with young handicapped children. Methodological limitations restrict the generalizability and interpretation of results from this pilot study.

Bristol and Schopler (1984) reported evidence of life-cycle changes in the stressors affecting families with autistic-like children. Their research indicates a shift from physical fatigue in the early years to concerns about emerging sexuality and growing independence in the adolescent years. The similarity of this trend to families with nonhandicapped children was noted by the authors. However similar these trends may be, the families with autistic-like children also faced stresses associated with the permanency of their child's handicap, battles for services, and life-planning decisions (Bristol & Schopler, 1984).

The stress reaction, chronic sorrow, and crisis theories used to investigate the impact of handicapped children on the family unit help explain the process of reaction to stress and the concomitant distress families experience, but not the process of adaptation. A majority of the studies represent a linear, cause-and-effect interpretation of stress and dysfunction within these families. That high levels of stress exist in some of these families as a function of life stage, child characteristics, economic conditions, and/or marital status does not necessarily mean that these families are not coping. The equivocal nature of the stress research and the dearth of information on the interaction of support and family characteristics allow only preliminary statements to be made about the impact of these children on family functioning. In contrast, research on adaptation and coping may provide a clearer conceptual framework for understanding parenthood in families with dependent members.

Adaptation to the Handicapped Child

Schilling, Gilchrist, and Schinke (1984) observed that "some families manage with resolve and competence while others barely survive the daily routine" (p. 48). The social competence of families, in large part, determines their relative success in seeking and using social support and coping strategies. Social competence is reflected in how families approach and resolve stressful situations. Within the past decade, researchers in the fields of sociology and psychology have investigated personal coping and social supports in families of handicapped and chronically ill children. More recently, investigations have been undertaken to describe the nature of the social networks available to families with special needs children. Data from these investigations provide information on variables perceived by families as important in their adjustment to life with a dependent child and those factors that correlate with enhanced ability to respond to stressor situations.

Intimate support from a spouse has been associated with enhanced adjustment to a disabled child. Friedrich (1979) administered a variety of stress, social support, and demographic measures to a sample of 98 mothers of handicapped children. Feeling secure in the marital relationship was the most significant variable associated with reduced stress of the mothers. This finding supports previous research with parents of handicapped children on the role of marital stability in facilitating adaptation to stress (cf. Farber, 1960; Gath, 1978) and the importance of mutual support inherent in a two-parent relationship (cf. Beckman, 1983; Bristol & Schopler, 1984).

The personal coping strategies of 100 parents of cystic fibrosis children were revealed in a recent study by Venters (1981). Parents employed a range of cognitive strategies to diminish the stress associated with their child's illness. Results indicated that two factors affecting family cohesion—communication and satisfaction—were also good predictors of successful adaptation to the child's illness. Effectively sharing the burden with family members and the family's ability to make philosophical sense out of the experience emerged as major coping strategies for these families. Venters determined that families functioned best when both internal and external supports were used to cope with and adjust to the child's chronic illness.

Bristol (in press-a) assessed the adaptation of families with autistic and nonautistic handicapped children. The Moos Family Environment Scale and the Coping Health Inventory for Parents (McCubbin & Patterson, 1981) were used to evaluate dimensions of family relationships and personal coping strategies. Families who supported one another, who were able to express their emotions, and who participated in outside social activities scored better than families who were more restricted and less supportive. Mothers reported that an education program offered the greatest support and that interpersonal relationships were valuable in coping with their child's handicap. Coping scores were significantly related to interviewer ratings of family adaptation. Highest stress scores were reported by mothers of high-demand children, who experienced diminished employment opportunities and unavailability of child care services.

In a follow-up investigation, Bristol (in press-b) studied family adaptation and informal social support. Adaptation was more strongly linked to perceived social support than to the severity of the child's handicapping condition. Mothers who perceived strong support from the husband reported fewer depressive symptoms, happier marriages, and better adaptation to the autistic child. Linking mothers to others who have similar children, either on an informal/local level or through a national support organization, was viewed as an important intervention strategy that might serve to reduce stresses in these families.

Social support, marital satisfaction, parenting, and personal stress were investigated in 56 families with spina bifida children and a cohort of 53 families with same age, nonhandicapped children (Kazak & Marvin, 1984). Measures of stress, marital adjustment, and social network dimensions were conducted using self-report and interview procedures. Mothers of handicapped children reported significantly more stress than all other parents in the sample. There were, however, no differences between groups on marital satisfaction. In fact, subscale analyses suggested that parents of the spina bifida children experienced greater satisfaction with levels of affection and degree of consensus. Stress in the spina bifida families was related directly to parenting issues. The handicapped children required more care, were less rewarding for the mothers, and contributed to elevated levels of maternal depression. Families of the handicapped children had significantly smaller, more tightly linked, and overlapping social networks than did their nonhandicapped counterparts. However, stress was not correlated with size of the social network.

Drawing on the entire data base, Kazak and Marvin (1984) noted the relative exclusion of the father from the parenting subsystem and his apparent integral role in the spousal relationship. They concluded that "while such a family structure deviates from the norm, and probably generates some further stress itself, it may also function as an efficient and adaptive solution to the pressures inherent in raising a handicapped child" (p. 74). Because network size was determined to be unrelated to any of the major stress measures employed in this study, Kazak and Marvin further concluded that network size reflects neither the quality nor the effectiveness of the network.

Gallagher, Cross, and Scharfman (1981) investigated the characteristics of parents who appear to have made a successful adjustment to the birth of a handicapped child. They hypothesized that social support would be a key factor discriminating between "successful" and "average" groups of parents. The data suggested that major sources of strength were internal supports (i.e., the personal characteristics of the parents and the quality of the husband-wife relationship). No significant differences were found between groups on stress, social support, or family roles. Both mothers and fathers agreed that the father should play a more active role in the family, but parents appeared to lack information on how to accomplish this role differentiation.

Division of roles and its impact on family functioning were pursued by Gallagher, Scharfman, and Bristol (1984) in a follow-up investigation of parents of preschool handicapped and nonhandicapped children. A rating scale was devised to assess actual and desired allocations of responsibility and the parents' degree of satisfaction with this division. Results revealed no significant difference between actual allocation of responsibilities expressed by husbands and wives with handicapped and nonhandicapped children. Additionally, there was a high degree of consensus between husbands and wives within each group on task allocations. As with previous research, mothers in both groups expressed a desire for greater involvement by the father. Adjustment to a preschool handicapped child appears to parallel adjustment to nonhandicapped children to a striking degree.

Socioeconomic status of the family is frequently identified as a critical variable associated with the availability of need-meeting resources. Rabkin and Streuning (1976) suggested that socioeconomic status can affect the magnitude of a stressor's impact, although not necessarily the frequency of its occurrence. Adaptation and coping strategies in disadvantaged families with handicapped children have not been reported in the literature. Rather, the economic variable has been studied from two vantage points—as an inherent stressor and as one that affects the family's ability to respond to stressor events (Bayley & Schaefer, 1960; Ramey, Mills, Campbell, & O'Brien,

1975). The relationship between available resources and stress is used to infer family ability to respond, but not how the family, in fact, does respond. In general, research investigations support the vulnerability of disadvantaged families to interpersonal and familial dysfunction, but have not yet focused on or revealed the processes of adjustment employed by these families.

Dunst et al. (1986) investigated the relationship of social support to personal and family well-being in 131 families of Appalachian and non-Appalachian handicapped preschool children. Self-report measures of stress and social support were administered to both groups of parents. Dunst and colleagues hypothesized that cultural and economic differences between the groups would manifest themselves in differential use of informal support resources. Their results indicated that social supports can mediate well-being, can lessen the distress typically attributed to the rearing of a handicapped child, and can do so with disregard for cultural, economic, and educational differences of the parents. More importantly, results of their research revealed that "social support generally accounts for more of the variance in terms of emotional-related problems than did the child's level of intellectual retardation" (p. 19). In addition, the findings also indicated that unavailability of social support did not adversely affect personal and familial well-being. One might surmise that parents find a way to cope and adjust, despite an apparently weak social support network.

The utilization of personal and professional social support networks was investigated by Suelzle and Keenan (1981). Parents of mentally retarded children in the preschool, elementary, teenage, and young adult years completed a mailed questionnaire. In general, parents of younger children utilized more services and support networks and were more supportive of integrated educational experiences. Parents of older children were found to be more isolated, less supported, and more in need of expanded services. The decline in unmet need for respite and counseling during the school-age years was contrasted with the great need expressed by parents of preschoolers and young adults who had completed school. This finding parallels the role of public schools as a provider of respite services (see Chapter 11).

Although additional studies have corroborated the tendency for families of handicapped children to have smaller social networks than families with nonhandicapped children (Friedrich & Friedrich, 1981; McAllister, Lei, & Butler, 1973), network size and density appear unrelated to the effectiveness of the network itself (Kazak & Marvin, 1984).

Despite this fact, many families with developmentally disabled children still face problems in identifying (Wikler, 1984), gaining access to (Salisbury & Griggs, 1983; Upshur, 1982b) and utilizing (Intagliata & Doyle, 1984; Wikler, 1981) social support resources. Many of these problems are related to attitudinal, geographic, economic, and training barriers (see Chapter 10).

It appears that many families of handicapped children are enduring greater levels of stress than exist in the general population. Given the lack of clear empirical support, it seems inappropriate to label these levels of stress as "extraordinary" or the compensatory responses and life-styles of the families as "deviant." Perhaps parents of handicapped children alter their perception of what constitutes a good quality of life to accommodate the realities of rearing special needs children. Thus, they cope and adjust because their tolerance for stress may have been toughened by the continuing demands of their child. They do so with the assistance of smaller, yet effective, social support networks. That they should continue to be restricted in their options for support is the central issue of this book. Clearly they should not.

Recently, researchers have suggested that families, as well as handicapped children, should be the targets of intervention services (Gallagher et al., 1984; Intagliata & Doyle, 1984; Kazak & Marvin, 1984; Lyon & Preis, 1983; Schilling et al., 1984; Sherman & Cocozza, 1984; Turnbull et al., 1983). Those designing these interventions have paid particular attention to the ability of parents to relate to others who do not share their experience of parenting a handicapped child. This is viewed as a critical skill that can serve as a buffer to interpersonal stress and to enhance the parents' image of themselves as competent parents (Intagliata & Doyle, 1984; Longo & Bond, 1984; Schilling et al., 1984).

An example of parent-focused intervention is a study conducted by Intagliata and Doyle (1984). They investigated the interpersonal problems-solving skills of parents of developmentally disabled children. Following systematic instruction, parents demonstrated a marked increase in their ability to generate effective strategies to solve interpersonal problems while maintaining their already begun level of competence in generating strategies for dealing with child-related problems. These researchers suggested that teaching parents of handicapped children how to identify and solve family problems is a viable strategy for enhancing family integration and should be considered for its role in supporting families with special needs children.

RELATIONSHIP TO RESPITE SERVICES

Respite services can best be understood in relation to the more global concepts of social support and family support services. Social support, as previously described, refers to the emotional, instrumental, and informational assistance provided by the individual's social network. Adaptation and coping are viewed as positive outcomes of this assistance. Social support may emanate from within the family unit or from influences external to the family. Family support, on the other hand, includes counseling, financial subsidy, architectural modifications, respite, special education, and generic services for the family and the dependent family member. Respite services are but one of many family supports that should be available to enhance the integration and self-sufficiency of families with developmentally disabled children.

Respite is an outcome that results from the provision of services to a dependent individual or his or her family (family is used here to denote providers of primary care, whether such occurs in the natural home or in a community residential facility). The services provide relief to the family from the caregiving responsibilities associated with the dependent family member.

Respite services can be described as having primary and secondary intent (Cohen, 1982; Salisbury, 1983). Services designed specifically to provide relief to the family (e.g., the handicapped child spending short periods with a designated alternative care provider) are generally referred to as primary respite care. Secondary respite occurs when the services being provided have the disabled child as their target (e.g., education, day care, work), but happen to provide the parents with temporary relief from child rearing as a natural concomitant to their provision (see Chapters 10 and 11; Cohen, 1982). From both vantage points, respite services produce a supporting outcome that can potentially mediate the effects of parenting stress (see Chapters 13 and 14).

Family and child needs must drive the design and development of respite services. This premise is fundamental to ensuring that the services that are provided help achieve their intended purpose. If parents are offered options that do not match their assessed needs, wants, or abilities to use them, then service outcomes will not reflect the true potential of the respite concept (Salisbury, 1984).

Respite care provided in the natural home is viewed as most desirable by parents (McGee, Smith, & Kenney, 1982; Chapter 4). Many communities have generated in-and-out-of-home respite service options that reflect a continuum of approximations to the natural home environment (Salisbury & Griggs, 1983; Upshur, 1982a). Yet, the breadth and depth of service options must be tailored to individual family, child, and community needs and abilities. Strategies for accomplishing elements of this process are described in this text.

Parents of both handicapped and nonhandicapped children experience stress related to the caregiving demands of their children. A major element in the parenting research with both populations is the expressed desire by parents (particularly mothers) for *time*. Parents of nonhandicapped children identify demands on finite time and energy, reduction in time for spouse and children, increased amount of time spent on housework, and insufficient time for social participation as major contributors to stress (cf. Hoffman & Manis, 1978; Knox & Wilson, 1978). Parents of handicapped children express the *same* concerns (cf. Bristol & Schopler, 1984; Dunlap & Hollingsworth, 1979; Korn et al., 1978). However, when time is afforded parental figures, it is not clear how this time is actually spent.

Research reviewed earlier suggests that mothers in both groups most often spend free moments doing home care, child care, and other maintenance activities (cf. Gallagher et al., 1984; Hoffman & Manis, 1978; Ruhe, 1984). Wikler (1981), in a study of respite care use, found that mothers of developmentally disabled children were deficient in their use of free time for personal development. They tended not to use the available respite time. When forced to take a block of time off from child care responsibilities, they did not know what to do with the time. Wikler postulated that women may be socialized to devote less time to self and to spend the greatest proportion of their energies on spouse and family. Findings of greater levels of depression in mothers of handicapped and nonhandicapped children lend credence to this supposition.

Yet, simply having respite services available does not ensure that desired, positive outcomes will occur. As discussed by the contributors to this volume, both process and outcome evaluation data are lacking. If parents and service delivery agents are to mount a convincing argument for the effectiveness of respite services for mediating the effects of parenting stress (Wikler, 1981), reducing requests for out-of-home placement (Lawson, Connolly, Leaver, & Engisch, 1979), and promoting economic self-sufficiency (see Chapter 10), then systematic efforts must be undertaken to evaluate the outcomes of present respite services. The decision processes employed by policymakers and funding organizations can best be influenced by the provision of outcome data, rather than rhetoric and emotional pleas (see Chapter 15).

The changes in family dynamics that occur with the provision of respite care can also create additional stress. Rodgers (1983) reported that when respite services were provided to families of deaf-blind children there were concomitant increases in marital dysfunction and stress. As seen from a family systems perspective, the husband and wife had previously ignored areas of marital conflict by using the handicapped child as a "scapegoat." When respite services enabled the child to be served in an out-of-home placement for short periods of time, the parents were forced to confront their problems directly. Rodgers and others argue that respite care must be supplemented with family counseling services to assist parents in adapting to the episodic fluctuations in family membership (Rodgers, 1983; Salisbury, 1984).

Respite care is the support service that families with chronically ill and dependent children most often identify as a priority (McGee et al., 1982). Relief and opportunity for social and vocational pursuits have specifically been identified as needed outcomes by parents of handicapped children (Cohen, 1982; Lyon & Preis, 1983; Seltzer & Krauss, 1984; Upshur, 1982a) and nonhandicapped children (Hoffman & Manis, 1978; Ventura & Boss, 1983) alike. Yet, opportunities for respite are not equally available to both populations (see Chapter 4). Thus, although respite has been shown to have the potential to mediate the effects of parenting stress (Cohen, 1982; Joyce, Singer, & Isralowitz, 1983), thus serving as a viable family support, problems in developing and implementing respite services still remain.

The similarities among parents of all children are far greater than are the differences. The greatest inequities between the handicapped and nonhandicapped populations lie in the availability and accessibility of resources to meet individual, as well as family, needs.

A CONCLUSION AND A BEGINNING

The purpose of this chapter is to establish a frame of reference for understanding the parenting experiences of families who are raising their handicapped child at home. The typical and unique stressors experienced by these families, within the context of smaller social support networks, suggest the need to augment the resources available to these families. The development of respite services, and in particular, respite care, is one strategy that may help mediate the effects of high levels of unresolved stress, and support the family's desire to maintain their child in the natural home. Each family is a unique entity, deserving of a range of family support services that they can match to the fluctuations in their needs and circumstances. Strategies for achieving a continuum of respite services are provided in the chapters that follow.

REFERENCES

Abernathy, V. (1973). Social network and response to the maternal role. *International Journal of Sociology of the Family, 3,* 86–92.
Ackerman, C. (1963). Affiliations: Structural determination of differential divorce rates. *American Journal of Sociology, 69,* 13–20.
Aldous, J. (1978). *Family careers: Developmental change in families.* New York: John Wiley & Sons.
Bayley, N., & Schaefer, E. (1960). Relationships between socioeconomic variables and the behavior of mothers toward young children. *Journal of Genetic Psychology, 96,* 61–77.
Beckman, P. (1983). Influences of selected child characteristics on stress in families of handicapped infants. *American Journal of Mental Deficiency, 80,* 150–156.
Beckman-Bell, P. (1981). Child related stress in families of handicapped children. *Topics in Early Childhood Special Education, 1*(3), 45–54.
Bell, C. S., Johnson, J. E., McGillicuddy-Delisi, A. V., & Sigel, I. E. (1980). Normative stress and young families: Adaptation and development. *Family Relations, 29*(4), 23–26.
Blacher, J. (1984). Sequential stages of parental adjustment to the birth of a child with handicaps: Fact or artifact? *Mental Retardation, 22*(2), 55–68.
Blackard, M. K., & Barsch, E. T. (1982). Parents and professional's perceptions of

the handicapped child's impact on the family. *Journal of the Association for the Severely Handicapped, 2,* 62–70.

Boss, P. G. (1980). Normative family stress: Family boundary changes across the life span. *Family Relations, 29*(4), 17–22.

Bossard, J. H. S., & Boll, E. S. (1956). *The large family system.* Philadelphia: University of Pennsylvania Press.

Bott, E. (1971). *Family and social networks.* London: Tabistock Publications.

Bradshaw, J., & Lawton, D. (1978). Tracing the causes of stress in families with handicapped children. *British Journal of Social Work, 8*(2), 181–192.

Bristol, M. M. (1979). *Maternal coping with autistic children: The effects of child characteristics and interpersonal supports.* Unpublished doctoral dissertation, University of North Carolina, Chapel Hill.

Bristol, M. M. (in press-a). Family resources and successful adaptation to autistic children. In E. Schopler & G. Mesibov (Eds.), *The effects of autism on the family.* New York: Plenum Publishing Corp.

Bristol, M. M. (in press-b). The home care of developmentally disabled children: Some empirical support for a conceptual model of successful coping with family stress. In S. Landesman-Dwyer & P. Vietze (Eds.), *Environments for developmentally disabled persons.* Baltimore: University Park Press.

Bristol, M. M., & Schopler, E. (1984). A developmental perspective on stress and coping in families of autistic children. In J. Blacher (Ed.), *Severely handicapped young children and their families* (pp. 91–141). New York: Academic Press.

Burden, R. L. (1980). Measuring the effects of stress on the mothers of handicapped infants: Must depression always follow? *Child: Care, Health and Development, 6,* 111–125.

Burr, W. R. (1970). Satisfaction with various aspects of marriage over the life cycle: A random middle class sample. *Journal of Marriage and the Family, 32*(1), 29–37.

Cairns, N. V., Clark, G. M., Smith, S. D., & Lanksy, S. (1978). Adaptation of siblings to childhood malignancy. *Journal of Pediatrics, 95,* 484–487.

Caldwell, B. M., & Guze, S. B. (1960). A study of the adjustment of parents and of institutional and noninstitutional retarded children. *American Journal of Mental Deficiency, 64,* 845–861.

Caplan, G. (1982). The family as a support system. In H. McCubbin, A. Cauble, & J. Patterson (Eds.), *Family stress, coping and social support* (pp. 200–220). Springfield, IL: Charles C Thomas.

Cleveland, D. W., & Miller, N. B. (1977). Attitudes and life commitments of older siblings of mentally retarded adults: An exploratory study. *Mental Retardation, 15*(3), 38–41.

Cobb, S. (1976). Social support as moderator of life stress. *Psychosomatic Medicine, 38,* 300–314.

Cohen, S. (1982). Supporting families through respite care. *Rehabilitation Literature, 43,* 7–11.

Crockenberg, S. (1981). Infant irritability, mother responsiveness and social influences on the security of infant-mother attachment. *Child Development, 52,* 857–865.

Cummings, S. T. (1976). Impact of the child's deficiency on the father: A study of fathers of mentally retarded and chronically ill children. *American Journal of Orthopsychiatry, 46,* 246–255.

Dorner, S. (1975). The relationship of physical handicap to stress in families with an adolescent with spina bifida. *Developmental Medicine in Child Neurology, 17,* 765–776.

Dunlap, W. R., & Hollingsworth, S. J. (1979). How does a handicapped child affect the family: Implications for practitioners. *Family Coordinator, 26,* 3–10.

Dunst, C. J., Trivette, C. M., & Cross, A. H. (1986). Mediating influences of social support: Personal, family, and child outcomes. *American Journal of Mental Deficiency, 90*(4), 403–417.

Duvall, E. (1972). *Family development.* Philadelphia: J. B. Lippincott Co.

Embry, L. (1980). Family support for handicapped preschool children at risk for abuse. *New Directions for Exceptional Children, 4,* 29–58.

Farber, B. (1959). Effects of a severely mentally retarded child on family integration. *Monographs of the Society for Research in Child Development, 24,* (2, Serial No. 71).

Farber, B. (1960). Family organization and crisis: Maintenance of integration in families with a severely mentally retarded child. *Monographs of the Society for Research in Child Development, 25,* (1 Serial No. 7).

Featherstone, H. (1980). *A difference in the family: Life with a disabled child.* New York: Basic Books.

Fotheringham, J. B., & Creal, D. (1974). Handicapped children and handicapped families. *International Review of Education, 20*(3), 353–371.

Fotheringham, J. B., Skelton, M., & Hoddinott, B. A. (1972). The effects on the family of the presence of a mentally retarded child. *Canadian Psychiatric Association Journal, 17,* 283–290.

Fowle, C. M. (1968). The effect of the severely mentally retarded child on his family. *American Journal of Mental Deficiency, 73*(3), 468–473.

Friedrich, W. N. (1979). Predictors of the coping behaviors of mothers of handicapped children. *Journal of Consulting and Clinical Psychology, 47,* 1140–1141.

Friedrich, W., & Friedrich, N. (1981). Psychosocial assets of parents of handicapped and nonhandicapped children. *American Journal of Mental Deficiency, 85,* 551–553.

Friedson, E. (1960). Client control and medical practice. *American Journal of Sociology, 56,* 374–382.

Gabel, H., McDowell, J., & Cerreto, M. C. (1983). Family adaptation to the handicapped infant. In S. G. Garwood & R. Fewell (Eds.), *Educating handicapped infants: Issues in development and intervention* (pp. 455–493). Rockville, MD: Aspen Systems Corporation.

Gallagher, J. J., Cross, A., & Scharfman, W. (1981). Parental adaptation to a young handicapped child: The father's role. *Journal of the Division for Early Childhood, 3,* 3–14.

Gallagher, J. J., Scharfman, W., & Bristol, M. (1984). The division of responsibilities in families with preschool handicapped and nonhandicapped children. *Journal of the Division for Early Childhood, 8*(1), 3–12.

Gath, A. (1973). The school age siblings of mongol children. *British Journal of Psychiatry, 123,* 161–167.

Gath, A. (1977). The impact of an abnormal child upon the parents. *British Journal of Psychiatry, 130,* 405–410.

Gath, A. (1978). *Down's syndrome and the family—The early years.* London: Academic Press.

Geismar, L. (1971). *Family and community functioning: A manual of measurement for social work practice and policy.* Metuchen, NJ: Scarecrow Press.

Hetherington, E., Cox, M., & Cox, R. (1978). The aftermath of divorce. In J. Stevens & M. Mathews (Eds.), *Mother-child, father-child interactions* (pp. 149–176). Washington, DC: National Association for the Education of Young Children.

Hill, R. (1949). *Families under stress*. New York: Harper & Row.

Hirsch, B. J. (1980). Psychological dimensions of social networks: A multimethod analysis. *American Journal of Community Psychology, 7*, 263–277.

Hobbs, D. (1965). Parenthood as crisis: A third study. *Journal of Marriage and the Family, 27*, 367–372.

Hoffman, L. W., & Manis, J. D. (1978). Influences of children on marital interaction and parental satisfactions and dissatisfactions. In R. M. Lerner & G. B. Spanier (Eds.), *Child influences on marital and family interaction: A life span perspective* (pp. 165–213). New York: Academic Press.

Holroyd, J. (1974). The Questionnaire on Resources and Stress: An instrument to measure family responses to a handicapped family member. *Journal of Community Psychology, 2*, 92–94.

Holroyd, J. (1982). *Manual for the Questionnaire on Resources and Stress*. Los Angeles: UCLA Neuropsychiatric Institute.

Howard, J. (1978). The influence of children's developmental dysfunctions on marital quality and family interaction. In R. M. Lerner & G. B. Spanier (Eds.), *Child influences on marital and family interaction: A life span perspective* (pp. 275–298). New York: Academic Press.

Intagliata, J., & Doyle, N. (1984). Enhancing social support for parents of developmentally disabled children: Training in interpersonal problem solving skills. *Mental Retardation, 22*(1), 4–11.

Jacoby, A. P. (1969). Transition to parenthood: A reassessment. *Journal of Marriage and the Family, 31*, 720–727.

Joyce, K., Singer, M., & Isralowitz, R. (1983). Impact of respite care on parents' perceptions of quality of life. *Mental Retardation, 21*(4), 153–156.

Kazak, A. E., & Marvin, R. S. (1984). Differences, difficulties and adaptation: Stress and social networks in families with a handicapped child. *Family Relations, 33*(1), 67–78.

Knox, D., & Wilson, K. (1978). The difference between having one and two children. *Family Coordinator, 27*, 23–35.

Korn, S. J., Chess, S., & Fernandez, P. (1978). The impact of children's physical handicaps on marital and family interaction. In R. M. Lerner & G. B. Spanier (Eds.), *Child influences on marital and family interaction—A life span perspective* (pp. 299–326). New York: Academic Press.

Lamb, M. E. (1978). Influence of the child on marital quality and family interaction during the prenatal, perinatal and infancy years. In R. M. Lerner & G. B. Spanier (Eds.), *Child influences on marital and family interaction: A life span perspective* (pp. 137–163). New York: Academic Press.

Lavigne, J. V. & Ryan, M. (1979). Psychologic adjustment of children with chronic illness. *Pediatrics, 63*, 616–627.

Lawson, J. S., Connolly, M., Leaver, C., & Engisch, H. J. C. (1979). Short-term residential care of the intellectually handicapped. *Australian Journal of Mental Retardation, 5*, 307–310.

LeMasters, E. (1957). Parenthood as crisis. *Marriage and Family Living, 19*, 352–355.

Lerner, R. M., & Spanier, G. B. (1978). *Child influences on marital and family interaction: A life span perspective*. New York: Academic Press.

Litwak, E., & Szelenyi, I. (1969). Primary group structures and their functions: Kin, neighbors, and friends. *American Sociological Review, 34,* 465–481.

Longo, D. C., & Bond, L. (1984). Families of the handicapped child: Research and practice. *Family Relations, 33*(1), 57–66.

Love, H. (1973). *The mentally retarded child and his family.* Springfield, IL: Charles C Thomas.

Lyon, S., & Preis, A. (1983). Working with families of severely handicapped persons. In M. Seligman (Ed.), *The family with a handicapped child: Understanding and treatment* (pp. 203–232). New York: Grune & Stratton.

McAllister, R. J., Lei, T., & Butler, E. W. (1973). The ecology of retardation: Two views. *Social Science and Medicine, 8,* 585–589.

McAndrew, I. (1976). Children with a handicap and their families. *Child Care, Health & Development, 2,* 213–237.

McCubbin, H. I., & Boss, P. G. (1980). Family stress: Coping and adaptation. *Family Relations, 29*(4), 429–430.

McCubbin, H. I., Boss, P. G., & Wilson, L. R. (1978). *Developments in family stress theory: Implications for family impact analysis.* Paper presented at the preconference theory and methodology workshop of the National Council on Family Relations, Philadelphia, PA.

McCubbin, H. I., Joy, C. B., Cauble, A. E., Comeau, J., Patterson, J. M., & Needles, R. H. (1980). Family stress and coping: A decade review. *Journal of Marriage and the Family, 42,* 865–870.

McCubbin, H. I., & Patterson, J. M. (1981). *Systemic assessment of family stress, resources and coping: Tools for research, education and clinical intervention.* St. Paul: Family Stress and Coping Project, Department of Family Social Science, University of Minnesota.

McGee, J. J., Smith, P. M., & Kenney, M. (1982). *Giving families a break: Strategies for respite care.* Omaha, NE: Media Resource Center, Meyer Children's Rehabilitation Institute.

McLanahan, S. S. (1983). Family structure and stress: A longitudinal comparison of two-parent and female-headed families. *Journal of Marriage and the Family,* 347–357.

Miller, B., & Sollie, D. (1980). Normal stress during the transition to parenthood. *Family Relations, 29,* 459–465.

Minuchin, S. (1974). *Families and family therapy.* Cambridge, MA: Harvard University Press.

Mitchell, R. E., & Trickett, E. J. (1980). Task force report: Social networks as mediators of social support. *Community Mental Health Journal, 16,* 27–43.

Neugarten, B. (1976). Adaptations and the life cycle. *The Counseling Psychologist, 6*(1), 16–20.

Olshansky, S. (1962). Chronic sorrow: A response to having a mentally defective child. *Social Casework, 43,* 191–194.

Powell, T. H., & Hecimovic, A. (1981). *Respite care for the handicapped: Helping individuals and their families.* Springfield, IL: Charles C. Thomas.

Price-Bonham, S., & Addison, S. (1978). Families and mentally retarded children: Emphasis on the father. *The Family Coordinator, 3,* 221–230.

Rabkin, J. C., & Streuning, E. C. (1976). Life events, stress, illness. *Science, 194,* 1013–1020.

Ragozin, A. S., Basham, R. B., Crnic, M. A., Greenberg, M. T., & Robinson, N. M. (1982). Effects of maternal age on parenting role. *Developmental Psychology, 18,* 627–634.

Ramey, C. T., Mills, P., Campbell, F. A., & O'Brien, C. (1975). Infant's home environments: A comparison of high-risk families and families from the general population. *American Journal of Mental Deficiency, 80,* 40–42.

Rapoport, R. (1963). Normal crises, family structure, and mental health. *Family Process, 2*(1), 68–80.

Raub, M. J. (1982). *How to start a respite program.* Sacramento: State of California Council on Developmental Disabilities.

Rodgers, J. (1983, November). *Respite care for families with deaf-blind children.* Paper presented at the annual convention of The Association for the Severely Handicapped, San Francisco, CA.

Rollins, B., & Cannon, K. L. (1974). Marital satisfaction over the family life cycle: A re-evaluation. *Journal of Marriage and the Family, 36,* 271–282.

Rollins, B. C., & Galligan, R. (1978). The developing child and marital satisfaction of parents. In R. M. Lerner & G. B. Spanier (Eds.), *Child influences on marital and family interaction: A life span perspective* (pp. 71–105). New York: Academic Press.

Ruhe, L. A. (1984). *The impact of handicapped children on family time budgeting, caretaking responsibilities, and the quality of life.* Unpublished master's thesis, Psychology Department, University Center at Binghamton, Binghamton, NY.

Russell, C. (1974). Transition to parenthood. *Journal of Marriage and the Family, 36,* 294–302.

Saenger, G. (1965). Factors influencing the institutionalization of mentally retarded individuals in New York City. In B. Farber & D. B. Ryckman (Eds.), *Mental Retardation Abstracts.*

Salisbury, C. (1983, November). *Research and training issues in the provision of respite care services.* Paper presented at the annual convention of The Association for the Severely Handicapped, San Francisco, CA.

Salisbury, C. (1984). *Lifecycle stress in families with a handicapped child.* Unpublished manuscript, Division of Professional Education, University Center at Binghamton, Binghamton, NY.

Salisbury, C. (1984, December). *Outcome evaluation of social support services.* Invited paper presented at the Governor's Conference on Family Supports, Albany, NY.

Salisbury, C. (1985). *Stress in families of young handicapped and nonhandicapped children.* Manuscript in preparation, Division of Professional Education, University Center at Binghamton, Binghamton, NY.

Salisbury, C. (1986). Adaptation of the Questionnaire on Resources and Stress-Short Form. *American Journal of Mental Deficiency, 90*(4), 456–459.

Salisbury, C., & Griggs, P. (1983). Developing respite care services for families of handicapped persons. *Journal of The Association for Persons with Severe Handicaps, 8*(1), 50–57.

Satterwhite, B. B. (1978). Impact of chronic illness on child and family: An overview based on five surveys, with implications for management. *International Journal of Rehabilitation Research, 1,* 7–17.

Schilling, R. F., Gilchrist, L., & Schinke, S. P. (1984). Coping and social support in families of developmentally disabled children. *Family Relations, 33*(1), 47–56.

Schonell, F. J., & Watts, B. H. (1956). A first survey of the effects of a subnormal child on the family unit. *American Journal of Mental Deficiency, 61,* 210–219.

Seltzer, M. M., & Krauss, M. W. (1984). Placement alternatives for mentally retarded children and their families. In J. Blacher (Ed.), *Severely handicapped young children and their families.* New York: Academic Press.

Sherman, B. R., & Cocozza, J. J. (1984). Stress in families of the developmentally disabled: A literature review of factors affecting the decision to seek out-of-home placement. *Family Relations, 33,* 95–103.

Skinner, D. A. (1980). Dual career family stress and coping: A literature review. *Family Relations, 29*(4), 43–52.

Spanier, G. B., Lewis, R. A., & Cole, C. L. (1975). Marital adjustment over the family life cycle: The issue of curvilinearity. *Journal of Marriage and the Family, 37,* 263–275.

Starr, P. (1981). Marital status and raising a handicapped child: Does one affect the other? *Social Work, 26,* 504–505.

Suelzle, M., & Keenan, V. (1981). Changes in family support networks over the life cycle of mentally retarded persons. *American Journal of Mental Deficiency, 86*(3), 267–274.

Tausig, M. (1985). Factors in family decision making about placement for developmentally disabled individuals. *American Journal of Mental Deficiency, 89*(4), 352–361.

Tew, B., Laurence, C., Payne, H., & Rawnsley, K. (1977). Marital stability following the birth of a child with spina bifida. *British Journal of Psychiatry, 131,* 79–82.

Tew, B., & Lawrence, K. M. (1973). Mothers, brothers, and sisters of patients with spina bifida. *Developmental Medicine and Child Neurology, 15,* 69–76.

Turnbull, A. P., Summers, J. A., & Brotherson, M. J. (1983). *Family life cycle: Theoretical and empirical implications and future directions for families with mentally retarded members.* Paper presented at NICHD conference on "Research on Families with Retarded Children."

Unger, D., & Powell, D. (1980). Supporting families under stress: The role of social networks. *Family Relations, 29,* 566–574.

Upshur, C. (1982a). Respite care for mentally retarded and other disabled populations: Program models and family needs. *Mental Retardation, 20,* 2–6.

Upshur, C. (1982b). An evaluation of home-based respite care. *Mental Retardation, 20,* 58–62.

Vance, J. C., Fazan, L. E., Satterwhite, B., & Pless, I. B. (1980). Effects of nephrotic syndrome on the family: A controlled study. *Pediatrics, 64,* 948–955.

Venters, M. (1981). Familial coping with chronic illness: The case of cystic fibrosis. *Social Science and Medicine, 15,* 289–297.

Ventura, J. N., & Boss, P. G. (1983). The family coping inventory applied to parents with new babies. *Journal of Marriage and the Family, 45,* 867–875.

Vickers, G. (1968). *Modern systems research for the behavioral scientist.* Chicago: Aldine.

Waisbren, S. (1980). Parents' reactions after the birth of a developmentally disabled child. *American Journal of Mental Deficiency, 84,* 345–356.

Warren, R., & Dickman, I. R. (1981). *For this respite, much thanks.* New York: United Cerebral Palsy Association, Inc.

Weintraub, M., & Wolf, B. M. (1983). Effects of stress and social supports on mother-child interactions in single- and two-parent families. *Child Development, 54,* 1297–1311.

Wikler, L. (1981). Stress in families of mentally retarded children. *Family Relations, 30,* 281–288.

Wikler, L. (1984, May). *Depression in mothers of older children with developmental disabilities: An exploratory study.* Paper presented at the annual convention of the American Association on Mental Deficiency, Minneapolis, MN.

Wikler, L., Haack, J., & Intagliata, J. (1984). Bearing the burden alone? Helping divorced mothers of children with developmental disabilities. In J. C. Hansen & E. I. Coopersmith (Eds.), *Family Therapy Collections Series: Families with handicapped members* (pp. 44–62). Rockville, MD: Aspen Systems Corporation.

Wikler, L., Wasow, M., & Hatfield, E. (1981). Chronic sorrow revisited: Attitude of parents and professionals about adjustment to mental retardation. *American Journal of Orthopsychiatry, 51,* 63–70.

Wilcox, B. L. (1981). Social support in adjusting to the marital disruption: A network analysis. In B. H. Gottlieb (Ed.), *Social network and social support.* Beverly Hills, CA: Sage.

Wright, J. S., Granger, R. D., & Sameroff, A. J. (1984). Parental acceptance and developmental handicap. In J. Blacher (Ed.), *Severely handicapped young children and their families: Research in review.* New York: Academic Press.

Chapter 2

BROTHERS AND SISTERS
ADDRESSING UNIQUE NEEDS
THROUGH RESPITE CARE SERVICES

Thomas H. Powell and Peggy A. Ogle

Recognition has been slow in coming that the sisters and brothers of children with mental retardation and/or other handicaps are important people in the total picture of human exceptionality. They have their own special needs which must be recognized and met. Their ability to contribute to the growth and happiness of their handicapped sibling is substantial. The investment is large, and they have the right to assistance and support.
—Allen C. Crocker (1983, p. 147)

- It's Saturday morning. "Mom! Dad! Ken messed the bed again! It stinks in this room! Mom!" As Mike and Ken's parents go into the boys' room to attend to what seems a never-ending problem, Mike says, "Won't this ever end? When will he grow up? I want my own room!"
- Debbie's 14-year-old brother, John, has autism. She has helped care for him for his entire life. This Friday there's a dance at her high school. She was invited and wants to go, but declined because her mother is chairing an event for a local chapter of the National Society for Children and Adults with Autism. If Debbie doesn't "babysit" John, no one will. She doesn't say anything to her mother.
- Every time they play together, it seems like an ice-hockey brawl. Melissa, who is 8 years old and severely mentally retarded, seems to enjoy breaking her younger sister's toys. Dolls with no arms or legs can be found everywhere.
- Last week at the "Stop & Shop" store, 7-year-old Karen, who is deaf and moderately mentally retarded, had a temper tantrum in Aisle 11 (cereals and breakfast foods). She screamed, kicked, and knocked down ten boxes of Fruit Loops. She had a temper tantrum right in front of everyone, including her 9-year-old brother Kevin. No amount of plead-

ing seemed to help. Kevin took off for the next aisle and left his father to deal with the problem. Later in the car on the way home Kevin said, "Let's not take Karen to the grocery store anymore."

• "Monica, I know I always ask you, but would you please watch Nancy while I run some errands this afternoon?" Nancy, 10 years old, was born both deaf and blind and is nonambulatory. "Please check her diaper in an hour." Monica just turned 13. "O.K., Mom, I think I'll take her to the park with me."

There are special problems and concerns of siblings who grow up with brothers and sisters with handicaps. A small panel of adolescent siblings shared some of their concerns with parents and professionals at parent meetings in Connecticut. Eileen's brother has severe mental retardation; Geraldine's sister has autism; Christopher's brother had Hunter syndrome and died 2 years ago; Ted's brother has a learning disability; Alice's sister was born with spina bifida. These five siblings spoke of their love for and devotion to their brothers or sisters. They spoke of their frustrations, embarrassment, joy, anger, and confusion. They told about their unique family system and the role each plays within that constellation. Most importantly, they taught about their special needs.

A common theme for all five siblings was their need for brief periods of relief, periods of respite. They spoke of their varying needs to engage in some activities without the constant demands of attending to their sister or brother with a handicap. "We love Ken, but it's really difficult to take care of him all the time. We feed him, play with him, take him to the bathroom, watch him, teach him. He's the constant activity in our lives" (G. Johnston, personal communication, May 7, 1984). "It's not like growing up with our other brothers and sisters. We need to be more understanding and careful with Susan" (E. Andrews, personal communication, May 7, 1984). "Being alone with Mom and Dad is real special. Maybe it's because we seldom are" (T. McConnell, personal communication, May 7, 1984). Those who listened to these siblings learned a great deal.

LIVING WITH A SISTER OR BROTHER WHO HAS A HANDICAP

It's not easy to grow up with a disabled sister or brother. It's not easy to be part of a family in which one member requires more than usual parental attention and family resources. It's not easy to identify with brothers and sisters who do not speak or play and who may break toys, have regular and intense temper tantrums, behave strangely, or are in the hospital a lot. Although it is not easy, most siblings survive the situation intact and develop strong positive feelings about their sisters and brothers and parents (Grossman, 1972; Mates, 1982; Schreiber & Feeley, 1965).

The special needs of siblings have received greater attention in the past few years. No doubt this is a result of the increased emphasis given to keeping children with handicaps at home and providing support to entire family systems. With this increased attention, there has been an increased recognition that siblings play a critical role in the overall development of handicapped children and that they are in need of special community services, especially respite care (Powell & Ogle, 1985).

SIBLINGS IN THE FAMILY SYSTEM

Families provide children with their first opportunities to explore, communicate, and interact with other human beings. Families are interrelated systems that support the interdependence of individual members. Each member of the family is a critical element of the system whose personality and interactions affect those of other family members. As one member of the family changes, so too will all other members.

In their analysis of sibling interactions and interdependence, Schvaneveldt and Ihinger (1979) assert the importance of considering families as systems. They outlined five basic assumptions in regard to sibling relationships:

1. Within most families, there exist three subsystems of interaction. Each of these subsystems (spouse-spouse, parent-child, and sibling-sibling) operates semi-independently within the family structure.
2. Siblings both initiate and receive social interactions. Family interaction is dynamic, with husbands and wives affecting each other, parents and children affecting each other, and siblings affecting each other.
3. Sibling interaction is a continuous process of development that occurs throughout the life-span.
4. The personality development and social behaviors of family members are partially determined by family composition and interaction.
5. Sibling groups have properties similar to other small groups.

As Powell and Ogle (1985) note, the sibling relationship is perhaps the most long-lasting and most influential relationship of one's life. It begins with the birth of a brother or sister and continues throughout one's lifetime. The duration of that relationship is certainly substantial. Unlike parental relationships that may last 40–60 years, the sibling relationship may last 60–80 years. Unlike any other relationship between people, the sibling relationship provides two people with physical and emotional contact at critical stages throughout their lives. Siblings provide a continuing relationship from which there is no annulment. This permanent relationship allows two people to exert considerable influence over each other through longitudinal interactions (Bank & Kahn, 1982).

In our current, quickly changing society, sibling relationships are becoming increasingly important. Bank and Kahn (1982) suggest that changes in American society have led to greater levels of sibling contact and emotional interdependence. In particular, these researchers note that the reduction of family size, greater family mobility, increases in divorce and remarriage rates, greater numbers of employed mothers, and increased levels of parental stress have resulted in greater reliance on one's siblings. Additionally, as individuals live longer, siblings provide a longitudinal source of support to each other, especially in later years.

Impact on Siblings

How do children with handicaps influence their brothers and sisters? The impact the handicapped child has on siblings is a major concern of many parents. Several authors (Lobato, 1983; McHale, Simeonsson, & Sloan, 1984; Powell & Ogle, 1985; Seligman, 1983; Simeonsson & McHale, 1981) have reviewed and analyzed much of the research on the relationship between handicapped children and their nonhandicapped siblings. Basically, this research shows that there can be both positive and negative effects for the nonhandicapped child.

On the positive side, some siblings report satisfaction in learning to live and cope with the demands of a handicapped child. They also experience genuine joy and pleasure at the smallest accomplishments of the handicapped child and feel a warmth and compassion for all people as individuals with unique needs and abilities (see Laureys, 1982; Lettick, 1979; Myers, 1978). At the same time, other siblings report negative effects, including feelings of bitterness and resentment because of the extra attention given the handicapped child. Some siblings also experience fears and anxiety over how to interact with the handicapped child or even guilt because of their own good health (see Featherstone, 1980; Myers, 1978; Zatlow, 1982).

It is helpful to envision the effects of a handicapped child on the sibling in terms of a continuum with very positive outcomes at one end and very negative outcomes (i.e., psychological disturbance) at the other. It is important to remember that this continuum of outcomes for siblings is not static. Simply because a sibling appears to have a very healthy, positive relationship at one time does not mean that at another time the same sibling may not express some very negative behaviors and feelings toward the handicapped child.

Many different factors seem to contribute to determining where the nonhandicapped sibling functions on this continuum at various points in time.

Comparison of the findings of research studies has revealed discrepancies, which can be attributed to differences in measurement instruments or research design or even to the different ages of the subjects studied. However, the discrepancies may also be related to the fact that the nonhandicapped sibling's adjustment is dependent on characteristics of the family in general, on characteristics of the nonhandicapped child, or on characteristics of the handicapped child (Lobato, 1983; McHale et al., 1984). Family characteristics, including family size, socioeconomic status, and religion, seem to be major factors affecting sibling adjustment. Additionally, parental attitudes and expectations, as well as characteristics of both the nonhandicapped and handicapped child, such as age, gender, temperament, and the type and severity of the child's handicap, also significantly influence the sibling relationship and affect sibling adjustment (Powell & Ogle, 1985). A discussion of these four major contributing factors follows.

Family Characteristics

Family Size　Taylor (1974) has suggested that siblings from larger families are generally better adjusted than those from smaller families. It seems natural that in two-child families where one child is handicapped, parents are more likely to rest all their hopes and expectations on their one nonhandicapped child. In larger families, however, these hopes and desires can be distributed to several children and thus ease the pressure on the one child. McHale et al. (1984) agree that children from larger families are better adjusted, provided the families have adequate financial resources.

Socioeconomic Status　Family socioeconomic status can also affect sibling responses to a handicapped child. Grossman (1972) found that siblings from middle-class families generally had a range of positive and negative feelings that were predictable from their parents' attitudes. Middle-class families often have problems in realistically adjusting their high expectations for their handicapped child (McHale et al., 1984). At the same time, middle-class families tend to be more financially secure and better prepared to utilize outside resources, such as camps, respite care services, and a wide range of professionals, in securing help for any family needs. Conversely, families of lower socioeconomic status often have limited financial resources. Thus, siblings, especially females, who are from poorer families may be overburdened with extra caregiving responsibilities that cannot be provided for through other channels.

Religion　Stubblefield (1965), in a review of the literature regarding the role of religion in parental acceptance of a handicapped child, noted that the birth of such a child often precipitates a theological crisis for many parents. Religious faith affects the parents' responses to the birth. Zuk, Miller, Bartram, and Kling (1961) established moderate but positive correlations be-

tween measures of religious background and maternal acceptance of a handicapped child. They found that Roman Catholic families tend to be more
accepting of a mentally retarded child than are Jewish or Protestant families,
and they explained such acceptance as deriving from the explicit definitions
supporting the home and family life decreed by the Roman Catholic church.

Parental Attitudes and Expectations

Siblings' perceptions of their parents' attitudes toward the handicapped child
can indeed be a powerful influence on the nonhandicapped child's adjustment. Caldwell and Guze (1960), in a study of the adjustment of parents and
siblings, looked at 32 families, half with a handicapped child living in the
home and half with a handicapped child living in an institution. They found
that, generally, the two groups were similar in adjustment. One area in which
the two groups were clearly different was the sibling's perception of the ideal
living arrangement for the mentally retarded child. One group felt that the
home was the appropriate place for the child; the other group felt that the
institution was the best living situation. The responses were consistent with
whether the child was at home or institutionalized.

Holt (1958) also conducted personal interviews with parents in the
homes of 201 families with mentally retarded children. Holt noted that 5% of
the parents reported that their nonhandicapped children felt embarrassment and
shame toward their sibling with mental retardation and that such feelings
were, to some extent, related to the parents' own adjustment.

Other researchers have stressed the importance of the parental attitude in
sibling adjustment. Grossman (1972) has suggested that one of the strongest
factors affecting the nonhandicapped sibling's acceptance of the handicapped
sibling is the feelings of the parents, particularly the mother. After working
with parents who were unable to participate in open discussions with their
nonhandicapped children regarding a sibling's handicap, she has proposed
that the manner in which parents interpret and respond to a handicap determines the impact on the siblings involved. Graliker, Fishler, and Koch, in
their study (1962) a decade earlier, found that nonhandicapped siblings
showed less disturbance in home, school, and social activities when both
parents had the same positive attitude toward their mentally retarded child
than did children of parents who did not share such a positive attitude. Clearly, parental attitudes exert a significant influence on a sibling's acceptance of
a handicapped child. Siblings are better adjusted when their parents are more
accepting of the condition of the handicapped child (McHale et al., 1984).
Such attitudes seem to interact with religious beliefs as discussed above.

Characteristics of the Nonhandicapped Sibling

It is difficult to separate demographic characteristics in families with a handicapped child from those birth-order characteristics found in other families

with nonhandicapped children (Lobato, 1983). However, the gender and age of the nonhandicapped sibling in relation to the handicapped child seem to contribute to the sibling's adjustment. As mentioned previously, several authors have found that older female siblings are most adversely affected by the presence of a handicapped child (Cleveland & Miller, 1977; Gath, 1974; Graliker et al., 1962; Grossman, 1972; McHale et al., 1984) perhaps because they usually assume child care responsibilities and these responsibilities may be compounded when one of the siblings is handicapped. Except for oldest females, who usually experience the most adjustment problems, siblings of the same gender as the handicapped child are affected more adversely by the presence of a handicapped child than are siblings of the opposite sex (Farber & Jenne, 1963; Grossman, 1972; McHale et al., 1984).

Other research on gender and age has shown that the greater the age differential between the handicapped child and the sibling, the more likely the sibling will be well adjusted (Schreiber & Feeley, 1965; Simeonsson & Bailey, 1983). It also appears that when the nonhandicapped sibling is older (particularly more than 10 years older), he or she will be better adjusted (McHale et al., 1984; Simeonsson & Bailey, 1983). Simeonsson and Bailey feel that the poorer adjustment found in siblings who are younger or closer in age may be attributable to identity problems. These siblings may have difficulty, for instance, adjusting expectations about what the "older brother" should do when that brother is handicapped and may not even be able to feed himself.

The sibling must learn to adjust his or her own identity in relation to a sibling who is handicapped and who does not perform as a person that age would typically perform. Simeonsson and Bailey (1983) have also proposed that the extent to which siblings perceive themselves as competent in relation to the handicapped child will help determine the nonhandicapped sibling's adjustment. In effect, then, they suggest that older children, being innately more competent, or other children who have been trained and who feel competent with the handicapped child may be better adjusted than those who do not feel such confidence.

Characteristics of the Handicapped Child

Type of Handicap   It seems that the particular type of disability involved is not a crucial factor in the adjustment of the nonhandicapped siblings. One exception seems to be that, in families with higher incomes, siblings seem to be less well adjusted when their sibling's handicap is ambiguous or undefined (McHale et al., 1984). Lobato (1983) has detailed a series of studies on siblings of children with Down syndrome, cystic fibrosis, hearing impairments, autism, cerebral palsy, and childhood cancers and notes that all the researchers describe similar results regarding the psychosocial adjustment of the siblings. Emphasizing that there must be factors other than the type of handicapping condition that determine adjustment for the nonhandicapped siblings, Lobato has suggested that these factors may include such characteristics of the nonhandicapped child as sex or age relative to the handicapped child. It is also likely, she asserts, that parental attitudes toward the handicapped child, as discussed above, have a strong effect on the nonhandicapped child's sense of well-being. Simeonsson and Bailey (1983) have also suggested that other factors, such as individual traits, temperament, or functional behaviors of the handicapped child, may transcend the influence of any particular disability.

Severity of Handicap   Siblings are more adversely affected by more severely handicapped children, according to Kirk and Bateman (1964) and Grossman (1972). Again, the state of a family's financial resources interact with the severity of the handicap. In families of lower socioeconomic status, where there are no financial resources for babysitters or tutors, siblings typically have more caregiving responsibilities. These responsibilities, which include such tasks as feeding and bathing, have been discussed by several authors (Battle, 1974; Fotheringham & Creal, 1974; Robson & Moss, 1970; Schaffer & Emerson, 1964) as having an effect on mother-child interaction, the self-concept of the mother, and on parental stress (Beckman-Bell, 1980). Parents of handicapped children must deal with these aspects of child care often in unusual circumstances and for an extended period of time (Battle, 1974; Beckman-Bell, 1980; Fotheringham & Creal, 1974). Indeed, Beckman-Bell (1980), in a study to examine the relationship between characteristics of infants with developmental disabilities and maternal stress, found that caregiving demands of the child alone accounted for 66% of the variance in perceived parent and family problems. It follows that such caregiving demands might also influence sibling relationships.

Age of Child   The age of the handicapped child also seems to influence the adjustment of the siblings. Both Farber (1964) and Miller (1969) have found that as handicapped individuals grow older, their siblings experience more difficulties.

SPECIAL CONCERNS: FAMILY ADJUSTMENT

All families face a number of critical transitional periods in their lives that create stress. The birth of a new child, school entrance, a change in those living in the household—all are periods of stress. For the family with a child who has a handicap, however, the stress of these times may be particularly acute. Mackeith (1973) has described four such periods:

1. When parents initially find out the child has a handicap
2. When the child with a handicap becomes eligible for educational services and thus faces academic expectations

3. When the family member with a handicap leaves school and faces the personal confusion and frustration of all adolescents
4. When parents age and can no longer assume the responsibility and care for the person with a handicap

These points in family life serve as a framework to help service providers identify periods in which family members, particularly parents and siblings, can potentially experience intense stress (Simeonsson & Simeonsson, 1981). Knowing when stress is likely to occur enables professionals to direct their services to alleviate or minimize problems for family members during these critical times. Stress need not have completely negative effects, but can be turned into a positive force.

Turnbull, Summers, and Brotherson (1983) describe a number of stress situations that may occur at different points in a family's life. They note, for instance, that initially after the birth of a child who is handicapped, parents are concerned with "obtaining an accurate diagnosis," "informing siblings," and "establishing routines to carry out family functions." During a child's beginning school years, parents must decide the merits of main-streamed versus specialized placement for their child. Perhaps arrangements for child care and afterschool activities need to be made as well. During the child's adolescent years, parents must make decisions surrounding such important concerns as sexuality and vocational planning. After the school years, parents may experience stress with their continuing financial obligations toward the individual and with decisions on living arrangements. If the handicapped individual leaves home, the parents must adjust their relationship with each other and, perhaps, jointly face their daughter's or son's emerging interest in dating or marriage. During later years, parents worry about placement and care for their handicapped child after their deaths.

Just as all families face times of decision, so too does stress occur at natural points in families with a handicapped individual. Transitions at these points may be more difficult, however, for families with handicapped members. Traditional symbols or rituals marking a transition may be delayed or nonexistent (e.g., no high school graduation ceremony). Further, critical periods for nonhandicapped siblings may occur simultaneously, forcing the family to deal with the differing needs of individual family members at the same time (Turnbull et al., 1983; Wikler, Wasow, & Hatfield, 1981). Turnbull and associates (1983) additionally note that when a family must relocate to secure special services for a child with a disability, intense stress may be felt by all family members. Likewise, parents and siblings may experience stress as a family member moves from an institution to a community home. For parents and siblings who were previously told by professionals that institutionalizing their family members was in the best interest of all, the stress generated by the new concept of community-based services can be considerable.

Simeonsson and Simeonsson (1981) suggest that families with persons who have handicaps are, first and foremost, similar to all other families who face today's societal pressures and demands. By circumstance, such families must also face the special demands of raising a handicapped child. They note that the overall effects of handicapped children on families are conflicting. Although some families are strengthened by the experience, others are burdened to the point of separation or divorce. It seems more likely, however, that families are both strengthened and stressed by the presence of a handicapped child. The degree of strength and stress experienced is what varies in families.

Although it is not clear what impact a disabled child will have on a sibling, researchers agree that siblings with a brother or sister who is disabled experience higher levels of stress than other siblings (see Powell & Ogle, 1985). This additional stress may, in fact, place siblings at risk for developing behavioral and emotional problems that may be long lasting (Cerreto & Miller, 1981; Trevino, 1979). Unfortunately, the research literature to date does not provide parents or professionals with a clear understanding of the nature of this impact. Research is clearly needed to consider the degrees and nature of effect of having a sibling with a disability.

In lieu of more precise research, parents and professionals can learn about the various degrees of impact by considering the statements made by siblings themselves. One consistent theme often expressed by siblings is the additional responsibility of being a part of a unique family system. Myers (1978) notes: "My role in those days was someone who was always around to help care for Robert. That was my mother's phrase. My father called me his 'good right arm.' Robert himself called me 'Dad' before he corrected himself and called me 'Bobby.' . . . I never felt I dressed like a kid, never felt comfortable with the clothes I wore, never felt I knew how to act as a boy or a teenager. I was a little man" (p. 36).

Zatlow (1982) expresses strong feelings about her brother Douglas who has autism. Although she shares a loving relationship with him, she reminds us of the extra responsibilities she faced as a result of his disability.

> There was no relief from Doug. Day in and day out, his needs had to be tended to regardless of our wants and desires. He always came first. . . . Because Douglas's presence dominated everything, there was no real time for myself. Under these conditions, childhood takes on an uneasy dimension. A sibling denied the fundamental right of being a child. An opportunity to have friends over does not often materialize because visits were dependent on my brother's moods and behavior. Going out was governed by my mother's need for my assistance in any way. My mother nicknamed me "the other mother" as I took my responsibility with seriousness and

maturity in excess of my young years. Unfortunately, the pattern became a way of life. (p. 2)

In a similar manner, Hayden (1974) recalls a particular caregiving episode that left a lifelong impression.

When Daddy spent a year in Korea, I became Mother's sole helper. My role as second mother to Mindy held some prestige and much responsibility. It took away from play time with children my own age. And, just as a mother serves as an example for her children, I was expected to be an exceptionally "good" little girl. The high standards my mother set for my behavior, though, had not only to do with my setting an example; her reasons were also practical. Mindy's impetuous behavior left her with little patience, energy, or time to put up with shenanigans from me. . . . The responsibility I felt for Mindy was tremendous. One year when my "babysitting" duties involved periodic checking on my sister, Mindy wandered away between checks. After a thorough but fruitless search of the neighborhood, my mother hysterically told me that if anything happened to Mindy, I would be to blame. I felt terrified and guilty. I was 7. (p. 27)

Fromberg (1984) describes several significant caregiving responsibilities for his brother, Steven, who has autism. He refers to himself as a "part-time parent" (p. 344) in which his brother was his responsibility when his parents went out. In addition to caregiving, Fromberg relates other concerns:

Though caring for Steve was often trying, it was not the most painful experience associated with him. There was a kind of constant pressure in our family regarding Steve. Whenever we went out, we monitored his behavior constantly, trying to avoid major problems and to smooth out less troublesome actions. Sometimes keeping Steve in tow was as much trouble for the family as a whole as it was for me alone. (p. 345)

When a sister or brother has a physical handicap, siblings are commonly recruited to provide care (Travis, 1976). In some ways, some physically handicapped and chronically ill children enslave their siblings through constant requests and demands. Seligman (1983) observes that "chronically ill children have been observed being verbally abusive toward their normal siblings" (p. 160).

Without some relief from these extra caregiving responsibilities, siblings may respond in negative ways. Travis (1976) notes that some siblings who have been excessively burdened with physical care duties often leave home at about age 16. She also reports that some siblings, resentful about such responsibilities, express their resentment through hasty and unkind physical care. Klein (1972) talked with Diane, a young college student, who described her feelings about extra caregiving responsibilities:

Because my older sister and I were the oldest children, we took on alot of responsibility for Cathy. We took care of her alot; we babysat with her alot. I can remember so many days when I was just so impatient, so indifferent. I wanted to go outside and play. I did not want to sit around and take care of Cathy. I can remember even sometimes while I was changing her clothes, she would start crying or become frustrated and maybe I would spank her. (p. 15)

Within all family systems, siblings play a unique and vital role to the well-being of other family members. It is not unusual for siblings in any family to provide some care to the other children. All brothers and sisters occasionally find themselves in the caring and nurturing role to their siblings. This only becomes problematic when the caregiving becomes excessive, intense, and chronic. When there is no relief, no "light-at-the-end-of-the-tunnel," no sharing or distribution of the responsibility, problems tend to arise. One way to avoid potential problems is to systematically provide regular periods of relief to siblings through respite care.

RESPITE CARE AND SIBLINGS

Respite care is an essential community-based service aimed at supporting families who have children with handicaps (Powell & Hecimovic, 1981). Respite simply refers to a brief period of rest or relief; respite care is a community service for families to provide periods of short-term care for individuals with disabilities. Although respite care has primarily been developed to assist parents, comprehensive respite care programs can have a profound influence on other family members, particularly siblings.

Respite care services provide siblings with opportunities to be relieved of the constant pressure of family life with a handicapped child. As previously noted, siblings, in ways very similar to parents, experience extra stresses and problems as a direct result of the disabled child. Regular periods of respite are needed to provide relief from these extra demands and to ensure that the sibling has an opportunity to participate in family and community activities with minimal interruption.

Respite care programs can serve a number of critical functions for siblings. In particular, respite care assists siblings in five major ways:

1. *Renewing relationships with parents*   Many children with handicaps require inordinate amounts of parental attention and time, often leaving little time for parents to spend with other children. Regularly scheduled periods of respite *can* provide opportunities for siblings to be alone with their parents and receive individual attention.

2. *Providing time for special activities*   Community-based respite care services can allow siblings to participate in a full range of school and community activities. Some siblings forego opportunities to join clubs (i.e., Scouts, 4-H, etc.) or participate in school events (i.e., dances,

sports) because of extra responsibilities at home. Regular respite care, in which these extra duties are relieved, can help ensure that siblings have time to participate in ongoing activities.

3. *Allowing time for themselves* Some forms of respite care are provided to families while family members remain at home (Powell & Hecimovic, 1981). In such situations, a respite care provider comes into the home to care for the disabled child while other family members remain at home. This type of service recognizes that siblings need time to themselves in their own home. This freedom provides time for hobbies, friends, recreation, and sports.

4. *Enabling short vacations* In some families the child's disability is so severe that family participation in typical seasonal events is minimized. Through respite care programs, families are able to participate in special events, such as vacations. Regular family vacations without the disabled child may be helpful in refreshing all family members and providing family activities that otherwise would be impossible.

5. *Keeping the family system intact* A global benefit of a regular respite care period—enabling the family system to cope better with the demands of a child who has a handicap—may help it remain intact. Breaks in caregiving demands can lead to better coping skills for all involved and may prevent early institutionalization of the child who is disabled.

The potential institutionalization of a family member may be a traumatic event for siblings. Respite care can relieve some pressures for parents and siblings and provide opportunities for siblings to experience the joys and benefits of living in a special family (Helsel, 1978; Klein, 1972; Powell & Ogle, 1985; Torisky, 1979).

Naturally, not all families will utilize respite care programs to facilitate these goals. It may be necessary for some families to be "coached" or encouraged to consider the many possible functions for a respite care program. Knowing how the respite care program can assist siblings may help families utilize these services more frequently.

Involving Siblings in Respite Care Programs

Community-based respite care programs typically involve parents in the overall design, management, and evaluation of services provided (Powell & Hecimovic, 1981). Likewise, siblings can and should play a critical role in all aspects of respite care programs. Four such roles are outlined below:

1. *Providing information on respite needs* Many respite care agencies conduct regular needs assessments on respite care concerns. Siblings should be actively involved in providing ongoing information on their respite needs so that these needs can influence the type and direction of

programs developed. For example, siblings may express a strong need for respite to allow them to have more freedom after school to pursue sports, clubs, and recreational activities. With this information the respite care program can be specifically tailored to address this need. Once respite services begin, siblings should be regularly contacted to ensure that services are indeed meeting their needs.

2. *Evaluating respite services* Respite care programs should establish systems in which the services are regularly evaluated (Powell & Hecimovic, 1981). Such an evaluation system should involve siblings in all phases. Siblings can evaluate overall services, respite providers, and program costs, as well as evaluating individual episodes of respite services. The comments of siblings should be actively sought by respite care agencies. Additionally, the impact of respite care on siblings themselves in terms of relieving their personal stress should be evaluated. If respite programs are successful, data must be presented on the value of the program in terms of particular outcomes for siblings.

3. *Serving on the board of directors* Most community based services are organized with a board of directors representing consumers and family members (Thiele, Paul, & Neufeld, 1975). Siblings, notably late adolescent and adult siblings, can be effective board members in helping direct the provision of respite services. Because respite service is directed at family members, siblings should be directly represented on boards to ensure that programs will be designed to meet some of their special needs.

4. *Training respite care providers* Siblings often provide a great deal of information about their brothers and sisters from a different perspective from that of parents and professionals. Some siblings can be actively involved in respite care training programs, providing an awareness about siblings' experiences and needs. On an individual family level, siblings can provide critical information about the disabled child and his or her favored activities, as well as effective methods of care and behavior management. Respite care agencies should encourage the participation of siblings in both formal and informal training of care providers.

Using Siblings as Respite Care Providers

Providing direct care for a brother or sister for free is quite different from providing care for someone else for compensation. Some siblings make excellent respite care providers for other families. These siblings bring a keen sensitivity to the needs of children and adolescents with disabilities. As noted earlier, many of these siblings have years of "on-the-job" training in their own homes. That is not to say that siblings will not need training. In fact, respite care training may be the only formal training a sibling will receive and may provide an important source of information that can influence many areas of his or her life.

In some cases, it may be advantageous for the sibling to provide compensated respite care for his or her own family. Paying siblings for the respite they provide parents may alleviate sibling stress. As care providers, siblings are thereby formally recognized for their contributions and rewarded for their extra efforts. Arranging respite care payment to siblings for regular caregiving services communicates a clear understanding of the services siblings provide and lets them know that they are not taken for granted. Payment naturally offsets their inconvenience as any job would. Although siblings can provide some respite care within their own home, this should be viewed as supplemental respite care and arranged with some caution. Some siblings, already feeling overburdened with direct care responsibilities, may not make the best respite care providers for their own families or others. Naturally, parents need to be judicious in selecting siblings to serve as respite care providers. The benefits of respite care for siblings, as mentioned earlier, need to be kept in mind when siblings are used for respite care. Using siblings as the sole providers of respite will preclude them from realizing the benefits of a respite care program.

Reasserting Natural Opportunities for Respite

Although sibling relationships are typically our longest lifetime relationships, there are many opportunities for brothers and sisters to have periods of time away from each other. Naturally, as siblings move from the preschool years to school age and adolescence, and then to adulthood, they spend less and less time together. The intensity of the sibling relationship will vary, depending on the opportunities to develop interests and friends outside the immediate family.

In some families in which a child has a handicap, it may be helpful if parents and professionals help siblings find natural forms of respite. Some respite care agencies may focus some of their resources on helping family members, particularly siblings, utilize generic opportunities for relief from everyday pressures and demands. Four possible suggestions are presented below:

1. *Clubs and sports* Siblings should be encouraged to participate in a full range of community events (e.g., Scouting, 4-H, Campfire, organized sports, service clubs) that are conducted away from the immediate family. In many cases, especially when siblings are young, it will be necessary for parents to facilitate the sibling's participation in these events.
2. *School* Simply going to school will provide respite periods for siblings. School may be the one place where siblings will naturally feel some relief

from the demands of the disabled child. However, in some situations siblings are regularly asked to help their disabled brother and sister at school. Well-meaning educators, unfamiliar with the demands placed on siblings at home, may inadvertently create extra stress at school. Siblings have been recruited to help transport, tutor, change diapers, feed, carry books, or discipline their disabled brothers or sisters at school. Needless to say, these extra demands are not natural brother-sister school interactions and should be discouraged. Siblings should be encouraged to establish their own lives, friends, and activities at school.

3. *Friends* Siblings should be encouraged to develop friendships and should be supported in those relationships. Some parents specifically arrange times when interruptions from the disabled child will be minimal so that friends can come to the house to play. Siblings should have sufficient time and support to allow them to develop friends and partake in natural friendship activities.

4. *Relatives* Another natural form of respite care is time spent with extended family members. Grandparents, aunts, and uncles are usually eager to help alleviate the strain and stress associated with raising a child with a disability. Giving the siblings opportunities away from the immediate family, but still within a supportive family environment, may be especially helpful. Spending the night or weekend with relatives will not only provide periods of relief but also may facilitate a special close relationship between the sibling and extended family members. Relatives may not recognize the importance and value of providing special time for the siblings and may need to be asked to provide this help to families.

Respite Care and Siblings as Adults

The sibling relationship for many people is the longest relationship they will ever have. Brothers and sisters grow old, with each sharing the stages of human development and growth. The adult who has a brother or sister with a disability faces a set of unique and sometimes complex challenges (see Powell & Ogle, 1985). One of these challenges may involve the need for comprehensive community-based respite care.

> Tony's parents died 3 years ago. At that time, Tony's brother Kevin, who has Down syndrome, moved in with Tony, his wife, and three children. Tony was initially faced with a conflict: how to meet with primary responsibilities to his spouse and children while at the same time meeting his inherited direct care responsibilities to his brother. After some period of adjustment, Kevin has become an integral part of Tony's family. Early on in their new relationship, Tony and his wife recognized their need for regular periods of relief. Kevin leaves their home for a few days of out-of-home respite care every month. He also spends 3 weeks a year with a respite provider so Tony and his family can go on vacation.

Even with the growing number of community-based residential programs, Tony's situation is not atypical in many family systems. When siblings and their families take on the direct care responsibilities for disabled brothers and sisters, their need for regular and intense respite care services will be great. Such situations should be a priority for respite care agencies.

IMPLICATIONS FOR FUTURE RESEARCH

Providing respite care as a systematic service to help siblings is a relatively new concept. There are still many unknowns and areas that should be subject to formal investigation and review.

Nonhandicapped siblings are affected by the presence of a handicapped child in both positive and negative ways. It seems that there is a continuum of positive and negative outcomes for siblings and that their position on this continuum is related to a number of variables that have been discussed in detail. We still do not know how to measure, however, where any individual sibling may be on this continuum. A sibling's status on such a continuum can, of course, change over time. Recent studies on siblings of children with handicaps have begun to focus on the actual relationship and the quality of interactions between siblings as well as on new variables, such as temperament.

An examination of these interactional factors should be the focus for the next phase of research on sibling relationships. Research must begin to consider the actual quality and the development of sibling relationships in natural environments and across the lifetime.

As Skrtic, Summers, Brotherson, and Turnbull (1984) note, one of the major weaknesses in our current knowledge of sibling relationships involving a person with a handicap is the lack of perspective on that bond in relation to the family system as a whole. We need to know, for instance, how sibling relationships differ in one- and two-parent families and how interactions with parents affect the interactions of the children at various times. We do not have any systematic information on the effects of respite care services for siblings. Furthermore, as Bell (1968) reminds us, interaction is a two-way street. We also need research on the effects the siblings have on their brothers and sisters with handicaps.

When a brother or sister has a handicap, will the effects on siblings be negative or positive? The complexity behind this question prohibits an easy or quick answer. Research that draws a single conclusion presents too simplistic a solution for the resolution of such a compound issue. On the basis of what we know in the 1980s, perhaps the best answer is, "It depends." It depends on a number of contributing factors, including parental attitudes and expectations, family size, family resources, religion, severity of the child's handicap, and the pattern of interactions between the siblings. With the use of new family-oriented services, such as respite care, professionals' understanding of the unique needs of families, especially of siblings, is increasing. It is to be hoped that these new community-based programs will help ensure that the experience of having a sister or brother with a handicap will be beneficial for all family members.

SUMMARY

Respite care services can serve a number of critical functions for siblings. Regular respite can: 1) provide time for renewing relationships with parents, 2) provide time for special activities, such as Scouts or sports, 3) allow time for the siblings to be by themselves and pursue their own interests, 4) enable the family to go on vacations without the constant demands of a child who is handicapped, and thus 5) help keep the family system intact by relieving some of the pressures that come with a child who is disabled.

Siblings can be involved in respite care services both directly and indirectly. They can be involved directly through serving as paid respite care providers for other families or even for their own family. They also lend an important perspective on any respite programs and can play a critical role in the overall design and management of respite services. Specifically, siblings can contribute valuable information regarding respite needs and the evaluation of respite services. They may also serve as excellent trainers of prospective respite care providers.

Natural periods of respite should also be encouraged as a strategy for the ongoing demands on siblings who have a brother or sister who is handicapped. Siblings can participate in sports and regular school activities away from the immediate family and should also be encouraged to spend time away from the home with friends and extended relatives.

Siblings are a critical link in the family process. In families with a child who is handicapped, the sibling relationship is a special one that can have both positive and negative effects for the nonhandicapped child. It is clear that these siblings experience additional levels of stress when their brother or sister is handicapped. Feelings of frustration, pressure, and resentment are often balanced against feelings of joy and compassion. Respite care services can be a critical component in providing relief from the demands of the child who is handicapped and thus supporting the siblings within the context of the family system.

"All in all, though, I feel that Robin has brought much good into the lives of our family. He has taught us a great deal about acceptance, patience, individual worth, but most of all about love."

—M. Helsel (1978, p. 113)

REFERENCES

Bank, S., & Kahn, M. D. (1982). *The sibling bond.* New York: Basic Books.

Battle, C. U. (1974). Disruptions in the socialization of a young severely handicapped child. *Rehabilitation Literature, 35,* 120–140.

Beckman-Bell, P. (1980). *Characteristics of handicapped infants: A study of the relationship between child characteristics and stress as reported by mothers.* Unpublished doctoral dissertation, University of North Carolina, Chapel Hill.

Bell, R. (1968). A reinterpretation of the direction of effects in studies of socialization. *Psychological Review, 75,* 81–95.

Cerreto, M., & Miller, N. B. (1981). *Siblings of handicapped children: A review of the literature.* Unpublished paper. University of California Los Angeles, Los Angeles, CA.

Caldwell, B. M., & Guze, S. B. (1960). A study of the adjustment of parents and siblings of institutionalized and noninstitutionalized retarded children. *American Journal of Mental Deficiency, 64,* 845–861.

Cleveland, D., & Miller, N. (1977). Attitudes and life commitments of older siblings of mentally retarded adults: An exploratory study. *Mental Retardation, 15,* 38–41.

Crocker, A. C. (1983). Sisters and brothers. In J. A. Mulick & S. M. Pueschel (Eds.), *Parent-professional partnerships in developmental disability services.* Cambridge, MA: Ware Press.

Farber, B. (1964). *Family: Organization and interaction.* San Francisco: Chandler.

Farber, B., & Jenne, W. C. (1963). Interaction with retarded siblings and life goals of children. *Marriage and Family Living, 25,* 96–98.

Featherstone, H. (1980). *A difference in the family: Living with a disabled child.* New York: Basic Books.

Fotheringham, J., & Creal, D. (1974). Handicapped children and handicapped families. *International Review of Education, 30,* 355–373.

Fromberg, R. (1984). The sibling's changing roles. In E. Schopler & G. Mesibov (Eds.), *The effects of autism on the family.* New York: Plenum Publishing Corp.

Gath, A. (1974). Sibling reactions to mental handicap: A Comparison of the brothers and sisters of mongol children. *Journal of Child Psychology and Psychiatry, 15,* 187–198.

Graliker, B. V., Fishler, K., & Koch, R. (1962). Teenage reaction to a mentally retarded sibling. *American Journal of Mental Deficiency, 66,* 838–843.

Grossman, F. K. (1972). *Brothers and sisters of retarded children: An exploratory study.* Syracuse, NY: Syracuse University Press.

Hayden, V. (1974). The other children. *The Exceptional Parent, 4,* 26–29.

Helsel, E. (1978). The Helsels' story of Robin. In A. P. Turnbull & H. R. Turnbull (Eds.), *Parents speak out* (pp. 94–115). Columbus, OH: Charles E. Merrill Publishing Co.

Holt, K. (1958). The home care of severely retarded children. *Pediatrics, 22*(4), 744–755.

Kirk, S. A., & Bateman, B. D. (1964). *Ten years of research at the Institute for Research on Exceptional Children.* Urbana: University of Illinois.

Klein, S. D. (1972). Brothers to sister/Sister to brother. *The Exceptional Parent, 2*(1), 10–16; 2(2), 24–27, 2(3), 24–28.

Laureys, K. (1982, November). Speech given at the National Society for Children and Adults with Autism, Washington, DC. Reprinted in the *Sibling Information Network Newsletter* (1984), *3*(1), 5.

Lettick, S. (1979). Ben. *Journal of Autism and Developmental Disorders, 9*(3), 293–294.

Lobato, D. J. (1983). Siblings of handicapped children: A review. *Journal of Autism and Developmental Disorders, 13*(4), 347–364.

McHale, S. M., Simeonsson, R. J., & Sloan, J. L. (1984). Children with handicapped brothers and sisters. In E. Schopler & G. Mesibov (Eds.), *The effects of autism on the family* (pp. 327–342). New York: Plenum Publishing Corp.

Mackeith, R. (1973). The feelings and behavior of parents of handicapped children. *Developmental Medicine and Child Neurology, 15,* 524–527.

Mates, T. E. (1982, July). Which siblings of autistic children are at greater risk for the development of school and/or personality difficulties? Paper presented at the National Society for Autistic Children, Omaha, NE.

Miller, L. G. (1969). The seven stages in the life cycle of a family with a mentally retarded child. *Washington Institution Department Proceedings of the 9th Annual Meeting, 2,* 78–81.

Myers, R. (1978). *Like normal people.* New York: McGraw-Hill Book Co.

Powell, T. H., & Hecimovic, A. (1981). *Respite care for the handicapped: Helping individuals and their families.* Springfield, IL: Charles C Thomas.

Powell, T. H., & Ogle, P. A. (1985). *Brothers and sisters—A special part of exceptional families.* Baltimore: Paul H. Brookes Publishing Co.

Robson, K. S., & Moss, H. A. (1970). Patterns and determinants of maternal attachment. *Journal of Pediatrics, 77,* 976–985.

Schaffer, H. R., & Emerson, P. E. (1964). Patterns of response to physical contact in early human development. *Journal of Child Psychology and Psychiatry, 5,* 1–13.

Schreiber, M., & Feeley, M. (1965). Siblings of the retarded: A guided group experience. *Children, 12*(6), 221–225.

Schvaneveldt, J. D., & Ihinger, M. (1979). Sibling relationships in the family. In W. R. Burr, R. Hill, F. I. Nye, & I. L. Reiss (Eds.), *Contemporary theories about the family.* (Vol. 1, pp. 453–467). New York: The Free Press.

Seligman, M. (1983). Siblings of handicapped persons. In M. Seligman (ed.), *The family with a handicapped child: Understanding and treatment* (pp. 147–174). New York: Grune & Stratton.

Simeonsson, R. J., & Bailey, D. B. (1983, September). Siblings of handicapped children. Paper presented at NICHD Conference on Research on Families with Retarded Children, North Carolina.

Simeonsson, R. J., & McHale, S. M. (1981). Review. Research on handicapped children: Sibling relationships. *Child: Care, Health and Development, 7,* 153–171.

Simeonsson, R. J., & Simeonsson, N. E. (1981). Parenting handicapped children: Psychological aspects. In J. L. Paul (Ed.), *Understanding and working with parents of children with special needs* (pp. 51–88). New York: Holt, Rinehart & Winston.

Skrtic, T. M., Summers, J. A., Brotherson, M. J., & Turnbull, A. P. (1984). Severely handicapped children and their brothers and sisters. In J. Blacher (Ed.), *Severely handicapped young children and their families: Research in review.* New York: Academic Press.

Stubblefield, H. W. (1965). Religion, parents, and mental retardation. *Mental Retardation, 3, 4,* 8–11.

Taylor, L. S. (1974). *Communications between mothers and normal siblings of retarded children: Nature and modification.* Unpublished doctoral dissertation, University of North Carolina, Chapel Hill.

Theile, R. L., Paul, J. L., & Neufeld, G. R. (1975). Deinstitutionalization. In J. L.

Paul, R. Wiegerink, & G. R. Neufeld (Eds.), *Advocacy: A role for DD councils.* Chapel Hill, NC: Developmental Disabilities/Technical Assistance Service, University of North Carolina.

Torisky, J. A. (1979). My brother Eddie. *Journal of Autism and Developmental Disorders, 9*(3), 288–290.

Travis, G. (1976). *Chronic illness: Its impact on child and family.* Stanford: Stanford University Press.

Trevino, F. (1979). Siblings of handicapped children: Identifying those at risk. *Social Casework, 60,* 488–493.

Turnbull, A. P., Summers, J. A., & Brotherson, M. J. (1983). *Working with families with disabled members: A family systems approach.* Monograph, The Research and Training Center in Independent Living, University of Kansas, Lawrence, KS.

Wikler, L., Wasow, M., & Hatfield, E. (1981). Chronic sorrow revisited: Attitude of parents and professionals about adjustment to mental retardation. *American Journal of Orthopsychiatry, 51,* 63–70.

Zatlow, G. (1982). A sister's lament. *Sibling Information Network Newsletter, 1*(5), 2, Reprinted from 1981, *Citizens Future.*

Zuk, G. H., Miller, R. L., Bartram, J. B., & Kling, F. (1961). Maternal acceptance of retarded children: A questionnaire study of attitudes and religious background. *Child Development, 32,* 525–540.

Chapter 3

RESPITE SERVICES AND OLDER ADULTS WITH DEVELOPMENTAL DISABILITIES

Matthew P. Janicki, Marty Wyngaarden Krauss,
Paul D. Cotten, and Marsha Mailick Seltzer

Sylvester C. is a 53-year-old moderately mentally retarded man who had lived from birth with his mother and father on a farm. He was referred for respite care services to a state mental retardation facility following the illness of his 90-year-old mother who was no longer able to remain in their home to care for him. Given her age and condition, the prognosis for her recovery was quite poor. The facility staff, following an assessment of the situation, concluded that an alternate care arrangement had to be made, because Sylvester could not remain on the family's farm. The staff noted that he did not need to be admitted to a long-term care setting, but rather a respite period during which a comprehensive evaluation could be made and an appropriate living arrangement found. After the evaluation of his functional skills, it was felt that he would be quite able to function in a personal care home and be enrolled in a work activity center during the day. Such a home and center were found in the community in which his sister lived, enabling him to maintain contact with his family.

A salient issue for policymakers, researchers, and service providers is the identification of services that maximize the quality of life for developmentally disabled persons and minimize their dependence on the most costly types of publicly supported services. For developmentally disabled persons of all ages,

51

the most costly long-term care service is in an institutional setting. Although studies have examined the factors leading to out-of-home placement among developmentally disabled youngsters and adults (Seltzer & Krauss, 1984; Tausig, 1985), little is known about the relative importance of specific services that would serve to forestall or prevent placement of elderly developmentally disabled persons in a nursing care facility or public institution.

Findings from work done in the area of gerontology suggest that informal support networks can serve as powerful buffers to institutionalization (Hooyman, 1983). It has also been shown that many elderly persons in nursing homes are functionally quite similar to those not in such settings (Brody, Poulshock, & Maschiocchi, 1978). The availability of family supports, in addition to "objective need" for care, appears to account for a significant portion of the variability of where elderly persons live.

Currently, a great deal of attention is focused on the need to provide supportive services to those individuals (usually family members) who provide the bulk of noninstitutional care to elderly persons. This issue is often termed "supporting the supports." One of the critical services needed by formal and informal care providers of elderly persons is respite care (Anglin, 1981; Janicki, Otis, Puccio, Rettig, & Jacobson, 1985; Seltzer & Seltzer, 1985). Despite respite care's importance for older persons with developmental disabilities, very little information is available about its provision or which respite care program models are appropriate.

There are two critical reasons for incorporating respite care as a unique service within the service delivery networks for older persons with developmental disabilities. First, for those elderly developmentally disabled persons who reside with their families, overnight respite care service is an important support service that may enhance the ability of family members to continue to provide care. In this context, respite care services can be conceptualized as a vital ingredient in "supporting the supports." Further, the available evidence suggests that the majority of elderly developmentally disabled persons do not live in age-specialized congregate care housing, but rather with mentally impaired adults of varying ages (Hauber, Rotegard, & Bruininks, 1985; Jacobson, Sutton, & Janicki, 1985; Seltzer & Krauss, 1985). Respite care services that provide temporary relief for caregivers may also promote the integration of older developmentally disabled persons into a variety of settings.

The second reason for considering respite care for older developmentally disabled persons stems from the role such a service plays for the elderly individual. Within the aging network of services, daytime respite care is often provided through the elderly person's participation in a social or recreational program for senior citizens. This approach to respite care is analogous to the use of day activity or sheltered workshops for developmentally disabled individuals. The availability of a variety of day programs is a standard component in the organization and delivery of services to the population impaired because of a developmental disability (Janicki, Castellani, & Norris, 1983). Whether considered a respite program for senior citizens or a day activity program for persons with developmental disabilities, the underlying goal is to provide relief from responsibility for informal or formal care providers while simultaneously offering age-appropriate day services to the elderly person.

In this chapter, the authors examine the following broad array of service concerns related to respite care, which are raised by the increasing size of the older developmentally disabled population residing in community settings: the size and scope of the need for these types of services, the character of the types of services needed, and how to address the needs. Examples from both the developmental disabilities service network and the aging services network are provided.

THE POPULATION OF CONCERN

Older Persons

In the United States, as in other industrialized countries, the size and continued growth of the overall elderly population are becoming a source of concern for administrators, program providers, and public officials. The nation's population of elders has doubled since the beginning of the century and is expected to triple within 50 years (Siegel & Taeuber, 1982). According to the U.S. Bureau of the Census, in 1960 there were approximately 16.7 million persons age 65 and over, comprising slightly more than 9% of the population. In contrast, the same age population numbered 25.5 million persons in 1980, representing slightly more than 11% of the nation's total population—a 55% increase in just 20 years.

Further, there has been a dramatic growth among older generational groups. In this same 20-year period the number of individuals aged 75 to 84 rose 65%, whereas the number of those 85 and older increased by 174%. Currently, over 60% of all older persons are between the ages of 65 and 74, 30% between the ages of 75 and 84, and about 9% aged 85 and older. Because women tend to outlive men, the majority of the nation's older population are female, and this disparity in longevity continues to increase with age (Rice & Feldman, 1985).

Most elderly persons live in their own homes (AARP, 1982). Only a small proportion (some 5% at any one time) of the overall elderly reside in nursing homes: however, this number increases to about 22% among the "very old"—those aged 85 and older. Living with a spouse is the most common community living arrangement for elderly persons. However, because females tend to outlive males, women and persons aged 85 or older are more likely to have some other type of community living arrangement. Studies indicate that only about 17% of all elderly persons live with either a nonspouse relative or a friend (Shanas, 1977). The same studies have indicated that those individuals of advanced age who live with others are at most need for such support services as respite care. This is in contrast to those individuals who continue to live by themselves; they tend to need a range of in-home support services, rather than out-of-home respite care (Dunlop, 1980).

These general characteristics of the overall elderly population are both similar to and different from what is known about the elderly developmentally disabled population. Conservative estimates of the size of the population of elderly developmentally disabled persons (defined here as age 55 and older) in the United States range between 200,000 to 300,000 individuals nationally (DiGiovanni, 1978; Jacobson et al., 1985), with women outnumbering men with increasing age. Further, the percentage of developmentally disabled individuals who are institutionalized increases with advancing age. A number of reports have indicated that between 40% and 60% of known older developmentally disabled persons reside in institutional long-term care settings (Cocks & Ng, 1984; Hauber et al., 1985; Jacobson et al., 1985; Janicki & MacEachron, 1984; Sutton, 1983). Most of those residing in community settings are in sheltered care living arrangements, such as adult homes, group homes, or foster family settings (Cocks & Ng, 1984; Hauber et al., 1985; Janicki & MacEachron, 1984; Sutton, 1983). Those developmentally disabled persons of advancing age who continue to live with their families represent only a small proportion of the overall known elderly developmentally disabled population.

For example, Sutton (1983) and Janicki and MacEachron (1984) reported that, of California's and New York's known developmentally disabled population who were in their 50s, some 17% and 13%, respectively, resided with a parent or guardian. The percent declined with age—11% and 5% for those in their 60s and 6% and 4%, respectively, for those 70 and older. Further, a survey conducted in Maryland of all known developmentally disabled adults residing at home revealed that adults age 50 and older represented only 5.1% of that state's total in-home population; the figure dropped to 0.7% for those individuals age 65 and older and to 0.2% for those age 75 and older (Black, Smull, Crites, & Sachs, 1985).

As more workers in the area of developmental disabilities become concerned with in-home and other support services for the elderly disabled population, questions arise as to appropriate functional and/or chronological criteria by which to identify or define the population (Jacobson et al., 1985; Seltzer, 1985). In the United States most services for the nation's elderly population are prescribed in the Older Americans Act of 1965 (PL 89–73, as amended). The Act defines eligibility for services using the chronological age of 60 and older. Within the field of developmental disabilities, studies indicate that in many instances the biological, psychological, and social effects of aging can appear in persons before age 60. This has resulted in considerable ambivalence in the use of a purely chronological definition for identification of elderly disabled persons. For example, there is accumulating evidence that individuals with Down syndrome may exhibit signs of premature aging as early as their late 30s and early 40s (Wisniewski & Hill, 1985). With most developmentally disabled individuals, however, their mid-50s appear to mark a period in life-span development in which the dimunition of some physical reserves and the onset of a psychological adjustment to being older are manifested (Janicki & Jacobson, 1986). Consequently, many developmental disabilities professionals acknowledge the early 50s (with the exceptions noted in relation to premature aging) as a time when life activities should be adjusted to reflect normative age patterns, interests, and physical capabilities.

Often, a distinction is made between developmentally disabled individuals who are "aging" (i.e., between the ages of 55 and 75) and those who are "aged" (i.e., over age 75). Aging in this sense corresponds to a period of life when an individual and his or her activities undergo changes that reflect differing orientations and roles as an adult. Being aged can be characterized by significant changes in physical, emotional, and psychological capacities.

Little information is available about the characteristics of elderly developmentally disabled individuals who receive respite services. However, as shown in Table 1, some preliminary data from New York's Developmental Disabilities Information System (Janicki & Jacobson, 1982) comparing elderly respite care receivers to nonreceivers show that, generally, elderly respite care receivers are more likely to be female, be more intellectually impaired, and be less capable or independent in basic self-care skills. Compared to developmentally disabled respite care receivers of all ages, elderly developmentally disabled receivers are more likely to be female, less intellectually impaired, more independent in mobility, and more capable in basic self-care skills.

In summary, older developmentally disabled persons represent a significant portion of the developmentally disabled population receiving publicly supported services and will continue to do so in the future. Currently only a small segment of these individuals live with relatives. However, as a group these persons will need more frequent respite care as they grow older and more frail. They are clearly at risk for possible institutionalization in the absence of support services both for themselves and for their primary caregivers. The next section examines the special needs and characteristics of this latter group.

Table 1. Comparison of older and younger developmentally disabled respite receivers and non-receivers

	All ages		Age 50 or older	
	Not receiving respite (18,269)	Receiving respite (1,158)	Not receiving respite (425)	Receiving respite (35)
Sex				
Males	58[a]	57	51	46
Females	42	43	49	54
Level of retardation				
Normal/above	21	7	14	6
Mild mental retardation	29	19	35	24
Moderate mental retardation	27	28	27	38
Severe mental retardation	15	25	19	24
Profound mental retardation	9	22	6	9
Undetermined	21	15	16	3
Free of impairment				
Hearing	94	90	89	85
Vision	91	85	87	91
Mobility	82	71	80	83
Independent in:				
Toileting	68	52	88	82
Eating	68	53	86	75
Dressing/grooming	49	33	63	55

[a]Percentages of those individuals residing with their families.

The Caregivers

Among the general population the main providers of personal assistance to older people typically are immediate family members, such as spouses and daughters (Gurland, 1978). However, many caregivers for the elderly are old themselves and are vulnerable to a number of the same problems experienced by the persons for whom they provide care. The primary family caregivers for the general elderly population are daughters. Most developmentally disabled persons, however, do not have offspring, and thus, a major difference between the mentally disabled population and the general elderly population is in the availability of younger family members to provide critically important support. The responsibility and burden of care for older developmentally disabled persons living at home consequently fall on their older parents or, in some cases, their siblings.

Seltzer (1985) notes that those individual variables that have been found to be related to the degree of family stress among caregivers in the general elderly population are often characteristic of the elderly developmentally disabled person. These variables include being unmarried, being more impaired, requiring personal care, and having a limited activity level. Thus, for those elderly developmentally disabled persons who are cared for by either their parents or a sibling, research findings suggest that these care providers are at risk for sustained stress in their caregiving role. Assuming that the majority of older adults who reside at home are in the 50 to 65 age group and that, in most instances their parents are 20 to 30 years older, the problem of care becomes one of a still older person providing substantial care for an older developmentally disabled person.

> *Mary K. is a 52-year-old woman who has Down syndrome and is moderately mentally retarded. She had been living with her parents all her life and had never been in a school or work program. Her mother, in her 80s, had become increasingly unable to care for the family because of a succession of illnesses. Mary's father, also in his 80s, was able to provide some help in the home during his wife's illnesses, but recently he fell and his injuries made it difficult for him to move about. A local senior center was notified about the needs of the family by a neighbor who was becoming increasingly concerned. A caseworker, following a visit to the home, made arrangements for a homemaker aide to come and prepare meals and provide housekeeping services on a daily basis. The senior center also notified the local Association for Retarded Citizens (ARC) agency about the family's plight. ARC made arrangements for Mary to receive periodic overnight respite at one of their group homes and to go to the senior center for their crafts and activities program three times a week. The family is now receiving some in-home supports, and the parents have made arrangements for Mary to move to the group home in the near future.*

As noted by Anglin (1981), parents in their 70s and 80s may need their own special support services to manage infirmities associated with their own aging. If they are simultaneously the primary care provider for an older developmentally disabled adult living at home, then care services must be directed at two generations (see the vignette of Mary K). It may be that the developmentally disabled adult is providing instrumental or emotional support for his or her parent(s). However, the need for adequate formal support services to such a family unit can be pivotal to the family's stability as a unit and to the individual's quality of life. Studies have shown that many older developmentally disabled persons living at home are the subject of a parental request for out-of-home placement. In a study of one state's waiting lists for residential services, almost 20% of developmentally disabled adults age 50 and older said to need a different residential care setting were individuals currently residing at home with their parents. The study also found that most of the requests for out-of-home placement were not for institutional care, but for community group home type settings (NYS OMRDD, 1985).

In order to avert or delay out-of-home placements for older developmentally disabled persons, especially those living with elderly parents, an enhanced combination of home care and day or support services for the developmentally disabled adult is necessary. These services, along with the typical social services provided by the disabled individual's day program, can assist aging parents in meeting the care and supervision needs of their developmentally disabled daughter or son. Indeed, a number of reports have indicated that respite or day care and other family supports are the most commonly requested services by parents or other in-community primary caregivers (Anglin, 1981; Black et al., 1985; Seltzer & Seltzer, 1985). Further, a preference for direct services, rather than fiscal assistance, has been found among caregivers of aged persons (Horowitz & Shindelman, 1984).

In addition to an elderly developmentally disabled person's parents, other caregivers, such as the extended family network, neighbors, and workers in community alternative care arrangements, can also provide respite care. In an extended family network, an elderly developmentally disabled person can often move in with other family members when temporary housing or relief for the primary caregiver is necessary. At times this may develop into a shared housing arrangement if the person has more than a minimum amount of skills and participates in a day program, thus providing some respite from supervision for the extended family members. Utilizing such an arrangement has other benefits as well; often space in a day program is limited and being able to remain in proximity of the program means that the older individual can remain enrolled in it.

Neighbors are often another source of respite care, particularly in smaller communities. Rural and less populated settings can be very supportive communities, and in many instances, a neighbor or church member may provide respite services in a time of crisis for the immediate family. Because the older developmentally disabled person is already known to a neighbor or church member and is readily viewed as an integral part of that community, respite care is often easier for both the older person and the caregiver.

Other caregivers include those individuals who work in a range of alternate care settings, such as group homes, or who serve as foster family care parents. At times these settings have a respite bed available that is dedicated for the use of developmentally disabled individuals of all ages. Or a vacant bed in the setting can be used as a respite care bed when overnight respite of an emergency or anticipated short-term nature is required. The obverse of this situation is often found in foster family care settings; foster family care providers agree to provide continual supervision for the developmentally disabled individual in their care. However, many states now recognize that even in these situations respite from the burden of care is necessary to avoid strain or provide the foster care parent time for personal business. In such instances, either another individual comes into the home while the foster care parent is away, or the developmentally disabled individual, by mutual agreement, is placed in respite care at another setting. In some instances, this respite can be achieved by the disabled individual's enrollment in a summer vacation or adult camp program.

THE RESPITE MODELS

The prevalent models of respite care developed for younger developmentally disabled persons (Salisbury & Griggs, 1983), with some variations, are also applicable to older developmentally disabled persons (see Figure 1). Respite

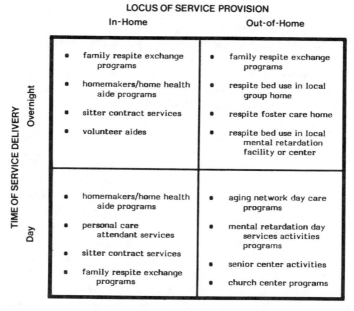

Figure 1.   Respite models by locus and time of service provision.

services for older persons can provide either time-limited overnight relief for the caregiver or extended daytime care for the disabled individual, coupled with the provision of a range of other support services. These basic models can also be generalized across various levels and types of impairment experienced by the older person, including persons who require intensive supervision due to an inability to care for themselves (e.g., individuals with Alzheimer's disease). What may differ is the manner in which daytime respite is provided, as discussed below.

Overnight Respite

This type of respite care is used for all age groups; it involves the provision of relief for a primary caregiver—either a parent, sibling, guardian, or a contract surrogate as in the case of foster family care—for one or more days including the overnight period. Such relief or respite may occur in the developmentally disabled individual's home, enabling the primary care provider to leave for a period of time, or may be provided in another site, such as a neighboring group home, a neighbor's house, a long-term care facility with respite capacity, a contract respite worker's residence, or other settings established for this purpose. Reasons for the parent/caregiver request for such service may include a family emergency, planned vacation, hospitalization, other caregiver commitment to be away, or simply a need for temporary relief from the day-to-day responsibility of care. Overnight respite care is discussed in more detail elsewhere in this volume.

Overnight respite can also take the form of a short stay in a health care or other type of long-term care setting for older developmentally disabled individuals who normally live by themselves, but because of a temporary infirmity or short-term need for nursing care cannot remain alone. The vignette of Tom S. illustrates this type of situation.

> *Tom S. is an 80-year-old mildly mentally retarded man who was admitted to a state mental retardation center at the age of 16 on the signature of two physicians who declared him to be "feebleminded." In 1979 he was referred to and accepted for admission in a supervised apartment complex, part of a complex of HUD-subsidized housing for elderly/handicapped persons in a small town. Before living at the complex he had been a foster grandparent as part of the Foster Grandparents Program at the retardation facility. He has continued to be involved in the program, as well as participating in a craft program for senior citizens. Recently, he had to have cataract surgery; because there would be no one to assume responsibility for his care immediately following discharge from the hospital, he was admitted to the infirmary at the retardation center for a short period of time. Once he was able to*

care for himself, he returned to his apartment and received some help from a neighbor.

Day Respite

This type of respite, also used for all age groups, is particularly relevant for elderly developmentally disabled persons. Day respite is becoming a prevalent model in the aging field, where it is usually referred to as "adult day care" (National Council on the Aging, 1984). In general, adult day care services, as sponsored by the aging services network, are described as an organized program of therapeutic, social, and health activities and services provided to adults in a congregate setting persuant to an individualized plan of care designed for the purpose of restoring or maintaining optimal capacity for self-care.

Generally, the aging network's model for adult day care includes the provision of medical, nursing, physical therapy, occupational therapy, and other types of services, such as podiatry, personal hygiene, nutrition, meals, and eye examinations, as well as a range of recreational and personal-social services. In many states, such programs are supported through funds obtained from the Older Americans Act (Palmer, 1982) and/or through state mental disability agencies (Goldstein & Egly, 1985). These programs can be categorized according to their primary function or focus: restorative, maintenance, or social (Palmer, 1982). Restorative models are particularly appropriate for individuals needing specialized medical care or follow-up and/or rehabilitative care. Maintenance models are applicable for individuals who need continuous supervision and assistance with basic personal and activities of daily living skills (ADLs). Social models are appropriate for individuals who need the structural and social support of being with age peers and participating in enriching and stimulating activities. Each of these models are needed by and thus generalizable to older persons with developmental disabilities.

Because the first two models generally represent long-term care service models for medically needy or psychiatrically impaired elders, rather than relief or respite services, the following discussion focuses on the social model. Of these three models, social programs have the most practical day respite applications for adults with developmental disabilities. These social day care programs serve those adults who need social stimulation and interaction, supervision, assistance with ADLs, and other areas of social functioning. In addition to providing structural settings in which these necessary services are provided to the elderly, these programs provide a valuable relief or respite to the caregivers of these elders. Further, the types of ancilliary activities available through these programs, such as opportunities for socialization, leisure-time activities, exercise, nutrition, and attention to health status, can be very beneficial to the older adult. Generally, these types of programs are provided as part of the local aging networks' comprehensive program structure and in many instances through senior centers.

In many communities, day respite services, including variations of the three models described above, that are appropriate for older developmentally disabled adults are available both through the locality's aging services network and/or the developmental disabilities services system. Such day services may be sponsored by the retardation system through agencies that also provide a selected range of residential, day, vocational, or family support services. Although these agencies typically target their services to the needs of the developmentally disabled individual, services may also be provided to parent(s) or other family members caring for an aging or aged mentally retarded persons. In other instances, parents can obtain social services and accompanying day respite care through the aging network's programs. In contrast to developmental disabilities agencies, aging network agencies supported by funds provided under the Older Americans Act are required to make available a broad range of support services, as well as in-home services, such as homemaker and home health aides, to the elderly person and/or the primary caregivers of these individuals. If both services networks are utilized, older mentally retarded adults who need a variety of types of support or assistance can obtain both the services provided by the developmental disabilities agencies and can participate in senior citizen center programs as a type of structured or formal day program.

Although many professionals in the field of developmental disabilities promote the use of generic senior centers by individuals with developmental disabilities, experience has shown that such service integration requires considerable investment of agency commitment and professional support. Many senior centers have reached out to older disabled persons and designed ways to integrate them into center activities. In other instances the social structure of the centers has served as a barrier to their more widespread use. Salamon and Trubin (1983) have noted that, in some centers, client behaviors that are problematic and/or create interpersonal tensions among the center's users contribute to social disharmony, rather than social cohesion. Although this characterization is not relevant for all senior centers, it highlights the need to develop administrative and programmatic linkages between the capacities of generic senior citizens programs and the needs of older intellectually disadvantaged individuals.

Janicki (1984) has described three potential barriers to the successful integration of elderly developmentally disabled persons into generic senior centers: "handicapism," economics, and inexperience and fear. The first barrier, "handicapism," is the expression of negative attitudes by center administrators, staff, and/or nondisabled center users toward age peers who are either mentally or physically disabled. This attitudinal bias manifests itself in center staff or users not wanting persons who are disabled in their programs.

The second potential barrier is economics. Limited monies are allocated to area agencies on aging and their providers. Service priorities may be established that preclude providing services for developmentally disabled individuals. Administrators of aging agencies argue that services to developmentally disabled individuals are the lifelong responsibility of the developmental disabilities services network, which has its own unique funding sources. One specific concern is that developmentally disabled persons might pose an increased demand on staff time and volunteer resources.

The last potential barrier, inexperience and fear, is rooted in a lack of knowledge by senior citizen center staff about how to provide services to "different" populations. Many aging services operators are neither trained nor prepared to provide services to someone who is developmentally disabled or otherwise disabled. They may overestimate the severity of behavioral problems commonly associated with developmental disabilities and therefore may be reluctant to include developmentally disabled persons in programs designed for elderly citizens.

There are similar barriers to the use of the developmental disabilities services system to accommodate the special care needs of elderly developmentally disabled persons. From a programmatic perspective, many retardation or developmental services providers in the community—and in insitutions, for that matter—are primarily oriented toward the service needs of children and adults. They are equally inexperienced in articulating and meeting the needs of older developmentally disabled persons. Although some program models exist, there is currently no systematic mechanism for disseminating information about those needs, and there is a clear lack of evaluation studies that could guide new program design. Further, the lack of staff knowledge regarding the aging process for persons with developmental disabilities is consistently noted as a major problem (Commissioner's Committee, 1983).

However, strategic mechanisms can be employed to overcome these potential barriers. For example, although negative attitudes toward disabled persons are prevalent in many sections of society, effective methods have been designed and employed to change those attitudes. Although such methods can be employed to reach those seniors who would not want to associate with age peers with disabilities, a more fundamental problem is inherent in these expressions of "handicapism." Many older persons, when in the company of a disabled individual, are confronted with their own mortality and growing frailness. Unless aging network programs attend to these latent fears, the problems of "handicapism" will remain. Economic considerations are more easily addressed. Mental retardation providers can develop staff-sharing agreements or supplemental funding arrangements that would provide the senior center programs with the additional resources needed to accommodate a small number of elderly developmentally disabled persons. The third barrier of inexperience and fear can be addressed by staff training and exchanges between aging and developmental disabilities providers. Senior center staff can attend training sessions conducted by developmental disabilities professionals, and developmental disabilities agency staff can attend training sessions conducted by gerontologists and aging services providers. Further, cross-employment on a part-time basis of personnel and professionals from both systems would also aid in the exchange of the relevant techniques of each field.

CONCLUSION

This chapter has examined the role of respite care services within the service delivery system for older developmentally disabled persons. It has also addressed a number of issues that need to be considered in the development of sound programmatic and policy guidelines for service growth. The increasing size of the elderly population of developmentally disabled persons creates a situation in which the need for respite care, as well as other support services commonly prescribed for older persons, will become more pressing. The potential value of respite care as a protective factor in forestalling out-of-home or institutional placement needs to be carefully examined through research. However, the evidence from work by gerontologists suggests that respite care is indeed a powerful form of support to both the elderly person and his or her care providers.

Major programmatic issues include the feasibility and consequences of integrating developmentally disabled elders with their nondisabled age peers in service networks that provide respite care. However, as discussed in this chapter, there are a number of potential and known barriers to such integration. Although attitudinal barriers are difficult to modify through administrative or programmatic decision making, it is possible to act positively in developing educational and training materials to increase staff capabilities in serving older developmentally disabled persons. In addition, more activity is needed to increase the production and dissemination of knowledge regarding the aging process for mentally retarded and otherwise developmentally disabled persons.

Particular emphasis needs to be paid to articulating the ways in which aging for this group is similar to and/or different from the aging process for nonchronically-impaired elders. Staff training activities need to be expanded for both gerontologists and developmental disabilities professionals. Neither of these two professional groups has received adequate preparation for meeting the needs of developmentally disabled persons as they age.

More attention needs to be directed at identifying support services considered critical by the care providers of older developmentally disabled persons. Respite care has typically been highly valued by families of developmentally disabled individuals, and it can be hypothesized that this service will only increase in its desirability over the life-span of caring for such persons. It is important, however, that the need for respite care be well documented in order to promote the development of sensitive and effective service delivery networks.

Greater access to the services available under the Older Americans Act for persons with developmental disabilities needs to be explored. Although many professionals in the aging services network assert that there are no disability-related barriers to the provision of services, there are too few examples of localities where such client integration has been tried and successfully achieved. It may be that professionals in the field of developmental disabilities are unaware of the potential uses of the Older Americans Act's provisions for their older clients. This lack of knowledge suggests that resource guides need to be developed and made available within the developmental disabilities service delivery field to acquaint case managers with the full range of services available. Lastly, based on the paucity of available demographic and service utilization data, it is clear that a substantially more focused research effort must be undertaken in this area.

REFERENCES

American Association of Retired Persons. (1982). *A profile of older Americans.* Washington: Author.

Anglin, B. (1981). *They never ask for help: A study of the needs of elderly retarded people in Metro Toronto.* Maple, Ontario: Belsten Publishing.

Black, M. M., Smull, M. W., Crites, L. S., & Sachs, M. L. (1985). *Mentally retarded adults and their families: A model of stress and urgency.* Baltimore: University of Maryland School of Medicine.

Brody, S., Poulshock, S. W., & Maschiochhi, C. F. (1978). The family caring unit: A major consideration in the long term support system. *The Gerontologist, 18,* 556–566.

Brown, D. L. (1972). Obstacles to services for the mentally retarded. *Social Work, 17*(4), 98–101.

Cocks, E., & Ng, C. P. (1984). Characteristics of those persons registered with the Mental Retardation Division. *Australian and New Zealand Journal of Developmental Disabilities, 9,* 117–127.

Commissioner's Committee on Aging and Developmental Disabilities. (1983). *Report of the commissioners committee on aging and developmental disabilities.* Albany: New York State Office of Mental Retardation and Developmental Disabilities.

DiGiovanni, L. (1978). The elderly retarded: A little-known group. *The Gerontologist, 18,* 262–266.

Dunlop, B. D. (1980). Expanded home-based care for the impaired elderly: Solution or pipe dream. *American Journal of Public Health, 70,* 514–519.

Goldstein, F. M., & Egly, S. R. (1985). Adult day care: An extension of the family. *Aging, 348,* 19–21.

Gurland B. (1978). Personal time dependency in the elderly of New York City. In Community Council of Greater New York (Ed.), *Dependency in the elderly of New York City.* New York: Author.

Hauber, F. A., Rotegard, L. L., & Bruininks, R. H. (1985). Characteristics of residential services for older/elderly mentally retarded persons. In M. P. Janicki & H. M. Wisniewski (Eds.), *Aging and developmental disabilities: Issues and approaches* (pp. 327–350). Baltimore: Paul H. Brookes Publishing Co.

Hooyman, N. (1983). Social support networks in services to the elderly. In J. K. Whittaker & J. Garbarino (Eds.), *Social support networks: Informal helping in the human services* (pp. 134–163. New York: Aldine Publishing Co.

Horowitz, A., & Shindelman, L. W. (1984). Social and economic incentives for family caregivers. *Health Care Financing Review, 5*(2), 25–33.

Jacobson, J. W., Sutton, M. S., & Janicki, M. P. (1985). Demography and characteristics of aging and aged mentally retarded persons. In M. P. Janicki & H. M. Wisniewski (Eds.), *Aging and developmental disabilities: Issues and approaches* (pp. 115–142). Baltimore: Paul H. Brookes Publishing Co·

Janicki, M. P. (1984, August). *Aging and aged developmentally disabled persons: A population in transition.* Paper presented at the Joseph P. Kennedy, Jr. Foundation Meeting on Programs for the Elderly Retarded Person, Bedford, MA.

Janicki, M. P., Castellani, P. J., & Norris, R. G. (1983). Organization and administration of service delivery systems. In J. L. Matson & J. A. Mulick (Eds.), *Handbook of mental retardation* (pp. 3–23). New York: Pergamon Press.

Janicki, M. P., & Jacobson, J. W. (1982). The character of developmental disabilities in New York State: Preliminary observations. *International Journal of Rehabilitation Research, 5,* 191–202.

Janicki, M. P., & Jacobson, J. W. (1986). Generational trends in sensory, physical, and behavioral abilities among older mentally retarded persons. *American Journal of Mental Deficiency, 90.*

Janicki, M. P., & MacEachron, A. E. (1984). Residential, health, and social service needs of elderly developmentally disabled persons. *The Gerontologist, 84,* 128–137.

Janicki, M. P., Otis, J. P., Puccio, P. S., Rettig, J. H., & Jacobson, J. W. (1985). Service needs among older developmentally disabled persons. In M. P. Janicki & H. M. Wisniewski (Eds.), *Aging and developmental disabilities: Issues and approaches* (pp. 289–304). Baltimore: Paul H. Brookes Publishing Co.

National Council on the Aging. (1984). *Standards for adult day care.* Washington, DC: Author.

NYS OMRDD. (1985). *A report on residential waiting lists.* Albany, NY: Author.

Palmer, H. C. (1982). Adult day care. In R. Vogel & H. C. Palmer (Eds.), *Long term care: Perspectives from research and demonstrations* (pp. 415–436). Baltimore: Health Care Financing Administration.

Rice, D. P., & Feldman, J. J. (1985). Living longer in the United States: Demographic changes and health needs of the elderly. In M. P. Janicki & H. M. Wisniewski (Eds.), *Aging and developmental disabilities: Issues and approaches* (pp. 9–26). Baltimore: Paul H. Brookes Publishing Co.

Salamon & Trubin (1983). Difficulties in senior center life: Group behaviors. *Clinical Gerontologist, 2*(2), 23–37.

Salisbury, C., & Griggs, P. (1983). Developing respite care services for families of handicapped persons. *Journal of The Association for Persons with Severe Handicaps, 8,* 50–57.

Seltzer, M. M. (1985). Research in social aspects of aging and developmental disabilities. In M. P. Janicki & H. M. Wisniewski (Eds.), *Aging and developmental disabilities: Issues and approaches* (pp. 161–173). Baltimore: Paul H. Brookes Publishing Co.

Seltzer, M. M. (1985). Informal supports for elderly mentally retarded persons. *American Journal of Mental Deficiency, 90,* 259–265.

Seltzer, M. M., & Krauss, M. W. (1984). Family, community residence, and institutional placements of a sample of mentally retarded children. *American Journal of Mental Deficiency, 89,* 257–266.

Seltzer, M. M., & Krauss, M. W. (May, 1985). *Programs for aging persons with mental retardation: Model program types and characteristics.* Paper presented at the 109th annual meeting of the American Association on Mental Deficiency, Philadelphia, PA.

Seltzer, M. M., & Seltzer, G. B. (1985). The elderly mentally retarded: A group in need of service. *Journal of Gerontological Social Work, 8,* 99–119.

Shanas, E. (1977). *The national survey of the aged.* Chicago: University of Chicago.

Siegel, J. S., & Taeuber, C. M. (1982). The 1980 census and the elderly: New data available to planners and practitioners. *The Gerontologist, 22,* 144–150.

Sutton, M. S. (1983, August). *Treatment issues and the elderly institutionalized developmentally disabled.* Paper presented at the 91st annual convention of the American Psychological Association, Anaheim, CA.

Tausig, M. (1985). Factors in family decision-making about placement for developmentally disabled individuals. *American Journal of Mental Deficiency, 89,* 352–361.

Wisniewski, H. M., & Hill, A. L. (1985). Clinical aspects of dementia in mental retardation and developmental disabilities. In M. P. Janicki & H. M. Wisniewski (Eds.), *Aging and developmental disabilities: Issues and approaches* (pp. 195–210). Baltimore: Paul H. Brookes Publishing Co.

Chapter 4

RESPITE CARE
A NATIONAL PERSPECTIVE

Mary A. Slater

During the past 2 decades, families with handicapped children have been increasingly encouraged to raise these children within a normal home environment. This encouragement has been predicated on philosophical as well as economic concerns. It is currently believed that handicapped children will achieve more normal levels of functioning simply by living within a mainstreamed supportive home environment. This concept, termed normalization, has had a profound impact on all levels of program development for the handicapped individual. Complementing this belief is a realistic financial concern for the rising costs of institutional care. In many states, the cost of institutional care ranges from $30,000 to $40,000 per child per year.

As families have attempted to raise their handicapped child at home, a number of concerns have arisen. Parents, particularly the mother, experience an increased burden of care. Handicapped children require special caregiving responsibilities daily and these responsibilities continue over prolonged periods. As parents and siblings expend substantial blocks of time in caring for, training, and transporting the handicapped member, other family functions are frequently neglected. Family members become socially isolated, with little time and energy available for normal social activities, such as visiting friends, relatives, and neighbors. Vacations tend to be forgotten. Special employment opportunities are rejected. Stress levels in the homes rise. Marital conflicts and neglect of normal sibling needs are of frequent concern. As time passes, many parents experience a loss of autonomy or feel a lack of control over one of life's major endeavors: raising a child. Families who have been unable to maintain their handicapped member within the home have identified a lack of dominance and control over their lives as the primary determining factor, with financial strains noted as a secondary concern

(Frohlich, 1975). In terms of psychological benefits, empowerment or maintaining control over one's major forces may be a greater source of fulfillment than financial independence (Boggs, 1984).

Respite care services have been initiated to provide at least temporary relief for these families. These programs were primarily initiated by grassroots efforts of families to meet a very practical need: relief from day-to-day caregiving responsibilities of the handicapped member. A number of program models have emerged; however, no theoretical or research knowledge was employed *to guide the development of these models.* Financial support was gathered from any available source. Federal, state, and local sources were tapped, and fees were charged where appropriate. Presently, these programs are located throughout the country. Yet, only limited information is available on these programs' type of models, availability, costs, staffing patterns, and implementation obstacles.

The purpose of this chapter is to provide an overview of current respite care efforts. Three major surveys are highlighted: 1) a nationwide survey of respite care programs conducted by the national office of the Association for Retarded Citizens (ARC), entitled "Characteristics of Respite Care Programs" (ARC, 1982); 2) state surveys of respite care programs; and 3) respite care services provided through state family support programs (Slater, Bates, Eicher, & Wikler, in press). Data from a limited number of program models are also included to indicate the possible effects of well-conceived and well-conducted programs on family members' internal functioning. Deficiencies in program models are summarized. The chapter concludes on a futuristic note by introducing the concept of "normalized family resources." This concept views respite care as one component of a community-based family support system, a system that focuses on aiding all family members to live as normal a life as possible.

NATIONAL ASSOCIATION FOR RETARDED CITIZENS

During 1982, the ARC conducted a nationwide survey of 568 respite care programs identified by state and local ARC units throughout the country. Several different models of services were identified by the more than 200 completed surveys (see Figure 1). Program models can be distinguished both on the basis of facility used and the process employed in providing respite care. Almost one-half of the programs provide services in the client's or provider's home. Home-based services offer the advantage of a familiar setting for the developmentally disabled individual and continuity of regular programs, such as educational, religious, and recreational services. This approach may be particularly beneficial for those handicapped individuals for whom transportation is a problem. A distinct disadvantage is that only one

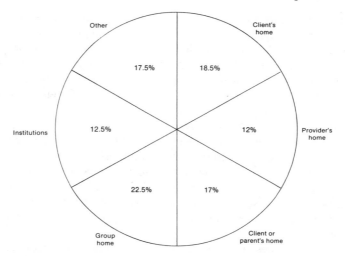

Figure 1. Percent of respite care models serving persons with developmental disabilities

family at a time is served by a home-based program. In contrast, when the developmentally disabled person is given care and supervision in the home of the provider, more than one individual with developmental disabilities may be served simultaneously. Frequently, the provider in the home is licensed for child care or certified as a foster parent. Disadvantages of this approach are attributable to the fixed site. Parents must transport the handicapped member to the provider's home, sometimes a difficult feat for the multiply handicapped individual. In addition, the handicapped individual may feel uncomfortable in unfamiliar surroundings. Some programs make respite available either in the provider's *or* client's home, depending on the family's preference.

Nearly one-quarter of the providers surveyed indicated that they provided respite care through group homes established to serve only respite clients. These group homes are usually operated by a service or volunteer agency (e.g., mental health/mental retardation centers, Association for Retarded Citizens, or United Cerebral Palsy) that maintains administrative responsibility, such as hiring and training staff members and processing admissions and scheduling. There are many advantages to this approach. Long periods of respite care are available in a least restrictive setting. Physical surroundings and daily activities may simulate a home-like environment. An adequately trained staff is available to serve developmentally disabled individuals who require intensive programming. The disadvantages of this approach are tied to the formal application procedures and the fact that there is generally a waiting list for it. Respite care clients may also be served in group homes primarily designed to meet the long-term community residential needs of developmentally disabled individuals. In this approach, one or two respite beds are maintained within the group home. Advantages and disadvantages are similar to those associated with respite group home care. Because only a few respite beds are available, there may be increased difficulty in obtaining the service.

Thirteen percent of respite care programs are provided by private or public institutions. Within these facilities, respite clients are served by the same staff and in the same setting as long-term residents. The major advantage of this approach is that difficult-to-manage and medically fragile clients may be served. Its major disadvantage is the restrictive nonnormalized setting. The disabled person may experience adjustment problems due to the marked differences between the institutional setting and the natural home environment.

In addition to these major approaches, a number of models were identified within the category of other approaches. Collectively, they constitute 18% of all respite care programs. Local volunteer and advocacy agencies offer respite care as part of their larger family support effort. Typically, the organization operates the respite program in its local headquarters. Drop-ins are usually accepted, and some programs provide evening care. The approach is designed to provide very short-term care that allows parents time for shopping and errands. The major disadvantage is the limited time-span and the service's inability to respond to emergency needs. To serve the client with chronic medical problems requiring 24-hour medical care and supervision, some pediatric clinics and nursing homes have arranged a respite service. The key advantage of this model is that it can accommodate clients who are refused admission to most other programs.

Parent cooperatives, another form of respite care, use members of developmentally disabled families who volunteer to serve as respite providers to other families. After a roster of volunteers is drawn up, the parent cooperative is usually coordinated by a staff member of a local agency or organization. The coordinator maintains records, ensuring that those who use respite care are also serving others. This approach is one of the most cost-effective as it requires funds only for the position of coordinator. Limited time is needed to establish the program because no extensive orientation or training sessions are required. However, as with all approaches considered, some disadvantages exist. Respite care is usually limited to overnight or weekend stays. Lengthy respite (longer than a weekend) is not practical. Burnout is a common problem because the respite providers are caring for members of their own family, in addition to other developmentally delayed persons. Without coordination, inequities are likely to occur, with some families overusing the service and others overproviding service.

Another form of respite is the residential camp. Camps accept placement requests for short periods (e.g., overnight/weekend), as well as extended stays (e.g., several days or weeks). Activities available for respite campers are usually recreational, such as hiking, boating, swimming, and cookouts. This approach is useful for those families who plan separate vacations for the developmentally disabled member. However, these programs are usually only available seasonally and generally do not meet parental needs for periodic respite care.

Funding/Cost of Services

The majority of respite care programs included in the 1982 national survey are funded through user fees and a variety of federal and state sources. Over 60% use a fee-for-service schedule, with the majority (74%) using a sliding scale. Maximum and minimum hourly and daily charges vary greatly. Average hourly rates range from a low of $1.00 an hour in group homes to $4.63 for care offered in a provider's home. Individualized respite services tend to charge higher fees than those programs serving groups. Fees for respite provided in public institutions are the highest, averaging $40.09 per day. It should be noted, however, that fees account for only 25% of operating costs. Federal, state, and local agencies are the chief funding sources for the remaining expenses. Specific funding sources vary. Federal funds were received by a number of programs through Title XX of the Social Security (N = 24), Title XIX of the Social Security (N = 16), and Administration on Developmental Disabilities (N = 18). State funds primarily came from mental health/mental retardation departments (N = 91), with developmental disability councils (N = 20) and state legislatures (N = 10) providing a limited amount. Local funds were obtained from community organizations, such as United Way (N = 37), private foundations (N = 22), and mental health/mental retardation centers (N = 20). (*Note: N* = number of programs receiving funds from these groups.)

Client Characteristics

Individuals with major developmental disabilities are served through current respite programs. Over 75% of programs in the 1982 ARC survey accept mentally retarded clients, with significantly fewer programs accepting individuals with cerebral palsy, epilepsy, and autism. Autistic individuals are served by the smallest number (less than 10%). Children of all ages are served, with individuals older than 18 years being most frequently involved.

Use of Respite Programs/Services Offered

According to survey, families tend to use short-term respite care (one day or less) on weekends and throughout the week during day and evening hours. The client's or provider's home are most frequently used for short-term care.

Group homes and institutions are most commonly employed for respite care lasting longer than a one-day period.

Types of services offered vary by length of care provided. Short-term programs provide basic services, such as physical care, self-help, transportation, and recreation. Programs that are designed for longer-term care may offer a range of services, including nursing care, speech therapy, physical therapy, education classes, and field trips.

Staff/Staff Training

The majority of respite care programs included in the ARC survey are administered by full-time or part-time professional staff, with a larger percentage reporting part-time than full-time professional staff. Social workers comprise the largest category of full-time professional staff. No information was provided on the prior educational background of the direct care personnel. However, over 70% of all respite programs require providers to participate in preservice training activities. Preservice training curricula cover a variety of topics related to developmental disabilities, including characteristics of developmentally disabled persons (77%), first aid (75%), basic service needs of developmentally disabled persons (74%), rights of developmentally disabled persons (64%), medications (60%), and fire safety (58%).

Implementation Problems

Eighty-three percent of the programs surveyed reported implementation problems during their early phase. The most commonly stated problem (34 programs or 39% of the sample) was the reluctance of families to use respite care. This may be a public relations problem, or parents may feel guilty leaving their handicapped member with a stranger. Another common problem is an inability to maintain an adequate number of respite providers (62 programs or 37%). It was difficult both to recruit and retain direct care staff. Staff retention was a particular concern in programs offering respite services in the client's or provider's home. Recruitment problems appeared to be related to the low wages and the time required for training and certification. Funding was another frequently noted concern. Funding was tenuous and present funding levels were inadequate to operate programs effectively (prepare promotional materials, pay direct care staff appropriate wages). Ten percent of the programs also noted problems serving emotionally disturbed residents with severe behavioral problems. Transportation was cited by 7% of the programs as being a problem for both client and provider. Bureaucratic obstacles were experienced by 6% of the programs; they had difficulty obtaining reimbursement from funding agencies, complying with zoning ordinances, and meeting licensing requirements.

In general, this national survey indicates that respite care programs do exist and that the most common form is community-based care provided in a home-like environment. However, these programs have many problems. Costs remain minimal for parents, but programs have difficulty finding a stable funding source. Mentally retarded and physically handicapped children are served, but those disabled individuals who have an emotional and/or behavioral disturbance are most frequently denied service. Staff are recruited and trained, but staff retention is a serious concern. Finally, and probably most important, parents appear reluctant to use the service. Speculations about the cause of this reluctance vary.

Although this survey provides a general overview of current respite programs many questions remain unanswered. How are individual states addressing the respite care issue? To what extent are individuals who need respite services actually receiving them? Is respite care effective in reducing family stress and enhancing family functioning? Are different forms of respite care (agency sponsored, parentally determined) more effective in enhancing family functioning? The following statewide respite care surveys provide some information on these concerns.

STATEWIDE RESPITE CARE SURVEYS

Statewide respite care surveys are available for three states: Massachusetts (Upshur, 1982, 1983); Indiana (Hagen, 1980, as cited in Upshur, 1982a); and California (Apolloni & Triest, 1983).

The Massachusetts survey was conducted in two phases. In Phase I, agencies with active respite care programs were surveyed. In Phase II, families with a handicapped child were contacted through the aid of statewide voluntary agencies; some of these families did not participate in respite care programs. Results of the agency survey component revealed that respite placement agencies were the most common form of assistance (51%). These agencies recruit and train community providers, matching client requests with providers. Care settings were the client's or care provider's home. Mentally retarded individuals were most commonly served. Austistic individuals and those with severe behavioral and/or medical needs were excluded most often. Three common implementation problems were noted: client reluctance to leave family, the family not returning at the agreed-on time, and lack of transportation.

The family survey, Phase II, revealed that agency-trained staff provide only a limited amount of total respite care. Families reported that 57.6% of daytime or evening care was provided by family network members. Only 5.9% had received respite care from a trained worker, and more importantly, 14% had no access to trained or untrained relief help. Service setting, whether the care was provided by a relative, neighbor, or respite worker, was almost always the client's home. Overnight care was also usually provided by a sitter, relative, or friend and took place in the family home. Over one-quarter used group or institutional care for overnight needs. However, 57.8% of these families reported they preferred overnight care to take place in their own home, but were unable to identify caregivers.

Families noted a number of problems in obtaining respite care. Inability to identify assistance was a problem for both day (30.7%) and overnight (20.1%) care. Reluctance to leave family members with a stranger and financial problems were other commonly noted concerns. From these family data it appears that simply having care available is not sufficient. Families require help in identifying respite agencies, feeling confident that the family member will receive quality services, and reducing guilt feelings about using respite as relief services.

Similar findings were obtained in a survey conducted in Indiana (Hagen, 1980 as cited in Upshur, 1982a). Although out-of-home residential placements were the most commonly available form of respite, families preferred home-based care. Regarding daytime care, 54% preferred home-based care conducted by a sitter, relative, neighbor, or friend of the family's choice. Home-based care conducted by a trained agency-provided worker was the second preference of families (42.1%). Preference for overnight care followed a similar pattern. Home-based care with a sitter of choice was the families' first choice (51.9%), whereas home-based care with an agency-provided sitter was the second most frequently noted choice (42.8%).

Problems within Indiana's currently operated system of respite care were similar to those of other states. Families were reluctant to use respite services, which were underfunded and provided inconsistently throughout the state. Clients with severe medical and/or behavioral problems were most frequently denied service. Family use patterns were also similar. Emergency, vacation, special events, shopping, errands, and simple leisure and rest periods were most commonly mentioned uses of respite care.

In California, parents are provided subsidized respite care through 200 state-contracted respite provider agencies. In a recently conducted survey of parents, respite care staff, and state agency personnel, a number of concerns were identified (Apolloni & Triest, 1983). Although service quality was rated as satisfactory by a majority of parents, providers, and agency staff, parents reported requiring a larger amount of respite time than present limits allow (present maximum limit of 35 hours). In contrast, agency staff noted that a large percentage of families (41%) did not use their full allocation. In addition, a sizeable number of families (26%) were unaware of the availability of services, and some did not feel comfortable leaving their handicapped member with a stranger (16%). Services were inconsistently provided across the state, with some agencies providing respite only in emergency situations and some only to mildly and moderately handicapped individuals. Finally, a high turnover rate of respite workers (50% per year) hampered the quality of care. Within this system parents have limited input into the nature and quality of respite provided, no financial reimbursement is available for family network members, and the concerns of the critically needy family (those with a profoundly handicapped, medically fragile, or behaviorally disordered child) are frequently ignored.

From these statewide surveys, it appears that even within states that offer agency-directed respite care, *family relief from the day-to-day care of the handicapped member is most frequently provided by family network members. Family members prefer this system, with agency-recruited and trained care providers consistently rated as the second preference.* In California, for example, where state-subsidized respite care is offered only through contracted respite care workers, over one-third of the families with a developmentally disabled child had not used the service. Many were not aware of the service, whereas others did not feel comfortable using it. In Massachusetts, less than 10% of the families had received respite care from a trained worker, with the majority employing extended family members.

NATIONAL SURVEY: STATE FAMILY SUPPORT PROGRAM

Presently, 20 states—Colorado, Connecticut, Florida, Idaho, Iowa, Maryland, Michigan, Minnesota, Montana, Nebraska, Nevada, New Jersey, North Dakota, Ohio, Pennsylvania, Rhode Island, South Carolina, Vermont, Washington, and Wisconsin—offer support services specifically designed for families with a developmentally delayed individual. The purpose of these family support programs is unique among programs for the disabled person. The needs of family members, not only those of the developmentally disabled individual, are the focus. During 1984, a detailed survey of these programs was conducted (Slater, 1984; Slater et al., in press). Data were gathered on a number of program parameters, including purposes/goals, legislation, eligibility, administration, amount of support, services offered, and evaluation findings.

Services Offered

To assist families in maintaining or returning the handicapped individual to the family, states have designed a variety of family support programs that vary by type of services offered, administrative management, amount of support, and eligibility requirements. A laundry list best describes the many services that may be available across states (see Table 1). The most common service is respite care, which is offered by 19 of 20 states. It appears that many families simply need a rest period in which they can focus on other

Table 1. Type of services provided by state

State	Diagnostic/Assessment	Medical/Dental	Home Health Care	Medications	Special Diet	Respite-Day Care	Individual Counseling	Therapy/Rehabilitation	Special Education	Recreation	Transportation	Special Clothing	Family Training/Counseling	Homemaker	Housing Modification	Special Equipment	Unusual Expenses	Constant Care Allowance
Colorado			X			X	X	X		X			X	X		X		
Connecticut		X		X		X	X	X	X		X	X	X		X	X	X	
Florida		X		X	X	X	X	X	X		X	X	X		X	X	X	
Idaho	X	X			X	X	X			X	X	X			X	X	X	
Iowa		X						X							X	X		
Maryland			X			X	X				X		X		X	X	X	
Michigan						X	X	X					X				X	

State																	
Minnesota	X	X		X	X		X	X			X			X			
Montana[a]		X			X							X					
Nebraska	X	X			X	X	X	X		X			X	X	X		
Nevada[b]					X					X				X		X	
New Jersey		X	X		X		X						X		X		
North Dakota		X	X		X	X	X	X	X	X	X				X	X	X
Ohio				X	X	X	X					X		X	X		
Pennsylvania[a]					X		X		X	X		X	X				
Rhode Island							X			X			X	X	X		X
South Carolina		X		X	X		X			X					X		
Vermont					X		X								X		
Washington[a]		X			X		X			X					X		
Wisconsin[a]	X	X	X	X	X	X	X	X	X	X	X	X	X	X	X		

[a]General support services provided.
[b]Income supplementations for families in financial need.

pressing family matters, such as shopping, completing errands, and taking a family vacation without the handicapped member.

Although the list of services looks quite diverse, the majority of these services have one common characteristic: They were not reimbursable through any prior program. Housing modifications, specialty equipment, and special clothing are all expensive, and many families were not able to be reimbursed for these expenses before the creation of a family support program. Similarly, medications, frequent medical/dental visits, home health care assistance, and special diets are usually quite expensive and may be only minimally reimbursable through most insurance programs. Counseling is another type of service that family members themselves may require, as well as the individual handicapped person, yet its costs are minimally covered by other programs. Some states are flexible enough to include a category of unusual expenses that allows a family to make a case for any type of service their handicapped member may require.

Three types of family support programs exist: 1) cash subsidy, in which families are given financial assistance to purchase services; 2) direct state-provided services; and 3) combination programs in which both cash subsidies and direct services are offered. *The cash subsidy programs offer families the most flexibility in choice of service and service provider. In the case of respite care, families employ sitters of preference. Direct service programs offer less family autonomy as only state- or agency-contracted services are provided.*

Efficacy of Services

Detailed data on the type, frequency, duration, and costs of services provided and requested are available on family support programs in Washington state, Michigan, and Minnesota. In-depth studies have been conducted on Washington's Home-Aid Resources Program since its inception in 1976. The FY 1978 report is described below (Home Aid Resources Program, 1978). Through this program two primary services—respite care and resource therapies (communication therapy, recreational therapy, physical/occupational therapy, and behavior management)—and two secondary service programs, skill development and specialized training, are offered. The program is a direct service type, offering assistance only through state-subsidized agency personnel. Respite care accounted for the majority of statewide expenditures (61.5%), with resource therapies (32.2%), program skill development (6.0%), and specialized training (0.3%) accounting for a significantly smaller proportion of funds. There were marked urban-rural differences in service utilization. Rural families used resource therapies primarily (resource therapy 56%, respite care 33%), whereas urban families demanded more respite services (respite care 85%, resource therapies 15%). On a statewide average, each family received respite care on 3.4 occasions for a total of 15.5 days annually. The average annual cost of respite care per family was $329.05, with one day of respite care costing $21.22. Out-of-home respite care was the most popular type of respite care, being employed by 41% of the clients and using 60% of the resource aid funds.

Data from Michigan's four pilot family support programs also suggest that respite care is a primary component of supportive services (Herman, 1983). These pilot programs use the combination approach in which families are offered both a cash subsidy and some state-directed services. Although a number of primary services were offered (professional services, in-home intervention, respite care, special financial subsidies, and parent training), respite care was commonly utilized and, in fact, was considered a universal service. Summary evaluation data revealed that three separate forms of respite care were offered: sitter (family chose sitter, project reimbursed family for cost), in-home (project provided sitter), and out-of-home. In counties in which families were provided the choice of respite care options, families chose sitter services over other forms of in-home or out-of-home care. In one program (Clinton-Ingham counties) that provided all three types of respite care services, family friends were chosen to conduct 69% of respite care, whereas foster parents provided 21% and home-based (agency-provided sitter) services accounted for only 10% of respite care. In another county (Macomb-Oakland) family expenditures by type of respite were $4,701 for sitter services, $380 for in-home respite, and $410 for out-of-home respite.

It appears that if families are given a choice in type of service delivery, they will attempt to live as normal a life as possible, following patterns of behavior similar to families without developmentally delayed members. When given an option, families tend to solve family problems through enlisting the aid of family network members. Satisfaction measures reinforce this conclusion. Fifty-eight percent of the families involved in the subsidy programs deemed direct financial assistance more worthwhile than trainer-provided services, and 81% of the respite care provided by a family friend was rated as "very satisfactory" as compared to 57% of the agency-provided respite care services.

Participants in Minnesota's Mental Retardation Cash Subsidy Program also rated respite care as one of the most beneficial services offered, with 73% regarding it as a "great" or "very great" help (Zimmerman, 1984). As with Michigan's findings, family members and hired sitters (30% and 27%, respectively) were the most frequently used form of respite. However, when families rated quality of service, subsidy-purchased services were more highly rated than those provided by family and friends. (Note: it is not clear whether families were reimbursed for respite care provided by family members or friends.)

Although many other statewide family support programs include respite care as a service component, no detailed statistical summary or evaluation data are available on the respite care component.

MODEL RESPITE PROGRAMS

In addition to the above national and statewide surveys of respite care programs, valuable information has been reported on a small number of model respite care programs. Ptacek et al. (1982) developed a community-based respite care program for families with multiply handicapped children residing in rural areas of Wisconsin. Through this program, children received respite care in the homes of foster parents who were trained and supported by a local pediatric child care center. The model was designed to provide intermittent relief to family members from basic caregiving responsibilities. Respite was available for family vacations, a few days at a time during the week, a weekend once or twice a month, and/or on an emergency basis. Parental satisfaction reports noted that the service met their expectations (84%) and the child's needs (90%) and that parents felt comfortable leaving their child (87%). However, parents also noted that different forms of respite care should be offered; particularly mentioned was *the need for home-based respite care allowing the youngster to remain in natural surroundings.* In addition, parents emphasized that respite care was just that, a rest period, and their interest in the program was not to receive information or advice on being a better parent.

Upshur (1982a) conducted a pilot home-based respite care model project for multiply handicapped individuals who had previously been denied respite services due to behavioral problems. Respite workers—former nurses, teachers, and paraprofessional social workers—were carefully recruited, were provided 60 hours of training, were given access to on-call emergency backup personnel, and were paid higher than usual stipends. Thirty-five multiply handicapped individuals, many with severe behavioral problems, were served. Only two clients were refused service. Families had an overall positive response to the service, noting that providers were adequately trained and offered a useful service. Project workers commented that if a project apartment or house had been available the two clients who had been refused services could have been served as well. This model indicates that, when well-conceived and conducted models of respite care are available, even those multiply handicapped individuals with severe behavioral problems can participate. In addition, the majority of these services can be provided in a very cost-effective manner within the individual's home community.

Although respite care is designed to alleviate the physical and emotional burdens associated with raising a handicapped child, few empirical studies have examined its effects on family functioning and plans for institutional care. One exception is a study conducted by Joyce and associates (Joyce & Singer, 1983; Joyce, Singer, & Isralowitz, 1983). Joyce et al. (1983) surveyed the effects of a 4-month respite care program on the participating family's internal relationships, social activities, emotional and social strains, and plans for institutional care. Agency-trained caregivers provided respite within the family home. Positive effects were noted. A majority strongly agreed or agreed that respite care had assisted their family in relating better to their disabled son or daughter. Family members reported getting along better with each other. Family stress levels had declined and time for social and leisure time activities had increased. Respite care appears also to assist parents in avoiding institutionalization. Over 90% of the families reported that respite care was a significant factor in helping them care for their disabled child within the home. A significant correlation (.51) was obtained between those families who considered institutionalizing their child and those not able to maintain their child at home without respite care. The child's age affected parental perceptions of respite care. Parents with younger children viewed respite services as more useful than those with older handicapped children. Perhaps parents with older handicapped members have developed personal resources to deal with the care of their disabled member. No relationship was obtained between number of hours of respite care and overall quality of family life score. It appears that even a modest amount of intervention can assist families in reducing stress levels. Finally, it is important to note that 30% of participating families indicated that they would be unable to maintain their child within the home without respite services. Respite care may be an easily implemented, cost-effective method of supporting families who attempt to maintain their handicapped member within the family environment.

PROBLEMS WITH CURRENT FORMS OF RESPITE CARE

To evaluate this present pattern of respite care services, we must examine the effects of various forms of respite care on the needs of families. Families with a handicapped member typically experience social isolation, added chronic and acute forms of stress, and a reduced feeling of autonomy. Yet, these families strive to live as normal a life as possible. In light of these needs the following deficiencies are present in one or more of the various forms of respite care currently offered.

Emphasis on Professional/Paraprofessional Services

Presently, the majority of respite care programs funded through federal, state, and local dollars focus on agency-provided care. Although this type of care does provide family members with temporary relief from basic caregiving responsibilities, the majority of families prefer to hire a sitter of choice.

This sitter is usually a relative, family friend, or neighbor who has had a positive relationship with the handicapped member. However, only a very few states, such as Michigan, and usually only through pilot programs, reimburse parents using sitters of choice. Respite care and more fully developed family support programs are based on the assumption that family enhancement will result from the purchase of additional professional and paraprofessional services. Inherent dangers exist in these policies. The role of the family and extended family members may be usurped and family dependency on the formal delivery system may be increased by providing direct services to the disabled individual (Moroney, 1979). Boggs (1984) has noted that although some financial assistance and paraprofessional services may be needed society should not preempt ". . . the values of mutual assistance, the person-to-person, one-to-one free association caring support and assistance that family members and neighbors give to each other through transactions that leave no market trace" (p. 60). It appears that families, when given a choice, elect to solve their day-to-day concerns in as normalized a fashion as possible. What is now needed is societal support for these endeavors.

No Relation Between Theories of Family Functioning and Program Development

Respite care programs have been designed to meet practical needs of families for relief; they have not been based on theories of family functioning. This lack of influence of theoretical research knowledge on program development may severely limit program effectiveness. Zimmerman (1984) underlined this concern in a detailed follow-up study of the Minnesota family support program. Family experiences with multiple stressors and family life cycle stage significantly influenced the extent to which the support program enhanced family coping capabilities. In addition, over half of the families anticipated placing their handicapped member in an out-of-home placement eventually. There is a need for effective respite care and more fully developed family support programs based at least in part on family variables and systematic family theories.

Limited Organizational Structure

Numerous administrative deficiencies exist in the majority of respite care programs. Programs are designed and developed with minimal parental input, funding is unstable, and families lack information about the types of care available. Families with the neediest children are most frequently denied services, and only minimal evaluation of care effectiveness is conducted.

In those states that have passed family support legislation, many of these deficiencies are minimized. However, most of these states give priority to those families who have already requested out-of-home placement, thereby forcing families to deplete their informal sources of support before they can receive formal supportive services.

Total Needs of Families Not Considered

Although families require relief from day-to-day caregiving responsibilities, they also require a wide range of additional formal and informal supports. In those states with cash subsidy programs many of these additional needs are being met. Families are provided a wide range of formal support services including training, counseling, and home health aid assistance. Furthermore, because families are allowed to determine both the service and service provider, parental feelings of empowerment are increased. However, these programs have failed to include one of the primary sources of familial supports: extended family members.

CONCLUSION

Knowledge about respite has been summarized from a number of sources: program providers, state agency statistics, family participants, and families with a member who has handicaps who may or may not have participated in agency-provided respite care. Depending on the source, answers varied greatly to such commonly asked questions as what is the most frequent form of respite care employed and who provides it. National and statewide surveys, such as the ARC and California studies, focused on agency-directed care. According to these studies, the most common form of care is offered in the client's community by agency-hired employees either in the client's or provider's home. Funding for these programs tends to be unstable and is derived from a variety of local, state, and federal sources, except in such states as California where respite care is considered part of regional services for the developmentally disabled. Additional implementation problems abound. Services are scattered, families tend not to use the services, staff recruitment and retention are difficult, and families with difficult-to-serve children (e.g., autistic, behaviorally disordered) are most often excluded.

Data from family-focused surveys indicate that the majority of respite care is not provided by agency-sponsored personnel, but rather by family network members, such as friends, relatives, and neighbors. Families responding to the Massachusetts survey, for example, reported that over 50% of all respite care was conducted by family members, with only 5.9% receiving respite care from a trained agency-provided worker. Similarly, families responding to the Indiana survey overwhelmingly indicated that families preferred home-based services offered by a sitter-of-choice (family, friend, hired babysitter).

These findings were reinforced by data gathered from recent state-sponsored family support programs. Through the majority of these 20 programs, families are provided a wide range of supportive services, with respite care being a popular service of choice that is frequently labeled a universal service. In Washington, for example, many families used over half of their service dollars for agency-sponsored care. However, when families were afforded a choice of type of respite care, such as in the Michigan program, in-home care with a family-chosen sitter was most commonly employed. Conflicting results were obtained, however, from the Minnesota survey. Although families noted that network members provided the majority of care, agency-trained workers were rated as providing a higher quality of care.

Respite care is designed to alleviate stress within the home. Yet, few studies have examined the relationship between respite care and internal family functioning. The study by Joyce and associates is one exception. Through this study families were provided in-home respite care by an agency-trained worker for a short-term period. After the services were terminated, families noted that respite care enhanced their relationship with the disabled family member, gave members needed time to participate in normal, out-of-home leisure-time activities, and was a significant factor in allowing the family to maintain the disabled member within the home.

In conclusion, it appears that respite care programs are needed. Existing programs do provide at least temporary relief. In states where family support programs exist, additional family needs are met. However, it is suggested that these efforts may not be sufficient support for families attempting to raise a handicapped child within the home. Although many formal sources of support and financial assistance are needed, the unit that must be supported is the family of the handicapped child within its informal support network. It is urged that the maintenance and, if possible, the enhancement of informal familial supports be given equal programmatic emphasis to the provision of formal support.

This concept is termed "normalized family resources" (Slater & Wikler, in press). It is based on previously identified needs of families with a handicapped child, stress theory, and experimentally based family support programs. Families with a handicapped child strive for the same personal and social support as all families. Within this model families are encouraged to live as normal a life as possible. More specifically, families are encouraged: 1) to promote the autonomy and psychological well-being of each individual member; 2) to foster normal, flexible, internal family relations; 3) to develop and maintain normal social supports with friends, neighbors, and relatives; and 4) to obtain needed support services where possible through normal generic service programs.

Working within a normalized family resource model, the family and extended family members become the focus of service. Relatives, friends, and neighbors are encouraged to assist family members. Negotiations, contracting, and sharing of information are encouraged among all members. Needed formal supportive services are identified. A wide range of services are delineated, ranging from respite care, babysitting, and transportation to more formal professionally provided services, such as occupational and physical therapy. Many services are provided by outside family resources, with extended family members providing a wide range of nonprofessionally based services, including respite care, in-home programming, and transportation. Training is offered to family and extended family members as requested.

The program is structured around the provision of four main components: 1) a wide range of formal supportive services; 2) use of informal social supports where appropriate; 3) development of an individual family plan that emphasizes the needs of all family members, delineating goals and objectives to meet individual family member needs, as well as to enhance overall family functioning; and 4) a commitment by professionals to allow family members to determine the primary goals and objectives of their individual plan. Providing family members with decision-making power, it is hoped, will lead to the increased feelings of empowerment and autonomy basic to optimum internal family functioning.

A number of previously conducted family support programs (e.g., Berger & Fowlkes, 1984; Moore, Hamerlynck, Barsh, Spieker, & Richard, 1982) have been successful in reducing family isolation, enhancing internal family functioning and, most importantly, maintaining the handicapped child as an integrated family member. The authors suggest that statewide family support programs and individually conducted respite care programs may become more effective in meeting the total needs of families through following many of these same principles.

REFERENCES

Apolloni, A. H., & Triest, G. (1983). Respite services in California: Status and recommendations for improvements. *Mental Retardation, 21,* 240–243.

Association for Retarded Citizens. (1982). *Characteristics of respite care programs.* Arlington, TX: Author.

Berger, M., & Fowlkes, M. A. (1984). A family network model for serving young children with handicaps. In M. A. Slater & P. Mitchell (Eds.), *Family support services: A parent-professional partnership* (pp. 56–64). Stillwater, OK: National Clearinghouse of Rehabilitation Training Materials.

Boggs, E. (1984). Feds and families—some observations on the impact of federal economic policies on families with children who have disabilities. In M. A. Slater & P. Mitchell (Eds.), *Family support services: A parent-professional partnership* (pp. 65–78). Stillwater, OK: National Clearinghouse for Rehabilitation Training Materials.

Frohlich, P. (1975). *The 1967 national survey of institutionalized adults: Residents of longterm medical care institutions.* Washington, DC: U.S. Department of Health, Education, and Welfare, DHEW Publication No. (SSA) 75-11803.

Herman. (1983). *Family support services: Reports on meta-evaluation study.* Lansing: Michigan Department of Mental Health.

Home aid resources program. (1978). Olympia: Washington Division of Developmental Disabilities.

Joyce, K., & Singer, M. J. (1983). Respite care services: An evaluation of the perceptions of parents and workers. *Rehabilitation Literature, 44,* 270–274.

Joyce, K., Singer, M., & Isralowitz, R. (1983). Impact of respite care on parents' perception of quality of life. *Mental Retardation, 21,* 153–156.

Moore, J. A., Hamerlynck, L. A., Barsh, E., Spieker, S., & Richard, J. (1982). *Extended family resources.* Seattle, WA: Children's Clinic and Preschool Spastic Aid Council, Inc.

Moroney, R. M. (1979). Allocation of resources for family care. In R. H. Bruinicks & G. C. Krantz (Eds.), *Family care of developmentally disabled members: Conference proceedings* (pp. 63–76). Minneapolis: University of Minnesota.

Ptacek, L. J., Sommers, P. A., Graves, J., Lukowicz, P., Keena, E., Haglund, J., & Nycz, G. R. (1982). Respite care for families of children with severe handicaps: An evaluation study of parent satisfaction. *Journal of Community Psychology, 10,* 222–227.

Slater, M. A. (1984, May). Survey: Statewide family support programs. Paper presented at the 108th annual meeting of the American Association on Mental Deficiency, Minneapolis, MN.

Slater, M. A., Bates, M. A., Eicher, L., & Wikler, L. (in press). Survey: Statewide family support programs. *Journal of Applied Research in Mental Retardation.*

Slater, M. A., & Wikler, L. (in press). Normalized family resources: Social work roles for families with a developmentally disabled child. *Social Work.*

Upshur, C. C. (1982a). An evaluation of home-based respite care. *Mental Retardation, 20,* 58–62.

Upshur, C. (1982b). Respite care for mentally retarded and other disabled populations: Program models and family needs. *Mental Retardation, 20,* 2–6.

Upshur, C. (1983). Developing respite care: A support service for families with a disabled member. *Family Relations, 32,* 13–20.

Zimmerman, S. L. (1984). The mental retardation family subsidy program: Its effects on families with a mentally handicapped child. *Family Relations, 33,* 105–118.

Chapter 5

PARENTS' PERSPECTIVES
FOCUS ON NEED

Editors' Note: *Two parents have graciously agreed to share their respite experiences through essays in Chapter 5 (Focus on Need), Chapter 12 (Focus on Providers), and Chapter 16 (Focus on Impact). The inclusion of parent perspectives in this text seemed fundamental to the topic at hand. Their contributions provide an important pragmatic base against which the research and models of other contributors can be juxtaposed. The reflections of these parents, representative of many such families, enable us to see how important the development and delivery of respite services can be to families with members with developmental disabilities. The contrasts and similarities provided by these two families bring to light many of the issues and findings discussed by other authors in this text. The editors greatly appreciate their openness and willingness to share their stories with us.*

Noreen Quinn Curran, the mother of Christine, reflects on her experiences in rearing a child with mild/moderate disabilities. She describes her situation in which respite services have been available in their area and are used to provide important opportunities for Christine, as well as for themselves. Clearly, the availability of respite services, in several forms, is viewed as an important dimension in maintaining a quality of life for all family members.

The situation of Harriet Horowitz Bongiorno, parent of Alan, provides a stark contrast to that of the Curran family. As the parent of a child with severe disabilities, Harriett did not have respite services available when Alan was born or as he was growing up. The importance of family supports is evident as one reads about Alan and his family. Her reflections illustrate the critical need to develop services in more sparsely populated areas and for those with children who have severe and profound disabilities.

Noreen Quinn Curran

Our daughter Christine is a 17-year-old young woman with Down syndrome. Her special needs are mild in some areas and moderate in others, her gross motor skills are good, and socially she is close to age level in her interests and activities. In other areas, especially academic, her needs are moderate. She describes herself as having "special needs in learning, but that's all," and has "Down syndrome, but only a little bit."

Christine continues to be mainstreamed in nonacademic classes in her high school program. In the community, she has been well mainstreamed in Boys' and Girls' Clubs recreation programs for a number of years, most notably the competitive swim team. She has worked at "the Club" as a swimming assistant/locker room attendant during her last 2 summers under the Summer Youth Employment Program.

Her interests are age-appropriate (e.g., she has "crushes" on a football player, watches "the soaps" avidly, and discusses her predictions about the mishaps to befall the stars). She wants to be an actress or model herself, someday. However, her conversation about these interests can become repetitive and wear down family members and others after a while.

Christine's recent desire for increased independence has been somewhat of a surprise to us. She clearly wants to "try her wings" as a teenager and be a separate entity from her parents and younger brother. Free of her parents, she goes to the shopping mall on Saturdays, shops, buys her lunch, returns on public transportation, and walks the few blocks home. She is immensely proud and protective of this weekly opportunity.

Another of Christine's characteristics is her ability to engage easily an unfamiliar adult in conversation regarding her interests. The one criteria she has for a respite care worker is whether they watch "General Hospital" or "Dallas." Christine seems to identify the young adult respite workers as her friends/confidantes/big sisters with whom she can share the activities and secrets of adolescence.

SYSTEMS INTERRELATIONSHIP

The Family

To understand the fabric of a family's need for and use of respite care, one needs to see the child within her "systems." The lack of opportunities for appropriate activities within each of the systems—family, peer groups, the school, and community—makes the need for respite services more acute for families. Building onto what is positive and already existing in the systems can make for respite services that are more natural and age-appropriate.

Christine's family is composed of two adults with fairly busy lives involving careers, personal interests, and family activities, and one sibling, Sean, 3 years younger, who is bright, popular, and creative. Time is spent together, but some time is needed apart for all members of the family. Unlike other family members, Christine seldom has the option to see friends independently outside her home.

In my association with other families, I see that their total family situation (e.g., parents' age, number of siblings at home, developmental parenting processes) has much to do with their need for and use of respite care. For example, if the parents are in their mid-40s and have a large well-functioning family with siblings close to the age of the adolescent with developmental disabilities, then respite care is not generally perceived as a needed service, as respite seems to happen naturally within the family. If, however, the parents are in their mid-50s and the other siblings have left home, (not at all an unusual situation), then respite care would most likely be welcomed as a needed service to relieve the parents for a while and to engage the adolescent/young adult in some constructive activities. Our family, being fairly young to have a young adult with special needs, having few family members, and with two active working parents, may have more than an average need for respite care—about 10 days per year.

Peer Group

Another system that provides for support and social contacts is Christine's peer group. Generally, her friends are not as independent as she is. They are more closely watched and protected and almost always have an adult close by. This does not provide them the optimum opportunity for relaxed socializing with each other except by telephone, which leaves them confined to home most of the time. Occasionally there may be a planned visit to one another's home, but the parents need to be ready to enjoy the sound of teenagers with special needs, as well as be available for assistance, should that be needed.

The School

The system that has really been a letdown for us is the public school. Christine attends a comprehensive high school, but little effort has been extended toward involving these young adults with mild/moderate special needs in the extracurricular school life. Therefore, when other teenagers are attending school dances, our teenagers are isolated at home; their main social activity is talking on the telephone about T.V. programs rather than participating in normal mainstreamed social activities with each other.

Community

The town recreation department provides a segregated program for adolescents and adults with special needs. But how appropriate is it for 17-year-olds with developmental delays to socialize and dance with 35-year-olds with developmental delays? There would be an outcry from parents of nonhandicapped children if this was the recreation program the town was providing their teenagers!

Our community does offer some appropriate socialization/recreation opportunities during the week or weekend through a quasipublic special needs recreation program. These "courses" are partially paid for by parents and partially by the town recreation department. The programs are staffed substantially by volunteer assistants, enhancing the integration effort. Fortunately, our daughter can walk or bike there and back herself, so little parental involvement is needed from 1:30 to 3:30 on Sunday afternoons—a brief respite. More of this kind of social/recreational opportunity, but for an extended time period (2 to 3 hours), would be very much appreciated by parents, particularly on weekends. Also, transportation services to and from activities would be an important addition to respite community services for many families.

FEELINGS

My feelings toward respite care have changed substantially over the 17 years of Christine's life, as have my views of what respite is and how it must adapt to changing needs.

As the "broker" of services for Christine, I was not always open to respite care, particularly by an outside agency. Early on, the "Supermom" syndrome had me in its firm grip, suggesting that only I or family members could care for our daughter and son. I had to learn to let go, to trust others to care for them as well as I, and sometimes better than I could (when I really needed a break)! Accepting my own limitations, physically and emotionally, has been an ongoing process. Finally, truly accepting that it's okay to need a break without feeling guilty, was a real breakthrough for me.

I believe that parents may need to go through some emotional processes and reality testing in order to request respite care.

1. The major caregiver needs to feel that he or she is *entitled* to respite. There needs to be an understanding that this parenting job is more demanding than more typical situations. Lack of adequate services "forces" parents and their child/adult with disabilities to spend more time together than is healthy for either one. This dynamic can increase the tendency toward dependency by the individual with disabilities and

overprotectiveness by the parents. Respite care can help promote healthier individual and family functioning.

2. We need to know our own tell-tale signs of fatigue/stress. For me, my daughter's repetitive conversations begin to annoy me; I have a decreased lack of interest in my own activities and become overly concerned about the details of her life. I know I need a break!

3. We need to believe that respite care will be a positive experience for all, or at least the family members (primary caregiver and person with special needs) who need it most.

4. Decide the time needed for respite, and make the call to the respite agency. Do it!

Harriet Horowitz Bongiorno

Eighteen years ago my husband and I were awaiting the birth of our first child with anxious anticipation. The Vietnam era was in full bloom and my husband, classified as 1-A, enlisted in the U.S. Army Band in hopes of avoiding being ordered to Vietnam as an infantryman. Following his basic training we were transferred to Fort Carson in Colorado Springs, Colorado, to spend the remainder of the 3-year enlistment period. Despite the 3-year enlistment, the future looked very promising for us. Our home, nestled among the foothills of the Rocky Mountains, provided us a safe, happy, and secure place to await the arrival of our first-born child.

Alan William was born on June 2, 1967, on a beautiful spring day. He arrived 2 weeks early and weighed 5 pounds and 12 ounces at birth. No two parents could have possibly been happier. Our son, our beautiful son, was born. Total joy was ours until a doctor informed us that something might possibly be wrong with Alan. Alan had been born jaundiced and had spots on his body called petechiae, which, according to the doctors, might indicate a lack of oxygen at birth. The next day the jaundice had lessened and the petechiae had lightened, and my son was placed in my arms to feed and cuddle and love. Any danger, it seemed, had apparently evaporated.

For the next few months the three of us led an idyllic existence. Loving parents carefully nurtured their pride and joy. As the months passed, however, it became increasingly apparent that Alan was not developing normally. Alan could not support his head, roll over, or sit up and made no attempt to crawl. I nervously read and reread books and articles describing the times when a child should reach each significant developmental milestone. The time for each stage came and went, and Alan did not progress. Diagnoses were sought from numerous pediatricians, neurologists, and therapists who collectively shrugged their shoulders and announced with varying degrees of sensitivity that Alan was "brain damaged" and as a result would be severely physically and mentally retarded. Alan was subsequently extensively tested and evaluated at the Children's Hospital of Philadelphia, and we were given the doleful news that Alan would, in all likelihood, make very little developmental progress in his lifetime. The only positive advice offered was to try to have another child as soon as possible in the hope that Alan might possibly develop a little faster by observing and emulating a sibling. Within a year Shelley was born, and we were four.

The birth of our daughter was a source of great joy . . . the lack of progress of our son was a source of profound and unspoken sadness. In desperation we sought help through a process called "patterning." With evangelical zeal, the Institute for the Achievement of Human Potential in New York touted the merits of the Doman-Delacato system of retraining the brain by manipulating the child's head, arms, and legs in a pattern to simulate crawling. The process of patterning and the satellite exercises that accompanied this process required the services of six volunteers per day for 7 days a week. Alan's program began at 9:30 in the morning and lasted until 3:30 in the afternoon. Our daily lives revolved around this rigid schedule for over 18 months. Alan's developmental increase was negligible. The overall effect on our family life was traumatic. The majority of my waking hours were spent either with the volunteers or carrying out the exercise program. My son's disabilities were all-consuming. Whenever or wherever a few spare moments existed they were spent trying to create some semblance of a normal childhood for our daughter. My husband and I had very little life of our own.

I felt totally isolated. While I was trying to cope with the problems of our severely handicapped child at home, Alan's father dealt with the problems by detaching himself from the reality of the situation. Howard taught elementary music during the day and was employed as a musician at various nightclubs 3 or 4 nights a week. His job kept him away from home a great deal. Although I believe that he loves Alan with all his heart, he could not bring himself to help with the routine care or the patterning program. Perhaps the reality of Alan's condition was too terribly painful for him to face, or perhaps he was not able to give of himself—I don't know. In retrospect, I tend to believe the former. In either event, I felt that I bore the burden of Alan's care alone.

When Alan was 14 months old we moved back to New York State and settled in a community 2½ hours away from our parents. Both sets of parents offered help—each in their own way. My parents visited us every third weekend and offered what relief and emotional support they could. As time passed, traveling became increasingly difficult for them because my father had developed heart and kidney problems. My husband's parents also visited us. Their support was financial, rather than emotional, and when they visited they were treated more like visiting guests than caring grandparents who had come to offer a helping hand. At one very low point in our married lives I can recall crying out in desperation and begging my husband to ask his parents to come take care of the children so that we could get away from our home situation for a few days. They responded to our cry for help by rejecting our plea and suggesting that we seek their help again in 3 more years, after they retired from their jobs and had more time to spend with their family. Perhaps Howard's parents, like their son, could not face the realities of Alan's condition and therefore declined. At that point, I felt as if someone had taken a knife and pierced my heart. We were distraught and very much alone in our agony. If two of those closest to us and to Alan had closed their hearts to our pleas, where then could we have turned?

Obtaining babysitters for Alan was another difficult task. During Alan's first 2 years, babysitters were not too difficult to find because Alan was small and we only left him for a few hours at a time. All that a sitter needed to do was give him a drink and put him to bed. But, as Alan grew larger and heavier, his need for total care became more pronounced, and finding competent babysitters became a far greater problem. We did not feel comfortable leaving Alan in the care of teenage babysitters due to their inexperience, and adult sitters were either too costly or shied away from caring for a handicapped child.

In the last 2 years the concept of respite care has been introduced to our community on a limited basis. Today our community is beginning to offer health care/homemaker services to parents who are in need of some aide or relief on a per-diem basis, and the local developmental center is attempting to alleviate some of the burden of the parents of severely handicapped children by allowing parents to place their child on a suitable unit (on a space available basis) for up to 30 days per year. Comparatively, our community may be offering much less in the way of support services than other locales, but it is making a start. If only they had started 16 years sooner . . .

We decided to place our son in a developmental center in 1971 when he was 4 years old. Although respite care comes too late for us, I view it as a Godsend to parents who may find themselves in a similar situation. One can only surmise, at this point, how respite care might have changed our lives. Alan's father and I have since divorced. Our divorce came many years later and was caused by other factors, but I often wonder how much of our marital disharmony originated in our early years together. Perhaps, if respite care had been available years ago, we, as a young couple, might have been afforded the opportunity to grow together, rather than apart. It is also conceivable that we might have been able to care for Alan for a longer period of time at home if there had been some form of outside support. One factor in making our decision to institutionalize our son was our inability to offer our daughter a normal life. Often she would sit by the window and watch the other children at play longing to join them. Too often she had been denied that privilege because Alan needed attention and could not be left alone for even the shortest period of time. What if respite care could have been provided so that more time might have been spent with our daughter? As far as our son was concerned, Alan might have learned to accept care from hands other than our own and perhaps might have been stimulated by new surroundings and new faces.

Overall, respite care, had it been available, might have strengthened a marriage, provided a sibling with a more normal early development, and, perhaps most importantly, offered a helping hand to a young couple who felt very much alone in their struggle to care for their severely handicapped child.

Part II

ISSUES AND MODELS FOR DELIVERING RESPITE SERVICES

Chapter 6

ISSUES AND MODELS IN THE DELIVERY OF RESPITE SERVICES

Joel M. Levy and Philip H. Levy

During the last two decades, there has been a concerted national movement away from the institutionalization of individuals with developmental disabilities. Spirited by a commitment to the theory of normalization ". . . making available to all mentally retarded people patterns of life and conditions of everyday living which are as close as possible to the regular circumstances and ways of society. . ." (Nirje, 1976, p. 231), the deinstitutionalization movement has dramatically affected the lives of persons with disabilities and their families. Fewer families are placing their children with developmental disabilities outside the home, parents who place their children with developmental disabilities do so at a later age, and some parents are receiving back into their homes the individuals with developmental disabilities whom they placed in institutions years earlier. In fact, in the state of New York, over 85% of all persons with a developmental disability are living at home and have never been placed in an institution or a community residence (Cuomo & Webb, 1984).

Clearly, despite enormous hardships and sacrifices, it is obvious that families prefer to keep their developmentally disabled member living at home as long as possible. However, the shocking fact is that home-based services currently receive less than 1% of the total federal budget expended for health and social services (Loop, 1980). Moreover, in most states, a disproportionate percentage of the social service and mental health budget is spent each year to support the placement of individuals with developmental disabilities out of their natural homes, whereas only a small amount is allocated to assist families in keeping their children with disabilities at home. This funding imbalance occurs despite the fact that, more often than not, the natural home is where many individuals with developmental disabilities belong, want to be, and can be better served in a more economically prudent manner.

With significantly more individuals with developmental disabilities living in their natural home or a community setting, society must now meet the challenge of creating a comprehensive array of services designed to meet the support and relief needs of their families and caregivers. A comprehensive system of family support services would minimally include respite care, homemaker services, case management, transportation, recreation, parent training, and information and referral. However, Castellani (1985) found that these services are often unavailable or inaccessible to people with developmental disabilities.

WHAT IS RESPITE?

Respite is defined as temporary short-term care provided to a developmentally disabled individual for the purpose of providing relief to the parent or primary caregiver. Its availability has repeatedly been cited by both parents and professionals as both a crucial preventive and emergency service, allowing families with members who have developmental disabilities the necessary relief to maintain family integrity and stability. Respite is utilized by parents to conduct errands, keep appointments, go on vacation, spend time with their spouse or with their other children, handle emergencies, or simply to relax. Respite is a temporary, intermittent service and can last from several hours to a 3- or 4-week duration.

Parents and family members may find relief from the day-to-day responsibilities of caring for their relative with developmental disabilities through both primary and secondary sources of respite. Primary sources of respite are those services with the main objective of providing families with a break from caregiving. Secondary sources of respite, although still providing relief to families, have other objectives as their primary goal. For example, the main goal of an educational program is to teach an individual a certain competency. Although a family may receive a break during the time when the person with a developmental disability attends school, it is not the primary objective of the school program to provide relief. It is important to distinguish between primary and secondary sources of respite so as to ensure adequate funding and recognition for formalized respite care.

A national survey (Wikler, 1980) was conducted to determine the needs of families with a developmentally disabled member. Respite care was one of the services most frequently identified as a need in this survey while also being cited as a service most often reported as not available.

This chapter discusses the critical issues related to the provision of respite care to developmentally disabled persons and their families; it includes a brief review of research on respite services; an examination of a variety of respite models; a description of the Young Adult Institute's Respite Project; an analysis of philosophical, staffing, fiscal, and legal concerns that can impede implementation of these services; and recommendations for future efforts in the development of respite services.

WHY IS RESPITE IMPORTANT?

Continuous care for a child or adult with a developmental disability often produces economic, social, and psychological stress for each associated family member. Although many families struggle to maintain a disabled person at home, lack of support, coupled with the disabled individual's need for constant care, produces undue burdens with which many families are unable to cope. This lack of support can lead to serious consequences, including child/spouse abuse, loss of employment, drug/alcohol abuse, marital and/or family discord, sibling truancy or delinquency, and hastening or forcing the family to make the reluctant and difficult decision to seek residential placement for the disabled family member.

The negative impact of a developmentally disabled member on family integrity and quality of life is substantiated in literature on developmental disabilities. Doernburg (1978) states:

> With the mother-handicapped child pair split from the integral life of the family, the father and other children manage with an exhausted part-time mother whose energies are disproportionately invested in one family member. Often the mother is unable to participate in the important "special events" in her normal child's life. (pp. 107–109).

In addition, some studies have shown a correlation between the existence of a disability and the incidence of child abuse. Chotiner and Lehr (1976) cite a national survey that states that 58% of abused children or children of Parents Anonymous members exhibited developmental problems prior to abuse. They noted that in research conducted by the Denver Department of Welfare, close to 70% of 97 abused children in the study had some previous mental or physical deviation.

Most people depend on the support and companionship of their spouse, relatives, friends, and neighbors during times of stress or crisis. For many families with a severely disabled relative, this support is either not available or may not be sufficient. The parents may be embarrassed by their disabled child's behavior or disability, or they may be rejected by family and friends because of the disabled child. Indeed, parents of a developmentally disabled child cite their sense of utter isolation—the feeling that they are all alone—as one of their greatest challenges.

Respite services are directed toward reducing strain, reinforcing and sustaining family integrity, and providing relief to forestall out-of-home placement for the disabled individual. Research, although somewhat limited, has indicated that respite support can have a positive impact on a family's ability to cope with caring for a disabled member.

Bristol (1984) has written about the importance of formal and informal social support in reducing the stresses that confront parents of children with disabilities. Informal sources of support include the availability and helpfulness of immediate and extended family, friends, neighbors, and other parents of handicapped children. Formal supports include the availability and helpfulness of support persons or support services ranging from paid respite workers to counselors, and respite programs. Bristol concludes that the availability of informal and formal sources of support is the major predictor of successful family adaptations. Moreover, Bristol's research with families of young developmentally disabled persons found that happier and more successful marriages were directly related to family members having adequate support from one another and from a peer group of parents of disabled children.

Research has also shown that parents perceive the receipt of respite as improving quality of life and relieving family stress (Joyce, Singer, & Isralowitz, 1983; Webb, Shaw, & Hawes, 1984), as well as precluding the need for out-of-home placement of the disabled individual (Apolloni & Triest, 1983; Webb et al., 1984). These studies validate the efficacy of respite services in enabling families to cope with the responsibilities of caring for a developmentally disabled member, and they provide objective support for funding and development efforts.

HOW IS RESPITE CARE DELIVERED?

Respite care can be provided in several ways, with the major distinction being that the service is provided either in or out of the family home.

In-Home Respite

In-home respite is typically provided by trained individuals who come to the families' homes either on a regular or an on-call basis. Following are some models utilized in the provision of in-home respite.

Homemaker Services Homemaker services are provided within the consumer's home by a trained and licensed homemaker. These services are available 7 days per week, at all times of day, in flexible 4–8 hour shifts. Homemaker services can be provided on an emergency or planned basis. Most parents utilizing the homemaker service leave the home while the services are being provided. Many states' departments of mental retardation and developmental disabilities have contracts with generic home health care agencies for the purpose of providing in-home respite.

Sitter/Companion Services The sitter/companion program offers short-term respite in the family home in a very similar manner to the homemaker service. The primary difference between the sitter/companion service and the homemaker service is that a family is usually matched with one sitter/companion who provides respite services on a regular and as-needed basis. This continuity of care permits the establishment of trust between the worker and the family and allows for the implementation of training and goal objectives during the provision of respite. In addition, the sitter/companion service typically employs an individual who is trained specifically to work with the developmentally disabled population.

Parent Trainer Services The parent trainer model is similar to sitter/companion services in that the provider of respite is trained in caring for a developmentally disabled person and the same person consistently provides the service. The distinguishing factor in parent trainer models lies in the source of caregiver recruitment. This model utilizes individuals who form part of a family's natural informal support network. Thus, relatives, friends, and neighbors are recruited, trained, and paid to provide respite services. Parents participate in the training program in order to ensure that specific information and strategies regarding care for their children are incorporated into the training.

Advantages and Disadvantages In-home respite care offers the following advantages:

1. The developmentally disabled person is not required to adjust to a new environment.
2. Specialized equipment utilized by the developmentally disabled person does not have to be transported.
3. The family does not have to arrange for transportation to the service.
4. The service can be provided at a relatively low cost.
5. Respite providers frequently provide care for other nondisabled children.

Limitations of in-home respite include the following:

1. The service may be inappropriate for disabled persons with extreme behavioral problems or severe medical needs.
2. It is more costly to provide care for one individual than to provide service in a group.
3. Liability issues arise concerning worker coverage while providing service in the home, transporting clients in workers' cars, potential abuse lawsuits, and medication administration.
4. Supervision of workers and monitoring of service quality are difficult

because of the diverse and dispersed locations in which respite is provided.

5. Respite workers must usually provide their own transportation to the family home. This can be costly for a college student who only works part-time and is difficult if the home is not convenient to public transportation.

Out-of-Home Respite

Out-of-home respite may be provided on a day or overnight basis in a variety of settings. Many out-of-home respite models are able to serve more than one developmentally disabled individual at a time. Below are some examples of out-of-home respite models.

Family Care Services   A number of states allocate one or more beds in the homes of licensed family care providers for the purpose of respite. This model is particularly suited for families who require respite for anywhere from one night to several weeks' time. Licensed family care providers receive training in developmental disabilities and usually serve additional individuals who are placed in the home on a permanent basis. Utilization of this model can sometimes be problematic due to a lack of available beds and the requirement in some states that the developmentally disabled person be admitted to a state institution or developmental center in order to be eligible for this service.

Parent Cooperative Services   In this model, families with a developmentally disabled relative agree to care for each other's relative reciprocally in their own homes. The advantages are that cooperative services can provide peer socialization opportunities for the disabled individual, and the service is provided free. Problems, however, arise because of difficulties in coordinating the exchange of services and in matching the age, functioning level, and care needs of the developmentally disabled persons to be served. In addition, many families already feel burdened and overwhelmed by the responsibility of caring for their own disabled relative and do not have the desire or energy to take on the responsibility for another person with a developmental disability.

Respite Provider's Home   In some cases, services are given in the private nonlicensed home of the person providing respite care. This model can be utilized for varying periods of time, ranging from during the day while parents are at work to several weeks while a family goes on vacation. Drawbacks to this model include the need for transportation to the provider's home and liability and insurance issues.

Day Drop-Off Centers   The day drop-off center uses space in a community setting that is allocated for the provision of respite services during a particular time period, either during the day or evening or on a weekday or weekend. Space may be located in a YM- or YWCA, a school, a community residence, a church or temple, a day treatment program, or any other community space. The respite care provided in this model is usually available on a regular basis with set hours (e.g., everyday after school or every Saturday evening) and provides services to a number of developmentally disabled persons at one time. Often, recreation and/or rehabilitation services are provided during the period of respite.

Intermediate Care or Community Residence Services Respite care is sometimes provided in an established Intermediate Care Facility (ICF) or a Community Residence (CR). Respite can be provided on a day, overnight, or extended basis and can be particularly beneficial for a developmentally disabled person who is in transition to an out-of-home placement. Barriers to use of this model are funding levels and the certified capacity of a residence, the need to match a person's age and functioning level to that of the individuals living in a residence, and the unavailability of residential beds.

Institutional Care Services Respite care is available in most state-run institutions or developmental centers, usually on an emergency basis. Some state institutions have allocated a certain floor or area specifically for respite, particularly to serve one or a number of low-incidence, underserved populations, such as those with autism, Prader Willi syndrome, or a dual diagnosis. Institutional care respite is beneficial because it is usually immediately available and employs a trained staff. Disadvantages include temporary relocation of the developmentally disabled person from the family home to an environment with many people; the frequent need to admit a person in order to receive services; and the reluctance of many families to place their relative, even temporarily, in an institution.

Respite Residence Model A number of communities have developed free-standing respite residences to provide temporary residential services for respite purposes. A respite residence can serve any number of people, depending on the certified capacity of the facility, and is particularly helpful to parents when they go on vacation, during periods of hospitalization, and as a form of crisis intervention. Problems can arise when there is too much diversity in age and behavioral and functional level of the developmentally disabled persons served. Thus, staff must be versatile and well trained in order to meet the varying needs of a continually changing clientele. In addition, the vacancy rate at free-standing respite residences can be high due to the as-needed basis on which service is provided. However, as long as these issues are adequately addressed in staff recruitment and funding methodologies, the respite residence model is very viable and beneficial.

Advantages and Disadvantages Out-of-home respite is particularly appropriate for families whose disabled relatives are: 1) adults or young adults, 2) in need of specialized medical or psychological care, and 3) in preparation for residential placement.

Conversely, out-of-home respite can be seen as less normalized, as it rarely reflects a natural home setting. As do parents of nonhandicapped children, parents with young disabled children are less likely than parents with older children to feel comfortable leaving their children in an unfamiliar setting outside the home.

There are advantages and drawbacks to each of the respite models discussed. Research has shown that an array of respite alternatives needs to be available to meet the varied support requirements of families. Cohen and Warren (1985) found in their review of respite literature that the following points regarding the provision of respite care were consistently highlighted:

1. Respite care is a highly needed service.
2. It is often used by families with limited natural support networks where the day-to-day care of a developmentally disabled child is particularly burdensome.
3. It can play an important role in reducing family stress, improving the mental health of parents, stabilizing the family, and reducing the likelihood of long-term placement.
4. Time is an important variable in relation to the effectiveness of respite services, with very limited amounts of services not likely to improve family functioning in any significant way.
5. Families prefer in-home services to out-of-home services, but about two-fifths of families report a definite need for out-of-home respite services.
6. Parents are generally very satisfied with the respite care services they have received, with the two frequently cited areas in need of improvement being time allotments and worker skills.

FISCAL ISSUES AND CONSIDERATIONS

Of the possible alternatives to institutional care, families who maintain their disabled child at home receive the least support both in dollars and services. The staggering costs of caring for a developmentally disabled child, coupled with the financial disincentives to maintain the relative in the natural home, force some families to make the difficult decision to seek placement for their child. This out-of-home placement could often be prevented or delayed if adequate family support services, particularly respite services, were available.

A small portion of current funding is allocated to support families caring for their developmentally disabled relative in the home. According to Moroney (1979), there are several reasons why the amount of funding is so low. A large part of these funds continues to be earmarked for institutions. Of the money that is allocated for community care, the largest proportion is used to support residential services. Finally, given the limited funding available to meet all the care needs of the developmentally disabled, priority is typically given to those disabled persons who are not living in the home.

Service delivery to persons with developmental disabilities is changing due to the recent successful efforts to repatriate individuals from institutions to community placements and to stem new admissions into institutions. This redirection is sound both philosophically from the perspective of normalization and fiscally from a cost differential analysis. However, funding allocations are still disproportionately skewed toward institutional care. Intagliata, Willer, and Cooley (1979) studied residential alternatives available to developmentally disabled persons in New York State and found significant differences in the annual cost of these services. Institutional care was the most expensive ($14,630), costing 7 times as much as care in the natural family home ($2,108), with group home ($9,255–$11,000) and family care home ($3,130) services averaging 4 to 5 times and 1½ times, respectively, that of natural family home care. If the commitment to provide services in the community is to be met, then funding allocations must shift correspondingly, with a substantial increase to assist families in maintaining their developmentally disabled relative at home.

Current funding systems for respite care vary from state to state. Many states have passed legislation to fund respite services, whereas other states have established statewide mechanisms for supporting a variety of respite care options. A recent analysis by Braddock (1984) indicated that state tax dollars constitute the largest source of funding for family support services. It is encouraging that states have taken the initiative to fund these services; however, this has resulted in wide disparities in family support allocations from state to state, with some states offering no services. In addition, these allocations still constitute only a small proportion of those states' total spending for services to persons with developmental disabilities, with funding often subsumed under other service categories.

Providing cash subsidies to families has also been explored as an alternative method to supporting home care of developmentally disabled persons. Initial reports indicate that cash subsidy programs can be effective in preventing residential placement and improving family life and the functioning of severely disabled children and are clearly less costly than out-of-home placement. However, if cash subsidy programs are to be successful, trained family support workers and a thorough case-management system must be in place. They cannot be successful if the services families need are not available for purchase.

Recent changes in federal Title XIX and XX funding sources are also having an impact on the provision and availability of respite services. Until recently, there were many financial disincentives and barriers that prevented the use of Medicaid funds for care of a disabled individual while he or she was living at home. Often, Medicaid would only pay the cost of care if the person were in an institution. The parents of Katie Beckett, a 3-year-old living in an institution and life-bound to a respirator, appealed to President Reagan to enable them to care for Katie at home where she would be with her family and the cost of care would be lower. This appeal resulted in the issuance of a landmark waiver that allowed Katie to retain her SSI and Medicaid eligibility while receiving care at home. In 1981, the Omnibus Budget Reconciliation Act, PL 97-35, was passed with the aim of reducing federal domestic expenditures. Section 2176 of this act permitted a waiver of Title XIX statutory requirements so that noninstitutional services could be financed through the federal/state Medicaid program. A waiver granted under this section may ". . . provide medical assistance to individuals . . . for case management services, homemaker/health aide services and personal care services, adult day health services, habilitation services, respite care and such other services requested by the State as the Secretary may approve." By 1983, 86 waiver requests had been submitted by 44 states. Forty-five requests from 35 states had been approved, and 30 were pending. Seventeen of 26 states with approved waivers requested support for respite care according to a study conducted by Greenberg, Schmitz, and Lakin in 1983.

As a result of fiscal limitations, some respite programs have established a sliding scale fee for services. Charging parents for service has the potential to increase service availability, but at the same time risks the exclusion of families who are on meager budgets and do not consider their need for a break (respite care) a legitimate family priority. According to Cohen and Warren (1985):

> Whatever financial resources do become available for the support of respite programs, the provision of respite care in some states will probably involve a financial contribution by middle class families toward the cost of this service. If a long-range point of view is taken, a strong case can be made against this practice both philosophically and fiscally. However, this practice may enable respite care legislation to be passed in some states where it might otherwise be unpassable. (p. 164)

DEVELOPING A COMMUNITY RESPITE PROGRAM

The Young Adult Institute (YAI), is a private not-for-profit agency that provides a full continuum of services to over 1,000 persons with developmental disabilities and their families in the New York metropolitan area. In 1983, YAI was one of three voluntary agencies selected in New York State to receive a legislative demonstration grant to develop a respite project. The goals of the YAI project were to assess the overall demand for respite care and determine the type of services that would meet this demand in the most efficient, effective, and economical manner; ascertain and evaluate the respite services that were currently being provided and identify the gaps in services; coordinate a countrywide network of respite service provisions that utilized the existing providers of care through service agreements; develop service delivery systems with input from consumers and social service providers to meet unfilled needs; oversee the implementation and administration of the respite services network to monitor and ensure that a full range of respite service options were available, accessible, and responsive to consumer needs; promote the knowledge and use of these services through an active outreach campaign; provide for the data collection, data analysis, and evaluation of respite services; and create a Respite Advisory Board to assist in the coordination and implementation of respite services. This section discusses the procedures utilized by YAI in implementing the Queens Respite network.

Before developing a community respite program, a thorough examination of the following issues is required.

1. What respite services are currently being provided in the area?
2. What are the needs of the community to be served, and has their input been incorporated in planning services?
3. What services can realistically be provided within the parameters of the projected budget?
4. Will respite care be provided in or out of the family home, or both?
5. Are the proposed services accessible to families?
6. What means of outreach will be utilized to make families aware of the services?
7. What criteria will be used for determining family eligibility?
8. How will staff be recruited, trained, and supervised?
9. Will workers be paid or recruited as volunteers?
10. What health and safety issues need to be addressed?
11. What liability and insurance issues need to be considered?

Needs Assessment

YAI staff initiated the Queens Respite Network by identifying existing sources of respite in the community. They found that services were limited to two sources, the Queens Developmental Center and voluntary-operated community residences. Emergency care was being provided through the developmental center, but only after the disabled individual was admitted to the facility. The admission procedures, which include a current medical and psychological examination and extensive family interview, can be very time consuming and arduous, especially for a family in crisis. In addition, many families were unwilling to utilize this source of respite because they did not want to admit their child under any circumstances to a developmental center.

Respite was provided in voluntary-operated community residences when a program vacancy occurred. However, residential vacancies are virtually non-existent, and the availability of this source of respite was negligible.

The next step in the project was to identify and assess the respite needs of the community to be served. A questionnaire regarding respite needs had been developed by the New York State Office of Mental Retardation and Developmental Disabilities (NYS OMRDD) for this purpose. YAI staff met with providers of services to persons with developmental disabilities in Queens County and received their cooperation in distributing the questionnaire to a random sample of the families they served. The results of this survey were published as part of a statewide report on respite services in New York (Webb et al., 1984); some highlights are presented below.

Of the families who responded to the survey, 64% expressed an unmet need for respite services, 55% indicated that respite services would help prevent or delay permanent out-of-home placement, and 72% preferred respite to be provided in their own home. The most frequently cited reason (44%) for not utilizing respite services was uncertainty about someone else caring for the disabled family member.

These findings established that parents perceive respite as a valuable and necessary service that will assist them in maintaining the developmentally disabled family member at home. In addition, the need to develop respite services in the county was substantiated by the number of respondents who expressed unmet respite needs. Based on the results of this survey, YAI staff determined that the majority of services developed would be directed toward the provision of in-home respite and that careful attention should be given to staff recruitment and training so as to reassure parents about staff capabilities.

Respite Advisory Board

Through the course of meeting with service providers to distribute the respite questionnaire, YAI staff recruited members for the Respite Advisory Board. This board, composed of parents and representatives from state and voluntary agencies, was organized to assist in the development, coordination, and implementation of the Queens Respite Network. The board is co-chaired by YAI and Queens Borough Developmental Services Office (QBDSO) staff and meets bimonthly. In addition, subcommittees have been formed on program planning, media and public awareness, legislative/governmental initiatives, and policy development.

Implementation of a respite advisory board is encouraged for those who plan to develop respite services. The Queens Respite Advisory Board serves a number of important functions, including generating consumer input, providing information on various respite models, organizing advocacy efforts, promoting the knowledge and use of respite services, contributing to the establishment of statewide respite standards and procedures, and ensuring that a full range of respite service options is available. For example, the board organized a group of parents to make a presentation to the State Legislative Mental Health Committee on the need for a permanent funding source for respite services; this effort led to a 3-fold increase in state appropriations for Family Support Services over the previous year's budget. In addition, the Respite Advisory Board helps prevent duplication of services and fosters cooperative efforts among the various providers of services.

Recruiting, Training, and Supervising Respite Workers

Parents are often initially ambivalent about receiving respite services. One parent expressed a common concern when she said, "Not only do we parents of handicapped children carry a load of guilt about our child's disability, but that guilt also makes us overprotective about our child!" (Stanzler, 1982).

In light of the fact that families are already likely to be experiencing high levels of stress and guilt, the key challenge of recruitment is to attract workers: 1) who are likely to stay with the program, minimizing the need for families to constantly readjust to new workers and 2) whom parents are able to trust to care for their disabled relatives.

Recruitment techniques often used by respite care programs include the following:

1. Preparing posters, flyers, and brochures for dissemination throughout the community
2. Making presentations at high schools, colleges, universities, churches, synagogues, senior citizen associations, and civic organizations
3. Submitting press releases and articles to local papers and community newsletters and public service announcements to radio and television stations
4. Placing advertisements in the employment sections of newspapers

YAI recruitment efforts targeted college students enrolled in social service programs at local universities and professionals working in the mentally retarded/developmentally disabled (MR/DD) field who might be attracted to the opportunity to use their skills to work on a one-to-one basis with disabled individuals. Program staff believed that these two populations would be likely to: 1) have an investment in helping families with developmentally disabled relatives, 2) have previous experience working with disabled individuals, and 3) view the experience gained through the position as a type of compensation in addition to salary. This perception would consequently increase worker motivation, self-satisfaction, and job performance and minimize employee turnover, tardiness, and absenteeism.

All workers were required to work a minimum of 5 hours per week, successfully complete a 16-hour training program, and make a minimum of a 6 months' commitment to a family.

Flyers were mailed to department heads at local universities and to directors of all agencies serving developmentally disabled persons in Queens, with a cover letter requesting cooperation in posting the materials.

Ten well-qualified part-time respite workers were hired, many of whom possessed several years' experience, either voluntary or professional, working with developmentally disabled individuals. The majority of workers were sophomores and juniors in college. Parents were consistently impressed with the workers' enthusiasm, confidence, and capabilities.

The 16-hour training program conducted by YAI staff served two vital purposes. One, of course, was to train staff to provide quality in-home respite care. Training for respite workers should minimally include the following: information on developmental disabilities and general medical problems; normalization; basic rights of people with disabilities; working with parents of developmentally disabled children, behavior management; language/communication; recreational activities; and first aid and emergency procedures. Training modules on communication skills were particularly helpful when workers found themselves listening to a parent desperately needing a friend or helper. Workers appreciated the opportunity to use role playing techniques for: 1) responding to difficult questions parents might ask, 2) saying "no" and setting limits, and 3) determining when it was appropriate to offer advice.

Second, the training sessions provided an opportunity for the respite coordinator to become acquainted with each worker's skills and personality. This "preassessment" was extremely beneficial to future matching of workers and families.

All respite programs must develop a system of matching families with respite care providers. A successful system should consider the following factors: time availability of the worker, where the worker lives, the worker's ability to handle particular behaviors, worker and family preferences; and the likelihood of the worker being accepted in the family's home.

One approach to matching families and workers is to separate respite workers into skill categories. The majority of workers would be matched with clients requiring basic sitter/companion services. Specially trained respite workers with skills in behavior management or medical needs would be available to care for more demanding clients and would be paid at a higher level. By offering higher salaries and periodic in-service training, YAI's program was successful in attracting workers capable of caring for autistic clients with extreme behavior problems. Workers responded positively to the challenge of working with difficult clients and to the opportunity to advance professionally.

Eligibility and Determination of Need

According to Cohen and Warren (1985), "the determination of need for (respite) services should be based upon the total gestalt of the family, with special attention to the needs of the primary caretaker" (p. 162). Whenever possible, a personal assessment should be conducted to determine the individual coping capacities of the parents, family functioning level, and existing informal support networks. YAI staff were often surprised at the disparity between the needs indicated by a statistical assessment (i.e., marital status, income level, degree of disability) and the actual coping level of the parent or family. Parental perception of their own ability to cope appeared to be crucial to determining the actual degree of need. In other words, some individuals cope more effectively than others, regardless of existing support networks. In fact, having extended family support nearby frequently appeared to *add* stress for some families, rather than to serve as a postive relief source.

Clearly, in establishing eligibility criteria for respite services, planners must realize that offering one standard allotment or type of service for *all* families is inappropriate. Criteria must remain flexible to meet the differing coping levels from family to family.

Liability

Because services were provided within a family's home, several unprecedented questions arose concerning agency liability during the implementation of the YAI Respite Network:

1. Are respite workers liable for client injury while providing service in a client's home?
2. Are respite workers insured to transport clients in their automobiles to community activities?
3. What training is required to certify workers to administer medication?
4. Are agency volunteers insured to provide service in client homes?

YAI was advised by the agency's legal counsel to maintain thorough documentation of all letters of recommendation, training attendance, and supervisory meetings for each worker to justify that all possible precautions had been taken to select reputable, qualified workers and to prepare them for their duties. All workers are required to complete a cardiopulmonary resuscitation course and are instructed to review emergency procedures with each family. Workers are advised not to transport clients in their own cars and that doing so would be at their own risk.

Initially, no workers were permitted to administer medication (including over-the-counter drugs), and families were obligated to make alternative arrangements for their children to receive medication. However, because this regulation restricted the use of respite by many families, two workers were selected to complete a state-approved medication course.

In light of the newness of respite services, all agencies are encouraged to investigate seriously the regulations applicable to their own locality and the boundaries of their agency insurance policy before sending respite workers into the field.

CONCLUSION

Respite services provide temporary short-term care for developmentally disabled persons for the purposes of relieving parents from their caregiving role and reducing stress within the family. Respite is considered by many families to be a survival, rather than a supplemental, service and gives parents the break they need to maintain their disabled relative in the home. Despite the fact that research strongly indicates that respite can positively influence a family's ability to function in a healthy, stable fashion, the provision of respite services remains fragmented and unsystematized.

Although limited in sophistication and scope, research on respite provision has substantiated that respite is a necessary service that can reduce the incidence of stress and strain experienced by families with disabled children. More longitudinal studies need to be conducted to document the peripheral impact of respite on other family members and the family as a unit before the true efficacy of respite can be determined. More solid data are also needed to determine the most efficient respite models and methods for dispensing services and the most cost-effective funding approaches.

Communities nationwide are experimenting with a variety of in-home and out-of-home respite models. This is an encouraging sign. To reach all populations, services must be flexible and broad-based, designed to serve clients of differing ages, functioning levels, and behaviors. Models must also consider in their design the varying needs of parents in terms of times and purposes for which respite is most often requested.

Inadequate funding mechanisms are the major barrier to respite provision. Strapped by budget limitations, agencies and parent groups struggle to provide even the most limited services and continue to advocate for a stabilized source for respite appropriations. Funding for respite varies from state to state, with the federal Medicaid waiver considered by some professionals to be the most encouraging resource for future funding.

The recent trend toward providing family support services, especially respite, offers the opportunity to expand the continuum of care to assist families in maintaining their disabled relative in the family home. It is the challenge and responsibility of parents, service providers, and government to engage in ongoing discussions that generate a broad array of available, accessible, economical, and responsive family support and respite services. Success is contingent on our meeting the challenge with creativity, enthusiasm, commitment, and an ever-present recognition of our goal—to maintain family integrity.

REFERENCES

Apolloni, A. H., & Triest, G. (1983). Respite services in California: Status and recommendations for improvement. *Mental Retardation, 21* (6), 240–243.

Braddock, D. (1984, February). *Statement on S.2053, The Community and Family Living Amendments of 1983.* U.S. Senate Finance Committee, Subcommittee on Health, Washington, DC.

Bristol, M. M. (1984, October). *Families of developmentally disabled children: Health adaptation and the double ABCX model.* Paper presented at the Family Systems and Health Preconference Workshop, National Council on Family Relations, San Francisco.

Calkins, C., Gibson, B., Grosko, J., & Bueker, J. (1982). *Respite care adapted for deaf-blind population: Training manual.* Kansas City: University of Missouri, Kansas City Institute University Affiliated Facility.

Castellani, P. (1985). *Prepared for the project: Financial incentives and disincentives to the involvement of families in the care and support of developmentally disabled sons and daughters.* Albany: New York State Office of Mental Retardation and Developmental Disabilities.

Chotiner, N., & Lehr, W. (Eds.). (1976). *Child abuse and developmental disabilities.* A Report from the New England Regional Conference, sponsored by United Cerebral Palsy of Rhode Island and United Cerebral Palsy Association.

Cohen, S., & Warren, R. (1985). *Respite care: Principles, programs and policies.* Austin, TX: Pro-Ed Press.

Cuomo, M. M., & Webb, Arthur Y. (1984). *The 1984–87 comprehensive plan for services to persons with mental retardation and developmental disabilities in New York State.* Albany: State of New York Office of Mental Retardation and Developmental Disabilities.

Doernberg, N. L. (1978). Some negative effects on family integration of health and educational services for handicapped children. *Rehabilitation Literature, 39*(4), 107–110.

Family subsidy programs evaluated. (1979). *New directions: The newsletter of the national Association of State Mental Retardation Program Directors, 9*(7), 2–4.

Greenberg, J. N., Schmitz, M. P., & Lakin, K. C. (1983). *An analysis of responses to the Medicaid home-and-community-based long-term care waiver program (Section 2176 or PL 97-35).* Washington, DC: National Governor's Association, Center for Policy Research.

Intagliata, J. C., Willer, B. S., & Cooley, F. B. (1979). Cost comparison of institutional and community-based alternatives for mentally retarded persons, Part I. *Mental Retardation, 17,* 154–156.

Johnson, B., & Morse, H. (1968). *The child and his development: A study of children with inflicted injuries.* Denver: Department of Public Welfare.

Joyce, K., Singer, M., & Isralowitz, R. (1983). Impact of respite care on parents' perceptions of quality of life. *Mental Retardation, 21*(4), 153–156.

Loop, B. (1980). *Family resources services and support services for families with handicapped children.* Omaha: University of Nebraska Medical Center, Meyer Children's Rehabilitation Institute.

Moroney, R. M. (1979). Allocation of resources for family care. In R. H. Bruininks & G. C. Krantz (Eds.), *Family care of developmentally disabled members: Conference proceedings* (pp. 63–76). Minneapolis: University of Minnesota.

Nirje, B. (1976). The normalization principle. In R. B. Kugal & A. Shearer (Eds.), *Changing patterns in residential services to the mentally retarded.* (Rev. ed.) Washington, DC: President's Committee on Mental Retardation.

Parents to receive subsidy payments (1976). *New Directions: The Newsletter of the National Association of State Mental Retardation Program Directors, 6*(1), 1–3.

Public Law 97–35. (August 13, 1982). Omnibus Budget Reconciliation Act of 1981.

Stanzler, M. (1982). Taking the guilt out of parenting. *The Exceptional Parent.* October 1982, 51–53.

Webb, A. Y., Shaw, H. W., & Hawes, B. A. (1984). *Respite services for developmentally disabled individuals in New York State.* Albany: State of New York Office of Mental Retardation and Developmental Disabilities.

Wikler, L. (1981). *Family relationships and stress.* Lexington: University of Kentucky Human Development Program (Title XX Training Project).

Chapter 7

RESPITE CARE PROVIDER TRAINING
A COMPETENCY-BASED APPROACH

J. Macon Parrish, Andrew L. Egel, and Nancy A. Neef

T he need for respite care is clearly documented (e.g., Cohen, 1982; Egel, Parrish, Sloan, & Neef, 1984; Meyers, Zetlin, & Blacher-Dixon, 1981; Salisbury & Griggs, 1983; Upshur, 1982a). In comparison with families without disabled members, families of handicapped individuals shoulder greater caregiving responsibilities (Farber, 1968; Mercer, 1966); experience more social isolation (Dunlap, 1969; Farber, 1968); and exhibit increased emotional distress (Cohen, 1982; Cummings, Bayley, & Rie, 1966; Erickson, 1968; Joyce, Singer, & Israelowitz, 1983). There is some evidence to suggest that the provision of respite care can decrease family stress (Wikler, 1981); enhance family functioning (Cohen, 1982); and reduce family requests for long-term residential placement (German & Maisto, 1982; Lawson, Connolly, Leaver, & Englisch, 1979).

The results of two recent surveys suggest that the availability of *well-trained* care providers may be an important determinant in a family's decision to rely on respite care services. Upshur (1982a) surveyed 300 families with mentally retarded and otherwise disabled members to establish a profile of needs for such services. Only 6% of the families indicated that they used trained providers. Many respondents expressed a preference for the availability of better trained workers who could provide respite care in their own homes. Indeed, the most common reason for dissatisfaction with services was the inadequate training of the respite care provider.

The contents of this chapter were developed under a grant (No. G008200404) from the USDE/OSERS/DPP. However, those contents do not necessarily represent the policy of that agency, and should not be viewed as an endorsement by the federal government.

In a more recent needs assessment survey, Egel et al. (1984) queried 75 parents of handicapped children. The parents frequently indicated that a lack of trust in others' abilities to care appropriately for their child's special needs was a major variable limiting their use of child care services. A number of parents expressed concern that available child sitters lack adequate training. Among the parents surveyed, 79% indicated that there was definitely a need for quality respite care services and that they were often unable to obtain acceptable respite care when they needed it. Almost all parents stated they would use the services of specially trained respite care providers if they were available.

The results of the surveys conducted by Upshur (1982a) and Egel et al. (1984) clearly indicate the need for more widespread and systematic training programs for respite care providers. Despite the consistent findings that families of handicapped children desire the services of specially trained child care workers, many individuals who deliver respite care have minimal, if any, training (Salisbury, 1984). As a case in point, Warren and Dickman (1981) found that 34% of respite care agencies surveyed did not have a training program, and another 39% offered less than 10 hours of training.

Unfortunately, most reports of respite care programs are solely descriptive and do not present detailed information regarding the content, length, or method of training. The length and scope of training provided appear to vary considerably from one program to the next. In her review article, Salisbury (1984) states that the length of training ranges from a few hours to 66 hours. The content of the training curricula sometimes consists of an introduction to the principles of deinstitutionalization and normalization; an overview of developmental disabilities; methods and schedules of dispensing medications; first-aid procedures for medical emergencies; use of adaptive equipment; methods of lifting, transferring, and positioning individuals with physical handicaps; management of behavior problems; completion of daily routines, such as feeding, toileting, dressing, and bathing; and strategies for prompting participation in leisure activities (e.g., Parham, Hart, Terraciano, & Newton, 1983; Powell & Hecimovic, 1981; Sloan, Neef, Parrish, & Egel, 1983; Upshur, 1982b; Warren & Dickman, 1981).

Although each of these topics is undoubtedly relevant to the provision of quality respite care, many training curricula only contain a subset of the content areas just listed. Furthermore, few if any training programs have incorporated topics addressing preparation for provision of respite care, maximization of educational strategies, self-defense tactics, and informing parents of the child's status on the parents' return (Sloan et al., 1983). Certainly one of the most important features of a respite care skills training program is that it be comprehensive in scope.

By far the most prevalent method of instruction has been inservice training centered around workshops (Salisbury, 1984). Some studies that have not specifically focused on the acquisition of respite care skills suggest that such inservice training may result in initial and maintained changes in staff and client behaviors (e.g., Gage, Fredericks, Johnson-Dorn, & Lindley-Southard, 1982; Watson & Uzzell, 1980; Zlomke & Benjamin, 1983). However, in a review of research related to the efficacy of inservice training, Ziarnik and Bernstein (1982) concluded that such training frequently does *not* lead to demonstrated improvements in staff or client performance. Furthermore, the effects of inservice training are often not only small in magnitude but also short-lived, raising questions about the cost-effectiveness of this training approach.

An alternative to inservice training through workshops is a competency-based training paradigm (e.g., Calkins, Gibson, Grosko, & Bueker, 1982; Lukenbill, Lillie, Sanddal, Hulme, Calkins, & McKibben, 1976). In such a paradigm, emphasis is placed on the acquisition and maintenance of *skills*, in contrast to a focus on the provision of general information designed to improve *attitudes* or to increase the trainee's *knowledge* base. The key features of a competency-based training model include identification and social validation of target skills; development of task analyses of such skills with corresponding operational definitions and assessment instruments; collection of baseline data regarding a trainee's level of proficiency in targeted skill areas before training; specification of learner objectives; provision of systematic training through lecture, modeling, and/or self-directed manuals; completion of behavior rehearsals; repeated measurement of trainee performance during and subsequent to training in both simulated and criterion situations; and, when necessary, provision of remedial training consisting of additional instruction, role plays, and performance-based feedback. Unfortunately, it appears that many training coordinators of respite care programs may not be well versed in the instructional technology that is prerequisite to the design and implementation of a competency-based training program. Furthermore, because of competing service-related and administrative responsibilities, many training coordinators may not have the time required to direct a competency-based training paradigm.

In addition to being comprehensive and competency-based, respite care training programs should be validated experimentally before widespread dissemination. Through repeated measurement of individual trainee performance during staggered baseline and training phases across a group of trainees, a competency-based approach to training readily permits a rigorous evaluation of whether the training package results in the acquisition and maintenance of targeted skills. In other words, the efficacy of a competency-based training model can be assessed easily through a single-subject experimental design in which each trainee serves as his or her own control (Hersen & Barlow, 1976;

Kazdin, 1982). Single-subject experimental designs obviate the need for large groups of trainees and for the assignment of some trainees to waiting lists or control groups in order to draw experimental comparisons. Furthermore, the imposition of single-subject experimental designs onto a competency-based training model allows for the detection of individual differences among trainees in their response to training and a consequent tailoring of the training program to the needs of each individual trainee. Through employment of single-subject methodology in conjunction with a competency-based training paradigm, an examination of the efficacy of training does not rely solely on activity measures, pre-post changes in trainee's attitudes and knowledge, trainee satisfaction with training, or the client families' satisfaction with trainee-provided respite care.

To date, most respite care training programs have been neither competency-based nor experimentally validated. In the absence of data regarding the effects of training, it has been impossible to investigate the relative cost-effectiveness of alternative training curricula; that is, to evaluate alternatives according to both their costs and their effects with respect to producing some outcome or set of outcomes. A cost-effectiveness analysis integrates the results of training activities with their costs in such a way that one can select those training activities that provide the best educational results for any given cost or that provide any given level of educational results for the least cost.

As Salisbury and Griggs (1983) point out, one of the most important considerations in the development of respite care services is that of cost. Ross (1980) concluded that few, if any, respite care programs can expect to receive stable federal, state, or local funding for program-specific needs. It is particularly unclear how the cost of training respite care providers is to be borne. In order to select training options that produce skilled providers for the least amount of money in the shortest period of time and to make a case for the allocation of government funds for the purpose of training, cost-effectiveness analyses are essential.

Another critical feature of a viable respite care skill training program is the extent to which the program is exportable to those not directly involved in its development. Over the years many critics have decried the tendency on the part of lay persons and paraprofessionals to rely solely on professionals, rather than on themselves or each other, for assistance (e.g., Morris & Hess, 1975). In the context of training respite care providers, such reliance not only significantly limits the lay person's accessibility to training through dependence on a few overly committed experts but also increases the cost of training because the fees of such experts are relatively expensive.

A well-designed training program is one that minimizes the degree of prior training, supplies and equipment, and ongoing technical sophistication necessary to implement it. Ideally, a training program is packaged in such a fashion that lay persons, with relatively little effort and without much, if any, direct training by the program developers, can acquire the skills necessary to direct the program. Furthermore, the optimal training program is one that can be conducted feasibly in service-oriented settings that may be lacking in time, space, money, and expertise. Without question, a critical test of any respite care skills training program is the extent to which it can be disseminated in a cost-effective manner and be maintained as well as adopted by community-based respite care programs without ongoing external expert assistance. To date, most designers of respite care training curricula have given far too little attention to packaging their materials for dissemination purposes.

The remainder of this chapter is devoted to specific issues and illustrations pertaining to the development and implementation of respite care skills training programs that are comprehensive, competency-based, experimentally validated, cost-effective, and exportable. At the conclusion of the chapter, suggested directions for future research into training-related issues are presented.

TRAINING CURRICULUM

The curricular content of most respite care training programs is designed by professionals based on their individual judgments of what providers should know about caring for developmentally disabled persons (Salisbury, 1984). It has been increasingly recognized, however, that the appropriateness and relevance of training goals are a judgment that only society or the ultimate consumers of the service are qualified to make (Wolf, 1978). Accordingly, there has been increasing demand for the social validation of intervention programs, including an assessment of the social acceptability of the *focus* of training, or whether the behaviors selected are important to individuals in the natural environment (Kazdin, 1977; Wolf, 1978).

Although the importance of conducting an analysis of respite care job requirements and establishing the ecological and social validity of training curricula is apparent, there have been few attempts to verify the relevance of the skills targeted for training (Salisbury, 1984). Clearly, if respite care programs are to have the desired impact on the client and family, the scope and focus of the training curricula must reflect a sensitivity to the needs and demands of those constituency groups.

Neef, Parrish, Egel, and Sloan (1985), for example, attempted to validate in several ways the content of an instructional package that was subsequently used to train respite care providers. Target respite care behaviors were derived from a survey of parents of handicapped children (Egel et al., 1984), a task analysis of a child care situation, and input from an interdisciplinary advisory board. Many of the parents surveyed felt that the respite providers were trained inadequately to care for their children. This was particularly true for the parents of the more severely involved children who exhibited a variety of special feeding and physical management problems. The three qualifications cited most frequently by parents as being essential for respite providers were: 1) patience and understanding, 2) dependability, and 3) special training and experience in working with handicapped children. Other qualifications deemed important by many parents included the ability to lift, transfer, and position physically handicapped children; a willingness to "take charge" and be both firm and consistent, and the ability to exercise good judgment in emergency situations.

These qualifications were subsequently operationalized and included in a task analysis of child care skills. Input regarding the content of the training curriculum was also solicited from relevant members of the community, including two additional parents of handicapped children, a speech therapist, motor development specialist, a pediatrician, a psychiatrist, a psychologist, two special education personnel, and two directors of county respite care agencies. Based on this input, each of the skill areas identified within the following four major categories was further task-analyzed: 1) Preparation and Parent Interaction (phone call, arrival, parent exit, parent return); 2) Child Behaviors (management of behavior problems; maximizing educational opportunities; managing mealtime, bedtime, and toileting routines); 3) Physical/Medical Management (positioning and handling, transfers, feeding, medication); and 4) Emergencies (seizures, choking, other medical and property emergencies). The resulting behaviors were then submitted to advisory board members, who were asked to rate those in his or her area of expertise, (e.g., the pediatrician reviewed target behaviors on medical emergencies) as to whether each was crucial, important but not crucial, or neither crucial nor important for respite care workers to acquire. Behaviors rated as neither crucial nor important were omitted. The respite care behaviors yielded through this analysis are presented in Table 1 and constituted the training curriculum.

In order to verify further that the training content was functional and relevant for job performance, parents of handicapped children and the coordinator of a county respite care agency participated in an evaluation of the overall quality of trainee performance in each of the target skill areas. Trainees were videotaped in a role-played respite care situation before and after training was provided. The two videotapes per trainee were presented in a random order to the judges, who were not informed as to which of the tapes represented pre- and posttraining performance. After viewing each tape, the judges were asked to rate the sessions on a Likert-type scale from 1 to 4 along 10 dimensions corresponding to the content of the training curriculum, as presented in Table 2. The assumption was that if the judges (service con-

Table 1. Target responses

I. Preparation/Information/Parent Interaction
  A. Phone call
    ____* name of parent
    ____* phone number
    ____* address
    ____* date/time needed
    ____* arrival time (1/2 hour early if first time)
  B. Arrival
    ____ arrives on time
    ____* name of child
    ____ age of child
    ____ ability level
    ____* handicaps
       (if physically handicapped:)
    ____ independence (mobility)
    ____* special precautions (positioning)
    ____* independence with eating
    ____* special precautions with feeding
    ____* special foods
    ____* special equipment
    ____* where kept
    ____* when used
    ____* how used and/or demonstration
    ____* medication taken
    ____* type
    ____* where kept
    ____* when given
    ____* dosage
    ____* how administered
    ____* communication system
    ____ new skills being learned
    ____ behavior problems
    ____ special management strategies
    ____ favorite toys and activities
    ____ daily routine
    ____ bedtime
    ____ mealtime
    ____ emergency phone numbers
    ____* parents

(continued)

Table 1. (continued)

_____*   fire/police/rescue squad/poison control
_____*   physician
_____*   neighbor or friend
_____*   emergency supplies (fire extinguisher, emetic)
_____   miscellaneous

C. After parents leave
   _____*   locks all doors
   _____   engages child in play/positive interactions

D. Parent return
   Reports any of the following that occurred:
   _____*   property emergencies
   _____*   medical emergencies
   _____*   seizure
   _____*   length
   _____*   behavior preceding onset
   _____*   patterns/sequence of movements
   _____   parts of body involved
   _____*   behavior following seizure
   _____   deviations from usual routine
   _____   behavior problems (frequent or severe)
   _____   description
   _____   frequency
   _____   strategy
   _____   positive behavior
   _____   miscellaneous (messages, etc.)

II. Child Behaviors
   A. Mealtime
      1. General
         _____   on time
         _____*   follows procedures described by parent
         _____   gives child small portions at a time
         _____   establishes rules at start of meal or after first occurrence of
                   problem
         _____   reinforces appropriate manners at least twice
         _____   converses with child on at least two topics
         _____   if snacks are given, small amounts and in accordance with any
                   established policies
      2. Feeding a child with oral-motor problems (scored per bite)
         _____*   puts child in proper chair and position
         _____*   if head hyperextended, repositions before feeding
         _____*   foods of appropriate texture

Table 1. (*continued*)

____*   food placed in appropriate location of mouth

____*   small bites

____*   pulls spoon straight out of mouth without scraping top teeth or lips

____*   provides jaw control

____*   feeds slowly (waits until previous bite is swallowed)

B.   Toileting (for child who is being toilet trained)

   ____   follows any procedures described by parents

       If none described:

   ____   prompts/takes child to bathroom at least once

   ____   provides assistance as needed

   ____   requires child to sit on toilet for 15 sec. or until eliminates

   ____   reinforces elimination on toilet

   ____   reinforces self initiations to use toilet

       If accident occurs (not resulting from seizure):

   ____   requires child to clean self and area, providing assistance only as necessary

   ____   requires child to sit on toilet for 15 sec. or until eliminates

C.   Behavioral problems (scored for each occurrence)

____*   consequates each incidence of inappropriate behavior (after maximum of 1 warning) within five seconds, using an appropriate procedure

____*   provides descriptive feedback

____*   after consequences, reinforces alternative appropriate behavior

____*   uses (appropriate) consequences consistently

____*   interacts positively with child at least 50% of observation intervals

____*   reinforces appropriate behavior at least once per hour

III.   Physical/Medical Management

A.   Positioning and handling

   ____   wears clothes that do not restrict movement

   ____   wears flat shoes

   ____*   changes child's position at least once per hour

   ____*   does not force joints to bend or extend

   ____*   breaks up abnormal patterns by flexing at nearest joint

       Before moving child: (scored for each occurrence)

   ____   clears path

   ____*   gets area or equipment ready

   ____   informs child

   ____   solicits child's help

(*continued*)

Table 1. (continued)

When transferring: (scored for each occurrence)

____*   lifts with back straight, bottom down

____*   controls child at key points when lifting

____*   carries child with back straight, bottom down

____*   controls child at key points when carrying

____*   maintains firm grip

____*   carries child facing outward

____*   does not rush

____*   takes short steps

____   changes directions by stepping around (not twisting)

____*   lowers with back straight/bottom down

____*   controls child at key points when lowering

In wheelchair: (scored for each transfer)

____*   hips flexed 90° or more

____*   child's head and trunk in midline

____*   seatbelt across hips and fastened

____*   legs separated 4 to 8 inches

____*   feet flat on rests and straps fastened

When positioning a child: (over wedge)

____*   arms forward and forearms touching floor (in supported sitting)

____*   hips flexed 90° or more

____*   sitter behind child providing support as needed (in side lying)

____*   child's back against wall/furniture

____*   head tucked forward

____*   top leg flexed 90° or more

B.   Medication

____*   correct medication

____*   correct dosage

____*   administered correctly

____*   on time

IV.   Emergencies

A.   General medical/property

____*   administers appropriate first aid (minor)

____*   takes appropriate steps to end emergency (minor)

____*   calls appropriate emergency personnel (major)

____*   reports all information requested

____*   follows any directions given

____*   monitors child throughout emergency

Table 1. *(continued)*

       ____*   gets child out of house within 2 min. (major property)
       ____*   calls parents when safe to do so and reports situation (major)

B.   Seizures

       ____*   helps child to floor within 5 sec. of onset
       ____*   rolls child onto side within 5 sec.
       ____*   moves furniture, hot/sharp objects out of reach
       ____*   loosens child's clothing
       ____*   removes child's glasses, hearing aid, etc.
       ____*   does not put anything in child's mouth
       ____*   does not restrain child
       ____*   stays with child during seizure and observes
       ____*   checks time within 10 sec. of onset
       ____*   if continues over 10 min., calls emergency personnel
       ____*   does not give child liquids immediately following seizure
       ____   if child voids, cleans child up after seizure
       ____   allows child to sleep
       ____*   if child sleeps, rolls onto side
       ____*   if child sleeps, check at least once every 1/2 hour
       ____   if child is confused, explains what happened

C   Choking

       ____*   if coughing, does not interfere
         if stops coughing/breathing,
       ____*   positions child correctly for back blows
       ____*   gives 4 back blows correctly
       ____*   positions child correctly for manual thrusts
       ____*   gives 4 manual thrusts correctly
       ____*   repeats above steps until obstruction dislodged or child starts coughing
       ____*   stops procedure within 5 sec. after child starts coughing/breathing
       ____*   after child stops choking, observes/finger sweeps child's mouth

D.   Educational Opportunities

       ____   uses at least two natural situations to try to teach the child something (involves clear S^D and consequence)
       ____   keeps requirements on child brief and non-demanding
       ____   helps child perform skills as needed for success

E.   Bedtime

       ____   engages in quiet time before bedtime routine
       ____*   on time

(continued)

Table 1. (continued)

____*	follows any procedures described by parents
____*	when finishes bedtime routine, leaves room within 30 sec. and does not talk with child after this
	If child gets out of bed:
____	returns without interacting
____	repeats as many times as necessary up to 4 times
____	If child gets up over 4 times, ignores
____*	checks on child at least once per hr. after child has gone to bed

*Responses deemed to be critical by an interdisciplinary advisory board.

sumers) observed clear differences in the quality of respite care performance before and after trainees acquired the target skills, this would indicate that the skills taught were those that were relevant or important to the provision of respite care. The results confirmed the validity of the training curriculum in that posttraining performance ratings substantially exceeded pretraining performance ratings in each of the target skill areas.

An additional consideration in the development of a training program is the *scope* of the curriculum. The curriculum must be sufficiently broad to encompass the skills necessary for providing respite care to a variety of clients, yet not so broad that the material cannot be acquired within a reasonable period of time. One approach would therefore be to focus on *generic* skills that would be applicable in a wide variety of situations (e.g., in providing care for children with a range of handicapping conditions). For example, in the training program developed by Neef and her colleagues, parent interviewing skills were emphasized (i.e., respite care providers were taught to solicit information from parents regarding the performance of requisite routines and procedures specific to the individual child). In this way, the acquisition of interviewing skills would enable the care provider to collect the information necessary to meet the idiosyncratic needs of the child.

If, for instance, the use of a particular piece of equipment was required, the care provider was to ask the parent to demonstrate its use and was then to practice the procedure in the presence of the parent. If, however, it is determined that such equipment is common to the population that is being served by a respite care agency, then it would be wise to include its use as part of the training curriculum. It is therefore recommended that ecological inventories be conducted to identify those skills that are most frequently needed and/or that are critical to the care of the target population being served. In addition, the involvement of service consumers in the development of the training curriculum is likely to result in a training program that is maximally relevant.

Table 2.   Mean consumer ratings of respite care trainees' performance on pre- and post-training probes

		Experiment 1		Experiment 2	
		Pre	Post	Pre	Post
1.	How completely did the sitter prepare for the evening by collecting all relevant information from the parent? 1 (very incompletely) to 4 (very completely)	2.3	4.0	2.2	3.6
2.	How appropriately did the sitter manage the child's behavior problems? 1 (very inappropriately) to 4 (very appropriately)	2.5	3.8	2.3	3.7
3.	In general, how would you rate the quality of the interaction between the sitter and child? 1 (poor) to 4 (excellent)	2.7	3.5	2.9	3.6
4.	How would you rate the sitter's ability to manage the child's routine activities (i.e., mealtime, bedtime, and toileting)? 1 (poor) to 4 (excellent)	2.9	3.7	2.3	3.5
5.	Overall, how would you rate the sitter's skill at handling the emergency situations which arose? 1 (poor) to 4 (excellent)	2.9	3.8	2.2	3.4
6.	How adequately did the sitter report all relevant information to the parent upon his or her return? 1 (very inadequately) to 4 (very adequately)	2.8	4.0	2.6	3.5
7.	How well did the sitter make use of routine situations to attempt to teach the child academic, self-care, and other skills? 1 (very well) to 4 (very poorly)	2.6	3.7	2.4	3.4
8.	If the child was physically handicapped: In general, how would you rate the sitter's skill at lifting, transferring, positioning, and feeding the child? 1 (poor) to 4 (excellent)	2.6	3.6	2.1	3.5
9.	Overall, how would you rate the quality of care this sitter provided? 1 (poor) to 4 (excellent)	2.7	4.0	2.6	3.7
10.	Overall, how comfortable would you feel having this person sit for your child? 1 (very uncomfortable) to 4 (very comfortable)	2.4	4.0	2.3	3.7

TRAINING APPROACHES

Several approaches have been used to train respite care providers, including "hands on" training provided primarily by the parent (service consumer), workshops or inservice training, and self-instructional manuals combined with role playing. Hands on training, in which parents bring their disabled children as participants in the training sessions (Griggs, 1983), offers the advantage that the parents who will be using the service can see that the trainees gain first-hand knowledge and experience in the care requirements of their children. An example of the successful use of this approach is the parent cooperative described by Ferguson and Lindsay (see Chapter 8). The disadvantage of this approach is that many parents may not be willing nor able to invest the energy for such a level of participation, nor is it reasonable to expect them to assume that responsibility in order to obtain the support services they need (MacMillan & Turnbull, 1983; Salisbury, 1984; Turnbull & Turnbull, 1982).

As previously described, the most common approach for training respite care providers—workshops or inservice training—is often costly and of equivocal effectiveness in facilitating the acquisition, maintenance, and/or generalization of skills. A number of strategies can be used to enhance the effectiveness of inservice training (Powers, 1983). These include: 1) systematic inservice training within the trainees' setting; 2) tailoring the program based on an assessment of the needs of individual trainees; 3) identification of content corresponding to actual job requirements; 4) involving the trainee in the planning, development, and evaluation of training strategies; and 5) use of strategies that address the milieu of the participants (Salisbury, 1984). As Salisbury (1984) points out, however, there appears to have been little transfer of the findings from research on inservice training to respite care provider training.

Neef et al. (1985), in a series of four experiments, evaluated an instructional package based on a self-directed training manual as a competency-based alternative to workshop training. In the first experiment, the effectiveness of an instructional manual in facilitating acquisition of respite care skills was evaluated. The manual consisted of four major content areas corresponding to the skill components delineated in Table 1: Preparation and Parent Interaction, Child Behaviors, Physical/Medical Management, and Emergencies. The format for each section consisted of behavioral objectives, an introduction, specific management strategies, examples of and rationale for these strategies, a reading comprehension quiz, an answer key with referral page numbers on which the respective material was addressed, and a remedial quiz with answer key.

Each section of the manual was presented sequentially to the trainees. If the trainee did not demonstrate mastery of the target skills during simulated (role-played) respite care situations after completing the respective section of the manual, in vivo remedial training was conducted. Such remedial training consisted of a review of the relevant material contained in the manual, after which the staff modeled the target skill and provided feedback as the trainee practiced it. The results of a multiple baseline design across skill areas showed that trainees' performance of the target skills increased substantially following presentation of the instructional manual, although some remedial training was necessary to achieve the mastery criterion.

The second experiment evaluated the effects of the manual presented in toto with a larger group of trainees and compared it to a workshop training approach. Workshop content was derived directly and solely from the information presented in the manual. Information pertinent to the successful completion of each item of the task analysis was presented orally and supplemented with videotaped vignettes depicting both proscribed and prescribed behaviors (negative and positive examples) and/or in vivo demonstration by the staff.

The results of this experiment indicated that the manual training approach compared very favorably in several respects with a workshop training paradigm. First, although both approaches were shown to be effective in facilitating the acquisition of a complex set of respite care skills, the instructional manual was far more *cost-effective;* the cost of assisting each trainee to reach criterion using the manual training package was $12.91 versus $43.41 with workshop training.

Second, the logistics of developing and leading workshops were far more difficult than those involved in developing and distributing a manual. Once the manual was produced and distributed, trainers simply provided remedial training as needed; workshops required the trainers to schedule sessions at times suitable for the majority of trainees, deliver the material repeatedly, and arrange make-up sessions.

Third, most of the individuals recruited for training stated a preference for reading the manual over participation in the workshops because of convenience factors. The manual was designed to allow each trainee to advance at his or her own pace and to refer repeatedly to numerous examples, as well as to test his or her own comprehension of the material.

Finally, unlike the workshop sequence, the manual served as an efficient tool for both remedial and initial training. The manual could easily be divided into sections that provided the trainee with more information and assistance in individual areas of deficiency. This advantage was also demonstrated in a third experiment; trainees, who had recently completed a respite care agency sponsored workshop but performed poorly on a subsequent evaluation of their skills, acquired the target behaviors with a conveniently administered manual-based training package.

Although the use of a training manual may thus offer some advantages, it requires active responding and therefore a greater effort on the part of the trainee than the passive participation that characterizes many workshops. Therefore, the provision of performance-based incentives (e.g., monetary rebates) may be an important feature of such training programs. In addition, some trainees may have difficulty acquiring information through printed media, and training manuals would not be well suited for these individuals.

EVALUATION

The construction of a training curriculum is only part of the process in developing a comprehensive model. A second, equally important, feature of any training program is the evaluation component. Assessment of trainees' skills both *before* and *after* training serves several important functions: The information can be used in tailoring the program to meet the needs of individual trainees, to document whether or not the trainees acquired the necessary skills following training, to identify areas in which remedial training may be required, and as a basis for making subsequent adjustments in the program to enhance its effectiveness.

Evaluation of trainees' skills before instruction is an important feature of competency-based training programs. First, it allows trainers to identify individual skill areas in which trainees are particularly knowledgeable or deficient. Such information may help guide the format of a training program by identifying areas requiring more or less emphasis. Tailoring the training program to meet the individual needs of trainees allows for more efficient use of the trainer's and trainee's time. Second, pretest data provide a standard against which the effectiveness of the training program can be judged. Posttest data alone would provide little information on the success of the training program. If, for example, trainees already possessed the requisite skills before instruction, posttest scores alone might lead one to conclude erroneously that the training program was both necessary and effective.

Comparison of pre- and postevaluation data enables trainers to determine whether trainees have acquired the target skills. Problems can arise if individuals are said to be trained when data are not available to substantiate that they have, in fact, learned the skills purportedly taught through the program. Attendance at or participation in a training program does not, of course, ensure that the necessary skills have been learned. Unless it is shown that trainees have mastered the requisite skills, they may not be prepared to provide satisfactory respite care. Unskilled care providers can not only damage the reputation of a respite care agency but can also jeopardize the safety of the children for whom they are responsible. Evaluation of trainee performance following instruction also enables trainers to identify areas in which remedial training may be required.

Thus, it is only through evaluation of trainee *performance* that a program can be judged to be effective. Unfortunately, few respite care training programs have provided evaluation data on trainee performance (Salisbury, 1984). Programs designed to teach different skills, however, have been useful in providing examples of the types of evaluation strategies that could be used with respite care training (cf. Fawcett & Fletcher, 1977; Fawcett & Miller, 1975; Fawcett, Miller, & Braukmann, 1977).

The most common method for assessing trainee performance is through the use of *written quizzes* (Upshur, 1982a; Warren & Dickman, 1981). Quizzes can include different question *formats,* such as multiple choice, true/false, or short answer. Each type of format has specific advantages and disadvantages, and readers are referred to Hopkins and Stanley (1981) or Mehrens and Lehmann (1969) for detailed discussions on how to construct items for each of the above question formats.

The *content* of the questions, regardless of format, should directly correspond to the material presented in the training program. If the target behaviors have been operationalized and validated, the task of designing appropriate questions is simplified. For example, a question relating to the performance of an emergency procedure for choking (see task analysis in Table 1) might be, "The child you are watching has just popped a button into her mouth. She is now coughing very hard, gasping, and looking scared. What should you do? 1) reach in her throat to get the button, 2) give her a drink of water, 3) pat her strongly on the back, 4) do not intervene." Questions should also require trainees to respond to situations that differ from the examples presented during training. Responses to such questions will indicate whether trainees have acquired a *generalized* skill that can be applied in a variety of contexts.

Using written quizzes for evaluation purposes has several advantages: They can be designed to sample responses to a wide range of management issues, require a relatively short time to develop and implement, and are easy to score. Despite these advantages, however, written quizzes do not allow for evaluation of how trainees would actually *perform* the skill in a respite care situation. In other words, there is no evidence to ensure that written responses will correspond to actual performance. For situations that require an immediate and accurate response (e.g., seizure, choking, ingestion of a poisonous substance), it is critical that the trainee have the opportunity to *demonstrate* the requisite skills in the context of actual or simulated situations.

A second method that has been used to evaluate skill acquisition is *role playing,* in which target behaviors are demonstrated in a setting that closely corresponds to the natural environment (Gardner, 1972; Jones & Eimers, 1975). Role playing, as a method of evaluation, has several advantages over written quizzes. The primary advantage is that actual performance of target skills can be evaluated under conditions that simulate the natural environment. Neef et al. (1985) found that respite care trainees who performed well in role-played situations also performed well in a respite care situation with a handicapped child. Despite these advantages, it may be impractical to rely solely on role playing to provide a comprehensive evaluation of trainee performance. Role playing must be conducted individually and is therefore time consuming; it may also require the use of resources that are not commonly available to respite care agencies (e.g., special equipment and materials or a room specially designed to simulate a home setting).

A practical and efficient alternative to relying exclusively on written examination or role playing for evaluation would be to combine the two approaches to take advantage of their strengths. This was the approach taken in the study by Neef et al. (1985). Initially, written quizzes were employed to assess trainees' mastery of the material presented through the self-directed instructional manual so that each trainee could review the areas in which he or she was deficient. Subsequently, participants were asked to demonstrate selected skills through role playing. Such an approach takes advantage of the versatility and efficiency of written examinations while using role playing to sample performance on selected critical skills. Thus, the advantages of role playing are accrued without the need for extensive resources.

Another alternative would involve having skilled care providers accompany and evaluate trainees in actual respite care situations. Using a *checklist*, for example, experienced care providers could directly observe and record the trainee's performance of each of the target skills. In this manner, on-the-job performance could be assessed under supervised conditions.

The above discussion highlights the importance of evaluating the effects of training and suggests methods for assessing trainee performance. Additional information can be obtained by soliciting *feedback from parents*. Salisbury (1984) noted that measures of consumer (i.e., parent) satisfaction are one of the most commonly used methods for evaluating respite care training programs (e.g., Neef et al., 1985; Patacek, Sommers, Graves, Lukowicz, Kenna, Haglund, & Nycz, 1982; Upshur, 1982a). Upshur (1982a), for example, employed a parent satisfaction measure to evaluate a home-based respite care program. She asked families using respite care to indicate their satisfaction with the service across several areas, including overall satisfaction, satisfaction with level of training, and ability to respond to medical and/or behavioral needs of clients.

Measures of consumer satisfaction are an important indicator of program success that can be used to validate the effects of training. However, satisfaction surveys are not by themselves sufficient to evaluate the effectiveness of a respite care training program because parents do not have an opportunity to observe performance of the service provider once they leave. In addition, parents may be reluctant to provide an honest assessment of the provider's performance, especially if they believe that a negative response might jeopardize their opportunity to obtain services in the future. Although steps can be taken to minimize this problem (e.g., by providing appropriate assurances, ensuring confidentiality, or inviting anonymous feedback), positive reports must be interpreted cautiously. Nevertheless, a thorough evaluation should include direct assessment of trainee performance, as well as consumer satisfaction measures.

FUTURE DIRECTIONS

To date, the literature regarding training issues is exceptionally sparse. A number of recommendations about future directions for the training of respite care providers can be provided, including content-related, methodological, and procedural suggestions.

Training of Coordinators in Instructional Technology

Hitherto, little effort has been expended in training respite care program coordinators in the design, implementation, and evaluation of competency-based training paradigms. Without doubt, a curriculum for training respite care coordinators in the provision of competency-based training is needed and should receive the highest priority. In the absence of such training, coordinators may find themselves to be overly dependent on training materials that are not well suited for the idiosyncratic needs of their agency or the trainees. In addition, without such training, coordinators may inadvertently emphasize the provision of information through lecture or pamphlets with no concomitant attempt to evaluate whether increases in knowledge are accompanied by acquisition of requisite skills.

Alternative Training Formats

Thus far, little attention has been given to the relative efficacy of alternative training procedures. As discussed earlier, competency-based paradigms are likely to be superior to workshops in promoting the acquisition of critical respite care skills (Neef et al., 1985; Ziarnik & Bernstein, 1982). Additional comparative analyses of different training strategies are needed.

Based on the results obtained by Neef et al. (1985), it appears that skill acquisition can be facilitated through the use of instructional manuals designed within a competency-based framework. With the exception of the finding that the inclusion of pictures in addition to written examples is preferred but does not have an incremental effect (Neef et al., 1985), little is known about the relative impact of various methods of presenting the manual content. For example, it is unclear whether a manual would optimally include negative as well as positive examples and, if both, in what order.

Furthermore, many respite care training programs consist of instructional packages. It is unclear whether each package component contributes positively to training outcome. For instance, there have been few, if any, studies specific to respite care skills training examining the effectiveness of videotaped versus in vivo modeling or of behavioral rehearsal and performance-based feedback components. In order to develop more streamlined, more cost-effective, and exportable training programs, additional component analyses are required.

Experimental Validation

The majority of respite care skills training programs have not been evaluated experimentally before their dissemination and use. The literature is replete with alternative experimental designs that can be employed to validate the effectiveness of a training curriculum before it is employed on a widespread basis. To date, most attempts to demonstrate the efficacy of various training procedures have involved either group comparison (Winer, 1971) or single-subject experimental designs (Hersen & Barlow, 1976; Kazdin, 1982). As mentioned previously, in the context of respite care skills training, single-subject experimental designs are likely to be found more suitable because they: 1) are more compatible with competency-based training curricula, 2) require fewer participants to complete the validation process, 3) obviate the need for a control group, 4) permit an examination of individual differences in response to training, and 5) thereby point directly to circumstances under which a training curriculum might need to be tailored.

Replicability

Most available descriptions of training programs are insufficiently detailed to permit replication. This lack of detail often severely limits the utility of the description and precludes the dissemination of the program described. The details that are most frequently missing include but are not limited to: 1) the initial steps involved in the design of the curriculum, 2) the structure and content of the curriculum, 3) the method(s) of recruiting trainees, 4) trainee characteristics, 5) the strategies utilized to evaluate the effects of training, 6) the evaluation data obtained, and 7) the costs of training. Truncated or vague descriptions may well be a function of the amount of space available in journals. Developers of training programs could provide needed details for interested parties through written manuals available from them or some central information source, such as the National Auxiliary Publications Service. In addition to ensuring replicability, the inclusion of substantive and methodological details may assist training coordinators in generalizing the program to their unique training objectives. Such details may also allow coordinators to determine which existing training programs, if any, are likely to be most effective given various types of trainees and training agendas.

Cost Analyses

Analyses of costs are particularly important at a time when funding for respite care skills training is difficult to acquire and/or maintain. With increasing frequency, government agencies and members of local boards are asking for data documenting that training programs are economical, as well as effective. Levin (1983) outlines a number of methods for analyzing the cost-effectiveness of educational programs. In many cases, a cost-absorption formula has been employed. Using this formula, expenses for personnel time, materials, and trainee remuneration are totaled and divided by the number of trainees successfully completing the training program. The resulting quotient yields the cost of training per trainee. The costs associated with specific training methods can then be compared in order to select the most economical training strategy. In addition, funding services can factor anticipated unit costs into their deliberations when examining proposed budgets for training programs and when deciding how much funding to allocate for a desired outcome.

Dissemination and Adoption

One of the most pressing needs is the development of a technology for promoting the dissemination and adoption of model training programs. Without this technology, the impact of model programs will continue to be limited in scope and duration, resulting in an unnecessary and expensive duplication of effort. Ideally, a respite care skills training program would first be devised and shown to be effective in an actual respite care situation. The generalizability of the training curriculum would then be established. Subsequently, the curriculum would be applied on a large scale, with continued evaluation of its effectiveness. In reality, a few model programs have been developed, some of these have been validated experimentally, even fewer have been demonstrated to be generalizable, and none has been subjected to the critical test of dissemination to and adoption by multiple agencies that are heterogeneous with respect to staff expertise, trainee qualifications, and priority given to training in terms of time and funding.

At this time, a technology for dissemination and adoption is not well developed. Program developers interested in such pursuits are guided more by conjecture than by evidence. According to Stolz (1981), variables considered to be critical to the dissemination and adoption process include: 1) the availability of data showing that the training curriculum is effective; 2) the design of a curriculum that is compatible with the goals of the recipient agency; 3) the dissatisfaction of the prospective adoption agency with its current training curriculum; 4) the ability of representatives of the potential adopting agency to visit and evaluate the ongoing model program; 5) the early involvement of those individuals who will direct the agency's training program in the adoption process; 6) availability of sufficient funds for dissemination; and 7) the involvement of an individual on the agency staff who is adequately trained to implement the curriculum, who is enthusiastic about the training effort, and who possesses the political skills necessary to maintain the training program if and when obstacles to continuance are encountered. Stolz (1981) suggests that the last variable is by far the most influential.

Feasibility

Although a few model training programs have been developed, it is questionable whether these programs can be implemented by training coordinators outside research settings. The feasibility of a particular training curriculum is a function of the skills and available time of the individual directing the curriculum. Many respite care program coordinators are primarily responsible for the maintenance of respite care services and therefore have definite constraints on their time with respect to recruitment and training. Data relevant to the issue of feasibility need to be collected. These data might pertain to the amount of training required for agency coordinators to become competent in the direction of the training program, the length and cost of training required for the trainees to reach a predetermined level of proficiency, and how often reevaluation of previously acquired skills and remedial training is necessary. In general, previous descriptions of training programs have not contained information that would allow readers to determine the feasibility of the training procedures employed.

Certification

Within recent years, increasing importance has been assigned not only to the provision of initial training but also to the establishment of certain minimum standards that must be achieved *and maintained* by respite care providers. For example, Oppenheimer and Upshur (1978), in the final report of the Respite Care Policy Development Project to the Massachusetts Developmental Disabilities Council, proposed that delivery of respite care be governed by a series of state regulations. These regulations would be enforced at the agency level through a contingency tied to funding; that is, the meeting of regulatory requirements would be a condition for funding.

More recently, Salisbury and Griggs (1983) recommended that individual respite care providers be certified and that all providers be required to earn a specified number of continuing education credits in order to be eligible for recertification. There are several advantages associated with the certification process. First, the determination of certification requirements might involve a survey of existing respite care resources and needs, the construction of an examination to assess the trainee's knowledge base, the completion of a task analysis of respite care skills, the development of a model training curriculum based on such a task analysis, and the hiring of individuals with expertise in monitoring and evaluation. Such activities, especially if coordinated at the state (if not federal) level, would likely result in increased pooling of resources and expertise and the development of more objective indices of competence. Second, a certification process that mandates the accumulation of continuing education credits may better ensure that respite care providers stay abreast of advances in service provision. Third, certification may raise the status of respite care and thereby attract more talented individuals to an area of service chronically beset with a staffing shortage. Fourth, certification might increase the probability that third-party payers and private insurers would partially cover respite care expenses. Fifth, if respite care providers were required to pay an annual certification fee, they might be more likely to provide respite care services in order to recoup their investment, rather than deliver services infrequently. Sixth, and perhaps most importantly, the monitoring and evaluation functions incumbent to the certification process would likely have some desirable reactive effects; that is, as a result of the ongoing certification process, providers may be more likely to uphold agreed-on standards of care.

SUMMARY

This chapter has presented guidelines for developing, implementing, and evaluating quality respite care skills training programs. The authors have suggested that more attention be devoted to the ecological and social validity of training curricula in order to ensure that training programs adequately address consumer (e.g., family) needs and demands. Curricula should also be comprehensive, focusing on generic skills that are applicable to a wide variety of situations and handicapping conditions. Training for respite care providers should be competency-based. Such a model will ensure that training focuses on *skill development*, rather than provision of general information.

Finally, respite care skills training programs should be experimentally evaluated to ensure that they result in the acquisition and maintenance of targeted skills. Additional evaluation data on consumer satisfaction with and cost-effectiveness of training are also crucial if the training program is to be widely adopted by community-based respite care training programs. Additional research, especially in the areas discussed in this chapter, is still needed in order to refine the methodology for designing and providing quality respite care skills training programs. The guidelines presented in this chapter, however, may enable agencies to begin developing and implementing training programs that are comprehensive, competency-based, experimentally validated, cost-effective, and exportable.

REFERENCES

Calkins, C., Gibson, B., Grosko, J., & Bueker, J. (1982). *Respite care adapted for deaf-blind population: Training manual.* Kansas City, MO: University of Missouri-Kansas City Institute, University Affiliated Facility.

Cohen, S. (1982). Supporting families through respite care. *Rehabilitation Literature, 43,* 7–11.

Cummings, S. T., Bayley, H. C., & Rie, H. E. (1966). Effects of the child's deficiency on the mother: A study of mothers of mentally retarded, chronically ill, and neurotic children. *American Journal of Orthopsychiatry, 36,* 595–608.

Dunlap, W. R. (1969). How do parents of handicapped children view their needs? *Journal of the Division of Early Childhood, 1,* 1–10.

Egel, A. L., Parrish, J. M., Sloan, M. E., & Neef, N. A. (1984, May). A survey of respite care needs and problems in the community. Paper presented at the Association for Behavior Analysis Convention, Nashville, TN.

Erickson, M. T. (1968). MMPI comparisons between parents of young emotionally disturbed children and mentally retarded children. *Journal of Consulting and Clinical Psychology, 32,* 701–706.

Farber, B. (1968). *Mental retardation: The social context and social consequences.* Boston: Houghton Mifflin Co.

Fawcett, S. B., & Fletcher, R. K. (1977). Community applications of instructional technology: Teaching writers of instructional packages. *Journal of Applied Behavior Analysis, 10,* 739–746.

Fawcett, S. B., & Miller, L. K. (1975). Training public-speaking behavior: An experimental analysis and social validation. *Journal of Applied Behavior Analysis, 8,* 125–136.

Fawcett, S. B., Miller, L. K., & Braukmann, C. J. (1977). An evaluation of a training package for community canvassing behaviors. *Journal of Applied Behavior Analysis, 10,* 504.

Gage, M. A., Fredericks, H. D., Johnson-Dorn, N., & Lindley-Southard, B. (1982). Inservice training for staff of group homes and work activity centers serving developmentally disabled adults. *Journal of the Association for the Severely Handicapped, 7,* 60–70.

Gardner, J. M. (1972). Teaching behavior modification to nonprofessionals. *Journal of Applied Behavior Analysis, 5,* 517–521.

German, M., & Maisto, A. (1982). The relationship of a perceived family support system to the instructional placement of mentally retarded children. *Education and Training of the Mentally Retarded, 17,* 17–23.

Griggs, P. (1983, November). An adaptive curriculum used in urban and rural settings. Paper presented at the 10th annual convention of the Association for the Severely Handicapped (TASH), San Francisco, CA.

Hersen, M., & Barlow, D. H. (1976). *Single-case experimental designs: Strategies for studying behavior change.* New York: Pergamon Press.

Hopkins, K. D., & Stanley, J. C. (1981). *Educational and psychological measurement and evaluation.* Englewood Cliffs, NJ: Prentice-Hall.

Jones, F. H., & Eimers, R. C. (1975). Role playing to train elementary teachers to use a classroom management "skill package." *Journal of Applied Behavior Analysis, 8,* 421–433.

Joyce, K., Singer, M., & Israelowitz, R. (1983). Impact of respite care on parents' perception of quality of life. *Mental Retardation, 21,* 153–156.

Kazdin, A. E. (1977). Assessing the clinical or applied significance of behavior change through social validation. *Behavior Modification, 1,* 427–452.

Kazdin, A. (1982). *Single-subject experimental designs.* Oxford: Oxford University Press.

Lawson, J. S., Connolly, M., Leaver, C., & Englisch, H. (1979). Short-term residential care of the intellectually handicapped. *Australian Journal of Mental Retardation, 5,* 307–310.

Levin, H. M. (1983). *Cost-effectiveness: A primer.* Beverly Hills, CA: Sage Publications.

Lukenbill, R., Lillie, B., Sanddal, N., Hulme, J., Calkins, C., & McKibben, M. (1976). *Respite care training manual.* Helena, MT: Developmental Disabilities Training Institute.

MacMillan, D. L., & Turnbull, A. (1983). Parent involvement with special education: Respecting individual preferences. *Education and Training of the Mentally Retarded, 18,* 4–9.

Mehrens, W. A., & Lehmann, I. J. (1969). *Measurement and evaluation in education and psychology.* New York: Holt, Rinehart & Winston.

Mercer, J. (1966). Patterns of family crisis related to reacceptance of the retardate. *American Journal of Mental Deficency, 71,* 19–32.

Meyers, C. E., Zetlin, A., & Blacher-Dixon, J. (1981). The family as affected by schooling for severely retarded children: An invitation to research. *Journal of Community Psychology, 9,* 306–315.

Morris, D., & Hess, K. (1975). *Neighborhood power: The new localism.* Boston: Beacon Press.

Neef, N. A., Parrish, J. M., Egel, A. L., & Sloan, M. E. (1985). *Training respite care providers for families with handicapped children: Experimental analysis and validation of an instructional package.* Manuscript submitted for publication.

Oppenheimer, J., & Upshur, C. (1978). *Summary of the final report of the respite care policy development project.* Unpublished manuscript prepared for the Massachusetts Developmental Disabilities Council.

Parham, J., Hart, T., Terraciano, T., & Newton, P. (1983). *In-home respite care program development.* Lubbock: Texas Tech Press.

Patacek, L. J., Sommers, P. A., Graves, J., Lukowicz, P., Kenna, E., Haglund, J., & Nycz, G. R. (1982). Respite care for families of children with severe handicaps: An education study of parent satisfaction. *Journal of Community Psychology, 10,* 222–227.

Powell, T., & Hecimovic, A. (1981). *Respite care for the handicapped: Helping individuals and their families.* Springfield, IL: Charles C Thomas.

Powers, D. A. (1983). Mainstreaming and the in-service education of teachers. *Exceptional Children, 49,* 432–439.

Ross, E. (1980). Financing respite care services: An initial exploration. *Word from Washington, 9,* 1–23.

Salisbury, C. (1984). Respite care provider training: Current practices and directions for research. *Education and Training of the Mentally Retarded, 19,* 210–215.

Salisbury, C., & Griggs, P. (1983). Developing respite care services for families of handicapped persons. *Journal of the Association for the Severely Handicapped, 8,* 50–57.

Sloan, M. E., Neef, N., Parrish, J., & Egel, A. (1983). Training manual for child care workers providing respite to parents of developmentally disabled children. Unpublished manuscript, University of Maryland, College Park, MD.

Stolz, S. B. (1981). Adoption of innovations from applied behavioral research: "Does anybody care?" *Journal of Applied Behavior Analysis, 14,* 491–505.

Turnbull, A. P., & Turnbull, H. R. (1982). Parent involvement in the education of handicapped children: A critique. *Mental Retardation, 20,* 115–122.

Upshur, C. (1982a). Respite care for mentally retarded and other disabled populations: Program models and family needs. *Mental Retardation, 20,* 2–6.

Upshur, C. (1982b). An evaluation of home-based respite care. *Mental Retardation, 20,* 58–62.

Warren, R., & Dickman, I. (1981). *For this respite thanks.* New York: United Cerebral Palsy Association, Inc.

Watson, L., & Uzzell, R. (1980). A program for teaching behavior modification skills to institutional staff. *Applied Research in Mental Retardation, 1,* 41–53.

Wikler, L. (1981, April). Stress in families of mentally retarded children. *Family Relations.*

Willner, A. G., Braukmann, C. J., Kirigin, K. A., Fixsen, D. L., Phillips, E. L., & Wolf, M. M. (1977). The training and validation of youth-preferred social behaviors of child-care personnel. *Journal of Applied Behavior Analysis, 10,* 219–230.

Winer, D. J. (1971). *Statistical principles in experimental design* (2nd ed.). New York: McGraw-Hill Book Co.

Wolf, M. M. (1978). Social validity: The cause for subjective measurement or how applied behavior analysis is finding its heart. *Journal of Applied Behavior Analysis, 11,* 203–214.

Ziarnik, J. P., & Bernstein, G. (1982). A critical examination of the effect of inservice training on staff performance. *Mental Retardation, 20,* 109–114.

Zlomke, L., & Benjamin, V. (1983). Staff inservice: Measuring effectiveness through client behavior change. *Education and Training of the Mentally Retarded, 18,* 125–130.

Chapter 8

THE RESPITE CARE CO-OP PROGRAM
PROFESSIONALLY GUIDED PARENT SELF-HELP

Janet T. Ferguson and Sally A. Lindsay

Saturday night, Bill and Donna M. went out for dinner and dancing. It was their 25th anniversary and the first one they have celebrated since their 13-year-old Nancy was born with multiple handicaps.

Nancy spent the weekend in respite care with the L. family. Saturday morning, as her dad rolled her wheelchair up the L's driveway, she chattered and giggled about staying overnight with 12-year-old Denise L.

The Ms and Ls are among 15 families in a Respite Care Co-op, in Kalamazoo, Michigan. These parents of developmentally disabled children and young adults provide each other with respite care and mutual support.

Ellie and Mitch L. have cared for Nancy before. She feels at home with them and in the other Care Co-op homes where she has stayed. For Nancy, respite care is like visiting extended family. It means staying with people who know, understand and like her—people who can share and get excited about her newly learned skills and can cope and be patient with her problems. Speaking is difficult for her, and respite care visits push her to use the new speech she is learning with her school therapist. Ellie and Mitch know how to encourage her and wait for her to finish her sentences. They learned this in the Care Co-op workshop sessions where co-op parents train and provide updated information to each other about the care needs of their developmentally disabled children.

The opening paragraphs (pages 143–145) of this chapter are adapted from Janet T. Ferguson, Sally A. Lindsay and Margaret A. McNees, "Respite Care Co-op: Families Helping Families," The *Exceptional Parent*, February, 1983, p. 9.

Care co-op parents enjoy the success of each other's children and share ways of dealing with their problems. Often, at first, parents hesitate to expose the less attractive behaviors of their children, or they fear that other parents cannot handle them. Some parents feel unsure about caring for the children of others. The Ms hesitated to plan overnight stays because Nancy is a bed-wetter. The Js worried about their 4-year-old autistic Andy, who impulsively hits others. The Ls were unsure whether others could manage their 9-year-old Nicki, who is moderately mentally retarded and hyperactive. One family spent an exhausting evening chasing Nicki, whose behavior ranged from flicking light switches on and off to emptying cupboards. At the next co-op meeting, with some guidance from the program coordinator (a social worker), other parents in the group shared their own experiences in caring for Nicki, and together they compiled a list of practical approaches found to work with him. This problem-solving approach has provided new ideas for each co-op parent who will be caring for Nicki—and also for Nicki's parents.

Nicki's list stays in his care folder, which accompanies him whenever he receives respite care. Each child's folder contains a parent-signed release for emergency medical care, the child's schedule, and special care information about eating, sleeping, medication, language, behavior, favorite toys and activities, and physical needs and appliances.

Families pay no money for care. Instead, care received is paid for with care given. The Ms will pay for Nancy's recent 36-hour stay with hours of care they give other co-op children. After Nancy's weekend with the Ls, both families reported their exact hours of care given and received to the parent who is currently serving as care manager. She recorded them in the co-op ledger. She keeps a record of each family's debit and credit hours.

Co-op families use respite care often—for fun, recreation, family needs or business, emergencies, vacations, or just rest. Care periods can be as short as 2 hours or as long as several weeks. Longer care is usually shared among several families with whom the child has stayed before and feels comfortable. During the first months, most co-op parents nervously use just 2 or 3 hours at a time. Later, overnight and weekend stays become popular. Some families save their hours for several longer vacations each year.

At first, parents new to a care co-op may not be sure how to spend their respite time. Free time has been a little out of their line! Soon after joining, one father complained, ''I don't know if I can use this Care Co-op—I can't afford to go out to dinner all the time!'' Others laughed, but agreed that they too were unsure about what to do with the respite time. At the coordinator's suggestion, the group spent some workshop time sharing ideas about inexpensive things to do as a couple, alone, or with their other children. Each couple developed a list of their own suggestions and shared it.

Most parents have some initial fears about joining a care co-op. At the frequent outreach presentations, in which a co-op parent and the coordinator introduce and talk about the care co-op, an interested but hesitant parent often asks, "I can hardly manage my own child. How could I ever handle someone else's too?," or "I don't know if I could ever leave my child at someone else's house," or "How would I know my child would get good care?" These concerns have kept some parents from joining a care co-op. But co-op members usually find that caring for other co-op children is not as difficult nor time consuming as they expected. And as they provide care, they gain skill and confidence. Most parents say that the respite time is well worth the effort of caring for another child. Also, most care co-ops make the rule that no parent needs to care for a child he or she is not comfortable handling. (Though the group usually urges everyone to try to work through any discomfort with a particular child.) Actually, parents tend to feel stronger and better able to care for their own disabled children after some experience in exchanging care with other co-op families.

The question of leaving a disabled child in care is a tough one for any parent using any kind of respite care for the first time. Support gained from other co-op parents seems to make it easier for these parents to get past that barrier. They soon realize that the same support they receive in caring for another child is there for the families caring for their own child. It is hard to feel guilty about leaving a child when he or she is obviously having a good time with people who enjoy him or her. In addition, co-op parents have learned that often the disabled child needs a break from them too!

THE PROGRAM

Definition

A parent respite care co-op program provides an agency- or organization-sponsored program structure and professional staff, which can support one or more parent-operated care co-op groups. It enables parents of disabled children or adults to join together to develop their own cooperative respite care service and support group as they need and want it. The concept is professionally guided and facilitated parent self-help.

Program Objectives

The care co-op program is based on the premise that the most productive use of respite care is family crisis prevention (i.e., keeping the caregiving parent healthy and able to cope). There are three program objectives:

1. To provide families relief or respite from chronic care often enough and for long enough periods to avoid caregiver exhaustion and to control family stress buildup

2. To make respite care readily available and without cost to families
3. To facilitate a parent mutual support system that will enhance parent self-confidence and coping skills

Background

This Program was first designed and developed at Family and Children Services of the Kalamazoo Area, in 1976–1977, by Janet T. Ferguson, MSW, under a grant from the Michigan State Developmental Disabilities Program. It was developed for and with families of developmentally disabled children and youth. Today, this program model is increasingly being used by agencies serving parents caring for children or adults with a variety of handicaps. It has also been adapted to meet the needs of caregivers of frail or impaired elders. Increasing experience suggests its suitability for caregivers involved with chronic care of any kind. This chapter discusses the respite care co-op program model as it was first developed in Kalamazoo and as it has evolved through use in other communities.

Because the care co-op program model involves professionally guided *parent self-help,* the original program was developed with co-sponsorship and close cooperation between Family and Children Services and the Association for Retarded Citizens (ARC) of Kalamazoo, whose basic principle is parent self-help. The agency provided the program funding and the professional staff (i.e., program "coordinator"), and the ARC board appointed four parents to an ad hoc board committee to work with the coordinator in developing the program. This ad hoc committee evolved into the steering committee for the program. Both agency and ARC executives were actively involved, with the ARC executive participating on the committee. Thus, in the first care co-op program, parent-professional teamwork developed both within the program and at the organizational level. (For financial and organizational reasons, the co-sponsorship did not continue beyond initial program development. But the cooperation and support have continued. Other programs developed since have recruited steering committee parents from other sources.)

The Parent-Professional Team

Parent-professional teamwork is the base and strength of the care co-op program. The program is built by parents and the coordinator working together through each step of development and operation. Putting this program together must be a team effort. *Neither parents nor professional can do it alone.* In both concept and practice, this cooperation is different from the usual approach to a human service problem.

Once the sponsor agency or organization has laid the groundwork—has established the program plan, goals and objectives, and budget and timeline; secured program funding; and appointed a qualified professional as program coordinator—the coordinator recruits four to six parents to serve on the steering committee. This is the beginning of parent-professional teamwork.

Program Resources—Contributions of Parents and Coordinator

The care co-op model turns to and recycles some old-fashioned resources, which, in recent times, have perhaps been overlooked. Co-ops are not new; co-op child care, schools, businesses and housing have been established in many communities. American folk tradition tells many stories of hard times when families helped each other. When life has been full of danger, stress, and uncertainty, people have often joined forces for the strength to cope. Often those who cooperated were those who survived.

For families caring for a chronically disabled person, life is indeed full of uncertainty, stress, and, at times, danger. So the care co-op model combines the *tradition of family cooperation* with *modern experience in social work* with groups, family problem solving, and community development. This program uses some of each component and combines them in new ways.

Parents and coordinator each contribute to the team effort their own particular skills, experience, time, and energy.

The coordinator contributes professional skills in:

1. Planning and organizing the new program
2. Supporting and enabling the steering committee and co-op group to develop the program
3. Program marketing—publicity, outreach and family recruitment
4. Program management
5. Interviewing and problem solving with families

The parents contribute:

1. Their motivation and energy to participate, which comes from urgent need for respite, desire to stay in charge of their own situation, and desire to help others
2. New energy gained from co-op mutual support
3. Their experience as caregiving parents—concern about their child's needs, caregiving skills, knowledge and expertise about their own child
4. Parent-to-parent trust, a major component of the care co-op
5. Continuing input about changing family needs, which keeps the program updated and on track
6. Time and labor to manage the respite care exchange, to provide respite care, and to serve on the steering committee

In working with the team, the coordinator's job is to help the parents learn what they can do, support and guide them in doing it, and build with them the care co-op program on the results.

Roles and Tasks

The *coordinator*, working in a parent-professional team, is responsible for the following:

1. Guiding and taking the lead in steering committee program development and program marketing
2. Recruiting and screening new co-op members
3. Supporting and facilitating parent operation of the care co-op (organizing, training for care, respite care exchange, and mutual support)
4. Handling program management and accountability

Parents, either on the steering committee or in the care co-op groups, are responsible for the following:

1. Assisting with program development and program marketing
2. Organizing the care co-op
3. Training each other for giving care
4. Managing the respite care exchange
5. Giving and receiving respite care
6. Providing each other with mutual support
7. Handling care exchange business and problem solving

Teamwork is a way of both conserving and effectively using the main program resources—the time, skills, and energy of parents and coordinator. It enables parents to provide each other with respite care and mutual support effectively. Team roles are defined so that both coordinator and parents do what each does best and avoid what the other could do better. For example, parents can provide care better, but the coordinator can lead program development better. Also team support avoids the parent burnout and discouragement that can be part of a strictly volunteer project.

Thus, on the one hand, the parent volunteers are not operating the program alone. Yet, on the other hand, the professional staff person is not providing respite care service *for* the parents. Instead, parent-professional teamwork provides yet a *third way* of serving that combines the skills of both.

PROGRAM DEVELOPMENT

The Process

The sponsor agency or organization *plans, organizes,* and *manages* the program under which any number of parent-operated care co-ops may be developed. The steering committee, guided by the program coordinator, *develops* the program. Together, they determine program policies and write their own program manual. They also decide their own ground rules and procedures for their co-op respite care exchange, which become the Handbook for each co-op group.

The team works together on program publicity, outreach, and family recruitment (i.e., program marketing). Often, using a slide-tape of the co-op in action, one parent and the coordinator show the program to interested parents or to professionals who can help them reach families. As parents raise questions or common concerns, the co-op parent explains how parents have built the care co-op to handle these same concerns.

In addition, the coordinator is in frequent contact with service network colleagues who work with disabled children or their parents. Ensuring that these colleagues understand the program concepts and plan, the coordinator keeps them informed as it develops. With each member of the service network, the coordinator tries to set up a mutually workable referral system. The co-op program needs key professionals—teachers, medical personnel, recreation workers, therapists, and social workers to help reach the families who could use a care co-op.

Since the program's inception, steering committees have felt strongly that parents should not screen other parents. Therefore, the coordinator, representing the co-op parents, visits interested families in their homes, at their request, to help them consider whether the care co-op would work for them.

Table 1 shows *roles and responsibilities* for parents and coordinator during the program development process. Note that the "lead" role changes depending on phase and activity in the process.

The Steering Committee

Steering committee members are usually the "pioneer" parents in a community—those few who enjoy being on the cutting edge and who become excited about helping to start something new.

In the original program, the steering committee consisted of four parents and the program coordinator. (Some programs have added a representative agency network professional to the committee.) As with most committees since, they met weekly for 2 months to carve out policies and procedures that could serve as a solid base of high care standards and well-defined care procedures. As their guide, they used this question: *What is needed to make these representative parents and their families feel comfortable taking part in a care co-op?* They tried to raise every possible question and concern and to build this program on their solutions to those questions. The concerns of the committee members were indeed the same as those of parents to whom they later introduced the co-op idea.

As with most parents who consider the Care Co-op, steering committee parents are usually hesitant at first. The original four began by stating that they would like to help develop this program "for others," making no prom-

Table 1. Roles and responsibilities

Steps in program development and operation	Sponsor agency administrator	Program coordinator	Parents
Phase I: Organization and planning			
Setting goals and objectives	Leads	Assists	
Establishing budget and obtaining funding	Leads	Assists	
Introducing program to key community people	Assists	Leads	
Locating and involving steering committee parents		Leads	Assist
Planning continuation funding	Leads	Assists	
Phase II: Developing program			
Developing program policies (program manual)		Leads	Assist
Determining respite care procedures (Co-op handbook)		Leads	Assist
Managing publicity and outreach		Leads	Assist
Interviewing and recruiting families		Leads	Assist
Forming Care Co-op group		Leads	Assist
Evaluating, revising, and expanding program		Leads	Assist
Phase III: Care Co-op operation			
Organizing Co-op group		Assists	Lead
Parents training each other to give care		Assists	Lead
Exchanging respite care		Assists	Lead
Sharing mutual support and problem solving		Assists	Lead

ises about joining the co-op themselves. After many hours of working together, discussing, and planning for a care co-op to fit their own needs, most began to feel a sense of commitment and ownership in it. Before enough families could be recruited to form the first co-op, the committee was impatient to get started. One father often said, "My wife and I haven't been out together since our son was born—and I *can't wait* for this Co-op to start!" As the manual was almost finished, a mother who had been outspoken about "doing this for other families" was asked whether she planned to join. "Are you kidding," she exclaimed. "Let others mess this up? . . . I'll be there!"

The group laughed, but most agreed. They would be right there making sure their co-op worked.

The steering committee parents usually form the core group of the first co-op, but the Committee also continues on in an advisory (to the agency) and policy making capacity.

Starting the Care Co-op Group

When at least five or six families are ready to join, the first co-op group is formed. With the coordinator's support, co-op members operate their respite care exchange. Each member trains the others to care for his or her child, and each both gives and receives care. Eventually, member families care for every child in the co-op. In addition, the group meets at least monthly to handle any care exchange business or problems, to provide new training, and to share experiences and information.

Safeguards

Today, the care co-op Program operates with a number of built-in safeguards that grew out of the penetrating questions raised by those first parents and others since then. Co-op parents trust the program because of the self-determining role of parents, the continuing support and guidance of the coordinator, the close relationship with other parents, and the following safeguards:

1. Specific program policies, care procedures, and care rules are determined by parents and followed day-to-day by each co-op group.
2. Every co-op family home complies with the health and safety checklist determined by parents.
3. The professional coordinator interviews, screens, and selects the families who join each co-op group.
4. In frequent group training sessions, each parent trains and provides updated information to other co-op parents about the care of his or her child.
5. Each child has a care folder, which his or her parents use for training others and which always goes with the child into care. It contains information about every part of the child's life and care, as well as specific emergency procedures and an emergency care release signed by the parent.

Yet, the strongest safeguard—the real glue that firmly holds the care co-op together—is the give-and-take of respite care, mutual support, information, and help to each other. The care co-op works on a friendly balance of "I give your child good care . . . I expect you to give my child good care.", and "I'm watching you . . . you're watching me!" The group becomes much like an extended family.

FAMILY PARTICIPATION

Benefits for Families

What does the care co-op program offer a family? More than the founding parents ever expected. They planned for reliable, safe, healthy, understanding care that would be easily available and without cost to parents, given by families trained to care for each child. Care co-ops offer those services, but parents have also found other benefits.

In addition, the co-op offers the *children or adults with disabilities* new friends and new experiences that help them grow. Their narrow home and school worlds open up as they visit with co-op families who know, like, and understand them. Often the visit provides a chance to show or try new skills for a new and appreciative audience or to "be a different person" for a while.

> Kerri, age 3, tended to control her mother's life and attention with clinging and crying. When left the first few times in co-op respite care, she had tantrums. Now, several months later, she often puts clothes in her bag and carries it to her mother, saying, "I want to go in the Co-op now!"

For the young adult with disabilities, respite visits can offer experiences that help prepare them for a future away from the family.

> Bill, age 19 and mildly retarded, enjoys visiting Ed and Angie, who are parents of a disabled preschooler and are both in their late twenties. Ed is a good role model for Bill, who often seems to return home standing a little taller after going fishing with Ed or riding along on family errands in Ed's pickup.

With co-op respite care, *brothers and sisters* finally have their turn alone with Mom and Dad. They also visit other families who live with and understand disabilities. They get to know other children who, like themselves, have a disabled brother or sister.

> When her family joined the co-op, Sandra was 10. She was painfully embarrassed when her parents would wheel her multiply handicapped older sister to her school Open House. She refused to bring playmates home and was tense and tongue-tied when other children asked her questions about her sister. In the co-op, she made friends with Lisa, whose family situation and severely handicapped sister were much like Sandra's. At monthly co-op meetings, the two girls were inseparable, and group sharing helped both families teach their daughters to live more comfortably with their situations. Today, Sandra, a high school senior, is an outspoken advocate for, and volunteer with, handicapped people.

Recently another co-op "sibling," 12-year-old Sam, was overheard telling neighborhood children who were laughing at a co-op child in his parents' care, "Don't stand there laughing! If he's doing something wrong, tell him. Teach him what to do!"

Through the care exchange process, *parents become a close support group.* Family members find mutual support in sharing experiences with other co-op families. For fathers, co-op meetings are often their first opportunity to talk frankly about their children. (Mothers are more likely to have shared problems and feelings with other mothers—in the doctor's waiting room or the school parent group.)

As the first care co-op began to meet, the fathers quickly became absorbed in talking with each other about their children. Some mothers heard for the first time their husbands telling of their own deep concern for their disabled children.

Families help each other identify needs, handle problems, and find services. Sometimes co-op parents act as knowledgeable advocates for other needed community services. In the original care co-op program's annual program evaluation, co-op mutual support and respite care were ranked by parents as being of equal value.

In the 9 years since the first program started, four severely disabled co-op children have died. Each time, the co-op families provided extensive support—sat with the family, brought food, spent many hours at the funeral home, and shared the continuing grief in the following weeks. The shared experience always seemed important to the entire group, for both the bereaved parents and the others (some of whom know well that their child could be next).

Parental Use of Respite Care

To stay healthy, co-op families learn to adjust their life-style to include respite care as a *routine of daily living.* In the care co-op, respite care is seen as a common-sense approach to the maintenance of family health, not as an occasional treat or for a one-time emergency. Co-op care, at no cost to parents, is almost always readily available as frequently and for as long a period as the family needs. So parents can plan enough respite time to make a difference.

But most co-op parents find that their own tendency to put off use of respite care—the "I'm OK today . . . I'll wait until I need it" syndrome—is an ever-present potential pitfall. The members of the co-op group continually deal with their own very human tendency to procrastinate. Newer members are also sometimes unsure about how to spend respite time and are even uncomfortable about using it. At first, there is the usual guilt about leaving the child with someone else. And some couples, after years of the child always being with them, may at first find time alone together something of a strain. Familiarity with these problems, friendly nudging, encouraging each member to remember to use care, and even group discussion of possible ways to use respite time, are all part of the mutual support co-op parents provide for each other.

The pay-off is two-fold: For the co-op family, maintaining the health of parent, marriage, and family requires regular use of respite care. For the co-op, as an organized group and a service, the more respite care is given and received, the stronger the co-op becomes and the better it functions.

Co-op parents at first anxiously use 2 or 3 hours of care—often waiting by the phone during the first respite time. Once past the early months, however, they use co-op care for hours, days, or weeks—sometimes for a family vacation—according to family needs. (A longer care period is usually shared between several families.)

At first, co-op care was planned for disabled children only. But most co-ops now provide care for *all* the members' children, handicapped or not. The original Co-op, now in its 9th year, has several times supported the family of a dying child, before and after the death, and parents of that child have remained in the co-op as long as they needed that support. From the caregiving experience and the group discussions, suggestions, and problem solving, parents have gained new care skills and new confidence with their own children, as well as with others. Care co-op members continue to explore and find new ways to make this program work for them.

Which Families Are Potential Care Co-op Members?

The Care Co-op Program is suitable for many, but not all, families who need respite care. For many, it can make more costly agency-provided respite care services unnecessary. It can be the "least restrictive" choice. But it cannot meet all respite care needs in a community.

The program works best as part of a continuum of community respite care services. It does not replace other programs. It is not a crisis program. Exhausted caregiving parents, families currently in crisis, chronic multi-problem families, or families with little energy or interest for managing their own family situations are usually not good candidates for a care co-op.

A care co-op best serves families who, though experiencing stress, still enjoy basic mental and physical health, who are still managing home and family, and who prefer remaining self-sufficient to seeking agency help. These are generally families who find appeal in parent self-determination, the opportunity to help others, parent-to-parent trust, the chance to tailor a respite care service to their own needs and to "watchdog" the care process, and the personal investment and sense of ownership in a care co-op. Many of this group of parents have never been to a human service agency or sought a crisis service. This does not indicate that they are free of problems or that, without respite care or support today, they would not become tomorrow's family crisis case. Yet, today, these families are most likely to be found through programs for special education, vocational training, recreation or Special Olympics, medical services, hospital intensive care units, or special therapies and parent organizations.

MAKING THE PROGRAM WORK

Program Marketing—Persuading Families to Participate in a Care Co-Op

The respite care co-op does not fix a crisis or cure acute problems. People do not come looking for it because they feel they need it. Yet, it can provide enough support and trusted respite care so the parent feels much less exhausted, stronger, healthier, and better able to cope and avoid crisis.

So how does a co-op team "sell" the care co-op to families it is intended to serve? How do they help parents get past the common resistance to using respite care ("We don't need it yet."), as well as additional fears about taking part in a care exchange?

On the one hand, parents are almost always skeptical at first. So are many professionals. Some parents take one look and exclaim, "Take care of still another kid? . . . That's no rest!" (They need to hear a co-op parent firmly say, "If you take care of two on Tuesday and then get all day Friday off, *that's a rest!*" and "It's just not as hard as you think it will be," . . . and then show why.) Others quietly shudder at the thought of other parents seeing their child at his or her "worst" or finding out how "badly" they cope. Some professionals quickly identify with these first reactions, and they protect or discourage their clients from getting involved.

But on the other hand, parents are drawn to co-op respite care without cost, to the opportunity to know other parents who are "in the same boat," and to helping others. However, before parents can imagine themselves in a care co-op, they need to hear about the program, see the slide-tape show, and most of all talk with the team—a co-op parent and the coordinator—together.

At outreach presentations, there is an instant common bond between the co-op team parent and the parents who are listening. Also, parents seem reassured to hear the coordinator and parent presenting together and obviously supporting each other.

As with any new and unfamiliar service, program marketing is a *major part* of putting together a care co-op program. In fact, publicity, outreach, and recruitment take a larger portion of program develpment time and effort than any other activity.

Program marketing is a process, an ongoing series of steps. It also requires a lot of repetition. Publicity efforts, such as a newspaper announcement, a flier, or a letter sent home from school, can be useful, but they are only a small part of the process. Marketing begins with introducing the care co-op concept to key colleagues and parents immediately after the agency decides to start the program. And it continues through the life of the program.

The marketing process for the Care Co-op Program involves the following components:

1. *Publicity* to the general community (radio, television, printed media), to the particular group of families the program hopes to serve, or to all professionals involved with those families (newsletters, fliers, and so forth)
2. *Outreach* to families or related professionals, often by a team of the coordinator and a parent showing and telling a group of parents and/or professionals or a family about their care co-op and their own personal experience with it
3. *Family Recruitment* in which the coordinator alone interviews the parents at home to help them clearly understand the program, to answer their concerns, and to consider with them whether the co-op would fit their needs and what their family might both give and receive in a care co-op

All three levels of marketing activity need to continue throughout the program operation. The family interview is the goal of the first two steps. In the first step of *publicity* the parent passively hears or sees the radio or television spot or the brochure. Publicity is needed to spread information and make the care co-op familiar, but it almost never results in a parent contacting the program. *Outreach,* however, involves face-to-face contact and a closer look for the parent at both the program and the team of co-op parent and coordinator. Still, the parent is passively listening and uncommitted.

In the *family recruitment* interview, however, the parent becomes actively involved. With the coordinator, parent and family consider their own needs and decide whether the care co-op might work for them. Without this personal contact focused on the family's needs, as well as meeting enough times with the coordinator so a trusting relationship is developed, most families will not join a care co-op.

Sometimes, of course, it is clear that the co-op is not right for the family or they for it. The coordinator then tries, if possible, to help them gain access to a more appropriate respite care service.

For potential co-op families (and also for community professionals), the marketing process needs to introduce the program and make it familiar; make it clearly understood—what it is, how it works, what if offers; make it trusted; and help the family clearly see and want what the co-op can offer it personally.

POTENTIAL PROBLEMS AND PITFALLS

The first pitfall of this program model is its seeming simplicity. When some professionals and many parents first hear about the care co-op, their response sometimes is, "What a wonderful idea! We'll just gather together a few parents and have them exchange care! . . . We know so many parents who could use this. They'll jump at the chance!"

The danger in such a simplistic view is that it may lead to a grant proposal or even a funded plan with an unrealistic budget, an inexperienced staff, insufficient staff time, an inadequate program development timeline, and no time or funding for program marketing.

To develop this program well takes time, effort, and skill. Most agencies need at least a year and an experienced coordinator working from half- to full-time in order to put together a program structure that will:

1. Reach and serve families throughout the service area
2. Last beyond the first few founding parents as an established service program
3. Serve a variety of unmet needs
4. Support several care co-op groups

The coordinator needs skills and experience in program development and program management, as well as in working with groups and with families. He or she needs to be innovative, a problem solver, and be able to grasp and try new approaches.

A well-developed system and process of program publicity, outreach, and family recruitment are required to make a new care co-op program become known and trusted enough that parents will join and take part and professional colleagues will help the program reach new families.

Other frequent pitfalls are those common to any newly developing program: 1) *the need for preliminary needs assessment* (What is the local need for respite care? Which families could use a care co-op?), 2) *the need for clear and specific program objectives* based on those needs (problems result when unclear objectives provide no definite program focus and no base for program evaluation), and 3) *the need to plan actively for future continuation funding from the start if the program is funded by a time-limited grant.*

Specific to this program are some problems that occur when the parent-professional teamwork concept is not fully understood or functioning. In small or large ways, the coordinator may be tempted to take over and do the job *for* the parents. This always weakens the program and can build in failure. More important, if this happens, the group ceases to be a "co-op," which by definition involves members equally sharing both tasks and rewards and mutually helping eath other.

With her first try, one coordinator did not locate parents for her steering committee. So she wrote the manual and handbook herself "to save time" and then tried unsuccessfully to recruit parents to use them. She missed the point that these books are necessary as the *record* and the *result* of the basic *parent decision-making process* about how they, as co-op members, will operate their own co-op and respite care exchange.

The concept that co-op *parents*—not a battery of teachers, nurses, therapists, or psychology students—will *teach other parents* how to care for their own handicapped children is sometimes rejected by both agency and parents in their initial planning for a new care co-op program. The following two program experiences show two possible responses to this issue and the results of each.

(A) The model program parents planned that they would train each other only until they had covered all that they knew. After that, they said, they would like the coordinator to bring in other professionals to complete their training. But the fact is that, in the 9 years since that program began, those parents have never found the limits of their knowledge about their own children! They continually train new families and provide updated information to their entire group about their children's care and training.

They have occasionally used a specialist to train them in such issues as cardiopulmonary resuscitation, wheelchair transfer techniques, and seizure management. In their care experience, they have found need to improve their skills in certain technical areas. However, this use of specialists has very different implications from having the sponsor agency organize and require professionally presented training as a condition of Co-op membership. In a care co-op, the parents remain in charge.

In this situation, the coordinator operated from two clearly understood care co-op program premises:

1. Co-op care exchange will depend on and function with the use of its basic resource (i.e., each parent's skills, experience, and knowledge about the care and training of his or her own child).
2. The need of the co-op for, and use of, parental expertise will give the parent new self-confidence, self-respect, and a sense of success and worth. This, in turn, will help the parent expand and increase both respite caregiving and parenting skills, take charge, and cope better.

The approach taken by this program encouraged these parents to invest time and energy enthusiastically in their own Care Co-op.

(B) In contrast, another agency developing this program assumed that they would need "a professional training component." They contracted with the local community college to train the parents in giving care. Although some parents came for training, almost none seemed interested in helping put together their own program. As the coordinator tried to recruit parents (*without* the team approach), she frequently heard from parents that they did not see why they "had to provide" their own care—that they would much prefer the agency to set up a respite shelter where they could leave their children. They wanted the agency to take care of them. Perhaps for some parents this approach would have met their needs. But in this situation, agency and staff—and therefore parents—missed the point, the real strength, and the pay-off for both parents and agency in this program: the parent self-help and the parent-professional team process.

The *process*—coordinator supporting parent decisions and planning about how the care co-op will meet their own needs—*is what builds the strength and structure on which this program functions and grows.* In the first efforts of the steering committee, the coordinator and parents are learning the teamwork relationship that they will use and depend on many times during the life of the program. Without strong parent participation in developing program policies and care exchange rules, there is no parent investment. With no parent investment, there are few parents interested in participating, and the result is usually no care co-op program.

Throughout the life of the progam, the more parents that can be involved in decision making about the program and in the respite care service itself, the stronger the program and each co-op group will become.

Finally, the need for program marketing presents pitfalls, particularly because many human service professionals are not accustomed to "selling" people on using a service program. For many professionals, program marketing is a new and unfamiliar human service skill that now becomes necessary as the funding situation increasingly demands innovation. The familiar old way of advertising a new service, and then waiting for potential users or clients to call, usually will not work for a new, unfamiliar, and noncrisis service.

Time and funding for the program marketing process need to be included in the program budget and timeline. A grant budget that does not include these costs is, at best, building in an inability to comply with the proposal timeline and target dates and, at worst, program failure.

THE PROGRAM IN THE SERVICE NETWORK

Characteristics of Interest to Funders and Service Providers

Cost   The care co-op program's operating budget is relatively low. After the start-up period, it can be decreased, maintained, or expanded according to plans for further program development.

At a time of severe budget cutbacks, the Community Mental Health Board, which has provided continuation funding for the original Respite Care Co-op Program, planned to eliminate this newest program from its funding contract with Family and Children Services. The Care Co-op parents testified before the Board that: 1) the Care Co-op was a major factor in keeping them from needing residential placement for their children, and 2) the cost of the entire Respite Care Co-op Program for 1 year equaled less than the amount the Board would be required to pay for just *one* of their severely multiply impaired children for 6 months at the state institution. Program funding was continued.

If the cost of a care co-op program is calculated, at least in part, on a per-care-hour basis, the cost decreases with increased use. However, care hours should not be used as the *only* basis for determining program cost-effectiveness. Actual service provided is best measured by *units of service* (one unit to equal one hour) including: child care periods, parent respite time co-op meetings for mutual support and problem-solving, parent-to-parent training for care, and the coordinator's initial interviews and ongoing contact with and assistance to individual families.

The program model is designed to sponsor *more than one care co-op group*. One coordinator working full-time could usually work with up to three groups (see the organizational plan in Figure 1). Beyond that number, a second staff person would be needed. To date, each group has seemed to reach an optimum level of functioning at between 15 and 20 families. In larger groups, families find it less easy to know each other well enough for the needed trust. Rather than growing larger, the co-op group needs to then divide, perhaps according to geographic location or child's age, and to continue on as two separate co-ops. Sponsorship of a number of co-op groups is a way to serve greater numbers and families with different socioeconomic levels, as well as varied geographical locations, life-styles, ages, or handicaps.

The major program cost is the professional salary for a skilled and experienced coordinator. Other *start-up budget items* include secretarial time, mileage, program marketing costs (slide-tapes, brochures, newsletters, and television and radio announcements, for publicity, outreach, and family recruitment), printing costs for the manual and handbook, and the cost of initial training and technical assistance for the coordinator in developing and operating the program.

A Professionally Guided Volunteer Service *The care co-op program is an alternative to paid professional in-home or out-of-home respite care.* It is intended to prevent the need for residential care. It can also help prevent most Co-op families from needing or using more costly agency-provided respite care.

The care co-op model uses parent time and energy to provide the respite care service. This uses a resource that is generally untapped by the service delivery system. In addition, unlike many volunteer projects, in a care co-op program, support by the paid professional enables the energy of the volunteer parent to be conserved, effectively channeled, and not over-used or burned out. One coordinator's paid time and energy enables the time and energy of a group of parent volunteers to provide the actual respite care service in one or more Care Co-ops. This is an 1) economical use of a professional salary and 2) conserves human resources.

In this program there is no cost to families for care. Parents pay for care received by giving care. As a result: 1) the agency never needs to ration or limit respite care hours or frequency of care, 2) there is no need for means

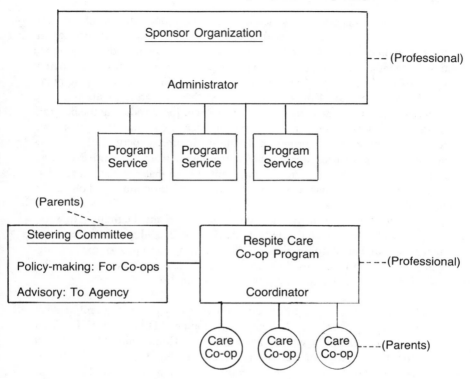

Figure 1. Respite care co-op program organization chart.

tests or categories, and 3) the agency needs no budget item for subsidizing cost of care because there are no fees.

The Program model is flexible and adaptable to each local situation and the needs of families to be served. It can provide in-home or out-of-home care for a variety of care needs, disabilities, geographical locations, economic and cultural differences, or family life-styles. It can work in rural or urban areas. It can also adapt to the changing needs of each co-op group.

The Care Co-op Program provides a least restrictive alternative for the local service network.

Dissemination of the Model

The care co-op program model is still experimental, and more remains to be learned about how to make it work to maximum potential and about what that potential might be.

The use of this program is increasing slowly, though steadily, for several apparent reasons: 1) the current financial climate in the field of services for the developmentally disabled that, for many, has discouraged new program development and has limited existing programs; 2) the inability of the parent agency's funding and program structure to become involved with disseminating the program model outside the agency's service area; 3) the time and experience needed to develop an effective system for introducing the program model and for providing training and technical assistance to agencies interested in utilizing this program; 4) the difficulties experienced by a few agencies that have tried to replicate the program from descriptive material only and without the program development system that has been developed; and 5) general unfamiliarity with building a service program based on parent-professional teamwork.

Despite this slow start, care co-op programs are beginning to serve families with children and adults with chronic disability or illness in an increasing number of communities. The following examples of existing Respite Care Co-op Programs illustrate how each new program has developed and adapted the model according to its local situation.

1. The model Care Co-op Program, sponsored by a private family agency and developed under a Michigan Developmental Disabilities (DD) Council grant, continues with funding from the Community Mental Health Board. The program, serving an urban and suburban area of 150,000, has developed one co-op group with a maximum of 17 families of children age 2 to 20 who have moderate to severe or multiple disabilities. Over a 9-year period, the program has had four staff changes. For 2 periods of several months each, it has functioned without a coordinator, that is, without parent-professional teamwork. During those periods, no new families joined, care exchanges diminished, and a few families dropped out. Agency budget cuts have curtailed staff time, so that although the one co-op group has continued to grow, as yet no more co-op groups have been developed.

2. A Care Co-op Program, sponsored by an early education and family service program of a private liberal arts college in New York State, serves a town of 25,000 and the surrounding rural area. Funded by a 3-year grant from a local private foundation, this program's first co-op group served 10 families during the first year and is growing. Member families have children age 3 to 10 with moderate handicaps (not all DD).

3. Another program, also sponsored by a private family agency and funded by the Michigan DD Council, briefly served a town of 30,000 and the surrounding rural area. The program was initiated by community interagency planning and was developed by a steering committee of six

parents, a coordinator, and two representatives of the interagency group. Two co-op groups were formed—one urban and one rural. (The area offered no other respite care and very few services for the DD population.) Strong parent interest gave impetus to both program planning and the development of both co-op groups. At the end of the grant year, the sponsor agency did not obtain continuation funding and the program ended. The parents tried unsuccessfully to maintain the co-ops on their own.

4. A federally funded respite care project includes several care co-ops in a New York State urban-suburban area. This adaptation of the program has substantially deviated from the original model. Variations include: 1) less involvement of parent-professional team, 2) use of mandatory professionally provided parent training classes instead of parent-to-parent training for giving care, and 3) no steering committee in an ongoing policy-making and advisory capacity.

5. In addition, the Respite Care Co-op Program model is being adapted to serve other populations. In Michigan, an Area Agency on Aging has received federal funding to develop a model program to serve caregiving relatives of frail or impaired elders, to disseminate program information through a series of statewide workshops, and to assist new programs with start-up. After 1 year, the model co-op consists of 11 families and is growing. The plan includes starting other co-ops in neighboring counties. This program has added a "helping member" component consisting of caregiving members who lose their own elders but want to remain in the co-op support group and assist with giving care.

CONCLUDING COMMENTS

In building the care co-op program model on professional skills combined with parent skills, and parent self-help combined with agency structure, the developers seem to have inadvertantly wandered into a kind of human services "no man's land"! Parent and agency resources have traditionally remained in their own spheres—1) the parent organizations (such as the Association for Retarded Citizens and other disability-related advocacy groups) and the parent self-help movement and 2) the public and private human service systems. There has been little communication between them. In a forward-looking community, staff members of both agencies and parent organization may meet occasionally at interagency meetings, but cooperation between systems, a joint effort of any kind, is most unusual.

This limited communication between spheres apparently is a result of different missions, objectives, funding, and systems of operation. Unfortunately, it leads to and perpetuates significant differences in perceptions of parent and family. For example, the roles and perceptions held of a parent who is both a member of the local ARC and a client of a case management agency (i.e., the way that parent is seen by each as functioning, coping, or contributing) may be so different as to be unrecognizable.

The care co-op program has experimented with cutting across the lines of these established spheres, combining the resources of each to produce a way of serving a need that is different from the services of either. This has opened up a realm of exciting possibilities. Both the parents and the professionals have needed to learn new roles and how to share program development and operational tasks. The usual result has been a new mutual respect and discovery by each of both their own and the other's expertise. Operating outside conventional boundaries has also stimulated energy, enthusiasm, and excitement, which have contributed to the operating premise that this model can be adapted successfully to almost any community or group of caregivers. The approach tends to be not, "Can a care co-op program work?," but rather, "What do we need to do to make it work here?"

In developing this program, the goal was to plan and construct a respite care service in which: 1) families could afford and use regular respite care as a family support service, 2) the amount of care available would not be tied to agency budget restrictions, and 3) each unit of service would not depend on use of staff time and tasks at every step.

As the idea of a cooperative respite care model was considered, the guiding question was: What might the majority of parents who are not yet in a state of exhaustion or family crisis do for themselves in developing and operating their own respite care? In addition to basic agency support to fund and stabilize the program, *what could coordinator and parents each best contribute* to the joint effort? This was the *first challenge* of this program model. It was met by the parent-professional team concept, combining parent self-help and professional guidance.

As the care co-op program has developed, a *second challenge* has arisen. Usually, neither the professional nor parents are aware of the particular skills and expertise of the other—the expertise that will support their own efforts as they learn to work as a team. So each new program involves a certain amount of mutual discovery. But also, the new roles and new relationships between parents and professional required by the program can raise a new set of problems both for the new team and for others in contact with the program.

For example, *parents* may see this program as only gathering together a few parents to exchange care. The need for program structure or marketing is usually not apparent to them, and even if it is, most are unsure how to accomplish either task. *The agency* may not trust that parents *can,* or would *want to,* operate their own respite care exchange. The *coordinator* may not understand the value and the pay-off for all concerned of assisting parents to *develop and operate their own care co-op* and so may inadvertantly take over important parent roles. Although professionally experienced coordinators, particularly those who have worked in community development or social work with groups, usually have little difficulty with the team concept, some coordinators, administrators, and funders do.

Why would professionally facilitated parent self-help be a concept foreign to the human service field, particularly to those serving developmentally disabled individuals and their families? A look at current practice suggests some potential reasons why.

Although human service philosophy usually speaks of enabling clients to develop their own potential for self-determination, practice is more apt to involve: 1) *doing for, not with* the client or parent and 2) the unspoken but common *assumption that the parent is weak, inadequate, and unable to cope.* The reasons for this are perhaps understandable. One learns to adjust one's perceptions and approach to the demands of daily practice and, for many professionals, practice involves large caseloads involving crisis situations. In addition, the practice of counting units of service to the disabled person but not to his or her parents further supports *a perception of the parents as insignificant.* It draws the focus away from the family interaction and keeps the agency staff unfamiliar with the real strengths and struggles of the parent. It carries the messages that service or support given to parents is unimportant and that parents have little to contribute.

Also, human services with a "crisis" mentality have helped to teach parents an *image of themselves as weak and inadequate,* an image that is daily reinforced in their own attempts to cope with chronic problems that usually have no solutions. Tired and frantic parents easily accept and do not challenge the "weak and inadequate" image, especially when it comes from a professional.

The care co-op concept that *parents are the experts* about the care of their own disabled children simply does not fit with the above assumptions.

For the Respite Care Co-op Program, the parent organization (with its experience in parent advocacy and self-help) and the human service agency (with its structure and systems for providing a program base, funding, and professional staff) each provide the half of the experiental and conceptual resources needed. The agency offers stability and funding mechanisms to develop and maintain the program structure; the parent organization and movement are more compatible with the care co-op self-help concepts.

So, the care co-op program needs both "worlds." Parents need help with the systems involved with building and operating a program structure. Professionals need help understanding and keeping in touch with changing parent and family needs, with what parents can and want to do for themselves, and with the strength parents can gain from supported self-help and mutual support.

However, neither the parent volunteer organizations nor traditional human service agencies have much experience in combining their expertise—in using professional skills to keep the parent strong and able to stay in charge. This is what the care co-op program tries to do. It is the job of the coordinator to make it happen. The parents and coordinator become partners—with a new kind of mutual respect and comfort in working together—each using his or her own particular skills to make the project work.

Each new care co-op program presents possible new directions for the parent-professional team to stretch to serve the needs. Both parents and coordinator need to continue learning how to use each other's considerable skills together to make this program work.

In using this model, much exploration still remains. The care co-op program model still operates in largely unfamiliar but fascinating territory. And there remains another question yet to be answered: Could guided self-help be used to serve other needs, in addition to respite care, and other populations besides parents and caregivers of chronically disabled individuals?

Chapter 9

THE COMMUNITY-BASED RESPITE RESIDENCE

FINDING A PLACE IN THE SYSTEM

Barbara Coyne Cutler

The need for respite care services is usually justified by presenting the most dramatic cases of families of children with severe handicaps (Cohen & Warren, 1985); yet the respite care models developed tend to exclude or serve least adequately the families of those children or adults most at risk of institutionalization (Apolloni & Triest, 1983). Persons with severe behavioral or medical problems, particularly adolescents or adults, fit poorly into a respite care system built on in-home care (Upshur, 1982). Providing respite care in the client's home rests on the assumption that parents need relief in the form of recreation outside the home. For many parents of persons with more challenging behaviors, however, relief means rest and quiet time at home without the presence of their handicapped member. These parents, when they are able to locate a respite provider who is willing to provide care in the provider's home, are often reluctant to leave their hard-to-serve children in a setting that has little or no professional support or back-up for potentially difficult or crisis situations.

Although surveys (Apolloni & Triest, 1983; Arizona Division of Developmental Disabilities and Mental Retardation Services, 1979; Hagen, Reasnor, & Jenson, 1980; Oppenheim & Upshur, 1978) show that persons with severe needs are being poorly served, these studies often draw their conclusions from the majority of their sample and make recommendations to provide services to the larger numbers of children with less severe handicaps. Despite

This chapter would not be complete without acknowledging the many parents who have shared their difficulties in finding appropriate respite care. They will recognize their stories and their contributions.

acknowledging that client behavioral and medical characteristics most frequently result in denial of service and noting that more than a quarter of their sample preferred out-of-home care, the Provider's Management (1978) study nevertheless recommended that models that provide care in the client's own home should be encouraged. The survey did not acknowledge the need to develop any systematic guidelines for residential respite for the hard-to-serve and older population. This survey is a typical system response to the needs of the population with severe handicaps.

It is not clear why the needs of persons with severe problems are not being addressed. Certainly, the cost and staff training needs in residential centers are greater; the maintenance of a year-round facility, however small, makes additional demands on agency staff and finances. These factors, combined with a view of residential respite centers as the most restrictive community models (Salisbury & Griggs, 1983) without regard for their appropriateness for hard-to-serve individuals, have discouraged the development of needed respite centers. According to Lash (1983), the "reality is, however, that unless the necessary services and supports are available in the community, the disabled individual can be just as isolated or even more isolated than he/she was or would be in an institution."

If we are serious about the ability of respite care to prevent institutionalization, then we must strive to meet the needs of families whose handicapped members are most at risk of institutionalization (Blacher & Meyers, 1983; Lotter, 1978), and to meet those needs appropriately, timely, and regularly. For the unserved and underserved, it is critical that a "zero-reject" system of respite care be developed. If the family can provide daily care to its handicapped member, the system should be able to respond with intermittent, periodic respite care (Cutler, 1979) of a quality that does not make parents feel that their children are being deprived of care and comfort during their absence; that is, the level and quality of care are at least equivalent to that provided routinely by the family. The question should not be, "Can we provide the hard-to-serve family with respite care?", but rather, "What is required to give this family the service it needs to maintain its severely handicapped member in the home?"

In most existing respite systems, the major gap is the lack of a community-based residential setting, the *primary* purpose of which is to provide respite service for the needs of specific clients. By definition, public long-term care facilities are clearly excluded from being considered as appropriate respite care centers. The few community residential respite programs that serve families who would otherwise be denied struggle to survive without adequate funding and the wide support of the respite community. When adequately supported and appropriately developed, however, such centers have much to offer not only to the most severely handicapped population but also to the less severely impaired clients and their families. They fill such gaps in services as certain types of emergency care, provision of hands-on training for providers, and relief for families who wish to take their respite care at home. Yet, there is little recognition of these benefits; instead these models are seen as costly and restrictive (Cutler & Helm, in press).

Although there are many similarities in the respite care needs of persons with severe behavioral problems and those with severe medical needs, the author's experience has been primarily with families of individuals who have been labeled behaviorally disordered, emotionally disturbed/retarded, and autistic and autistic-like; this chapter addresses issues of center-based respite care from that perspective. In 10 years of organizing respite programs; providing information, referral, and advocacy for potential respite clients; and accessing services as a consumer, a number of explicit needs and problems have emerged.

FAILURES OF EXISTING MODELS OF CARE

Popular models of respite care serve or are capable of serving the majority of families of developmentally disabled persons. In general, however, it is not the majority of families who are at greatest risk of institutionalizing their handicapped members.

Who Does the System Fail?

Potential clients with severe behavioral problems of all ages are poorly served, if at all. Families exposed to the constant strain of behavioral difficulties are often physically and emotionally exhausted (Cutler & Kozloff, in press; Horejsi, 1979). Planned vacations are not on their agendas. Many families report that what they really need is rest, sleep, and some quiet time with other family members. They want a few days off, totally and at home. They do not want nor need to cope with yet another person (the in-home respite provider) while their child continues to seek out the parent for the care and attention the parents normally provide in the home setting. Moreover, some overstressed parents do not have the physical and/or financial resources to remove themselves from the home (Cutler, 1979). Although there are some preschool and latency-age children from whom the parents require regular out-of-home relief, it is generally the aging parents of the older child—the adolescent or adult with severe problems—who are most likely to need out-of-home respite care (Blacher & Meyers, 1983). However, aging parents of persons with less severe problems can also benefit from out-of-home care by learning that a hitherto unresponsive service system is developing the capacity to serve their adult children in residential settings, thus mitigating the universal fear of "Who will take care of my child when I am no longer here?"

Adolescents and Adults with Severe Behavioral Problems Adolescents and adults with severe impairments demand much of their aging parents. Those parents who had escaped sleeping problems when their children were younger learn that the evening no longer brings a quiet hour or two. They are in fact on duty every waking hour that their children are in the home. Moreover, their sons and daughters usually depend on them completely to fill those waking hours with routine activities and companionship. Parental effort is expended and/or demanded from the time the client arrives home from the school or day program until the parents fall exhausted into bed. (Thus through lack of services, the severely handicapped individual's total dependence on the parents is reinforced.)

If a respite care worker is found who is willing to sit with the handicapped adolescent or adult to allow the parents to leave the home, a restrictive form of care—that is, babysitting the handicapped adult—is provided. Parents have complained that respite sitters do less with their hard-to-serve children than the family routinely does; for example, the parents may return to find the sitter and client sitting in front of the television where they left them when ordinarily someone in the family would have engaged the handicapped member in some routine activity, such as a trip to the park or store or making popcorn. The after effects of such "respite" are often that the parents feel sad or guilty and are less likely to use respite care despite the family's need for it.

The adolescent or adult can benefit from more age-appropriate activities as part of his or her respite care. Because the respite worker is likely to be closer in age to the client, there are more normalization opportunities available to the client in the company of the respite worker than the parents can provide. Although the sitter-companion model works well for the higher-level, more socially appropriate client (Lash, 1983), this model is not generally considered for the low-functioning and/or behaviorally disordered client because the respite worker is not secure in his or her ability to manage the client's behavior problems. The exception is the in-home care provider who is also the client's teacher or trainer in the client's regular day program; these workers have current knowledge of and experience in managing the client's difficulties and are capable of engaging the client in productive home and community activities (Goldenberg, 1984).

Although a higher rate of compensation could attract more respite providers to serve the more challenging clients, a higher pay scale is not the answer. Without adequate training, skills, and support for the respite worker, adequate services for the families of clients with severe problems will continue to be limited. When traditional sitting service is the only available respite service, adolescents and adults are deprived of an important learning experience. They need the opportunity to experience living temporarily in another setting, cared for by people other than their parents, in preparation for the time when they will leave their family home (Boggs, 1979).

Aging Parents   Aging parents also need the experience of seeing their adult children well cared for by others in other settings and of seeing that their children can survive that experience at least comfortably and even with some pleasure. Parents want to see that there are programs concerned with their children's individual needs, and strengths, likes, and dislikes and that can provide a warm social environment with their children's peers. Parents do realize that they will not live forever, and they want to help their dependent adult children learn to trust and be comfortable with other caregivers. But parents need experiences that will inspire that trust.

Parents who have known 15 or more years of repeated rejection and increasing isolation have fewer and fewer outside contacts (Suelzle & Keenan, 1981) and lack the energy to continue to reach out for supports that have been seldom there (Morton, 1978). Joyce, Singer, and Isralowitz (1983) assume that parents of adolescents have formed their own networks of stable resources over time. For at least the families of adolescents and adults with severe handicaps, however, parental expectations of receiving appropriate services and supports are low, and families have made some adjustment to lives of restriction (Bayley, 1973). For example, the widowed mother of a 30-year-old woman with severe handicaps has not had respite care in 10 years. Because of the constant care and the difficulties in managing her daughter she regrets that she has seen little of her grandson, who is shy and awkward on the rare occasions he sees her. Thus the parents of persons with severe handicaps can be deprived of both the assurance that their handicapped children can in fact be well cared for by others and the pleasure that should be theirs to find in yet another generation.

The system also underserves single parents (Wikler, 1983) and other sole caregivers of persons with severe handicaps. There are also some single parents of children with less severe handicaps but without a network of resources to support them in emergencies. Furthermore, single parents are only entitled to the same amount of respite care provided to two-parent families (Warren, 1983), despite the obvious additional physical and emotional burdens of the single parent.

The lack of appropriate, familiar respite care in emergencies can test parents' coping abilities to the breaking point and lead to long-lasting damaging effects (e.g., the parent who once felt in control can come to question seriously her (or his) ability to manage over the long run and may fear the next unexpected emergency). A death or illness in the family can create agonizing problems for parents, who are forced to leave their children with strangers in unfamiliar and unsupported settings for an extended period without assurances that the respite provider has the resources to manage the child well.

"Overprotective" parents include those parents who have had bad experiences with the system either through rejection or provision of inadequate services (Bruininks, 1979). Their children may have had difficulty fitting into the school system, may have been excluded from recreational and other community programs, and may have had painful respite experiences. Parents of children with behavioral disorders have received calls to come take their children home from the respite setting, or if the child survives overnight, weekend, or even the afternoon, the returning parents have been greeted with a list of complaints about the child's behaviors. Frustrated and disappointed, parents wonder if it is worth the effort to try to obtain respite. Many of these parents were honest about their children's problems and still they are confronted (sometimes crudely) with the fact that their child is hard to manage. They know their child is difficult. Because of their experiences and despite their needs, they are reluctant to seek out respite care. They still need services, but they also need assurances that their children will be cared for and well managed.

Some "overprotective" parents are cautious. For example, they would like to see the place where the service will be provided and meet some of the people responsible for their child's care. Such caution in parents of nonhandicapped children is acceptable. Yet the parents of handicapped children are expected to be grateful for any service that is provided. One respite agency director who worked hard to find a place in a residential program for 2 weeks was annoyed because the parent wanted to see the program. The parent had no car, and that agency assumed the burden of getting the parent to the program. The director of the agency was upset that the parent did not trust her judgment. Yet trust is built on experience. This parent needed the opportunity to evaluate the program and learn that the director had chosen well. Often, agencies dealing with reluctant or cautious parents or with parents who have been "burned" by the system assume that parents are unwilling to separate from their children and that they really do not want any respite care. Professionals too often label parental concerns as guilt and anxiety (Blacher, 1984). Yet one Massachusetts program, founded by parents, reported that parents' acceptance of the program was high when they had the opportunity to see the setting and meet with staff, and when they could use short periods of 1–2 hours, an afternoon, or even a single overnight respite at the start of their relationship with the agency. Once reassured by short periods of positive experience, they were able to trust the program and to use more extended and needed periods of respite care (a weekend, a week or longer). Perceived mistrust, suspicion, and stress in separating may actually be the parents' natural and responsible caution about leaving their children who are significantly dependent on others for their welfare and who are poor in directly communicating their own needs, if they can communicate at all, in programs whose ability to care for their children is still unproven.

Low-income, inner-city parents have some difficulty with the cultural implications of respite, of having strangers come into their homes or sending the child away for relief. Respite may need to be translated to these parents as a service mainly for the child, no matter how desperately the parents may need relief for themselves, in order for parents, relatives, and neighbors to accept the value of such service.

When the system fails the handicapped member and the family there is a tendency to blame the victim, the unserved and underserved families in need of respite (Horejsi, 1979). Clients with severe handicaps are too few, too difficult, and too costly, and they do not fit into the existing service system (Cutler, 1983). The families are too overprotective, too distrusting, and unappreciative of professional efforts to locate services. Yet, families who live daily with their handicapped member know what they need and feel. They need professional and community support in finding and developing services appropriate to the special needs of their handicapped family member; they need professional acceptance of their concerns, needs, and feelings (Donnellan & Mirenda, 1984; Vincent, Brown, & Davis, 1983; Wikler, Wasow, & Hatfield, 1983).

How Current Models Fail

A number of models of respite care have been developed: in-home care provided by respite workers and home health aides and out-of-home care provided by individual respite workers, respite foster families, and an occasional bed in a group home. Some of these services may partially meet some of the respite needs of the client with severe handicaps, but most tend to underserve or exclude the severely handicapped client because: 1) the settings and services are inappropriate to the clients' needs, 2) the staff are either inadequately trained and/or have little or no timely back-up or support for crises and difficulties, and 3) the amount of respite time allocated to people with severe needs is inadequate (Cutler, 1985).

In-Home Models of Care   Some parents who have tried in-home care have reported that the worker was inadequately prepared (Cohen & Warren, 1985; Upshur, 1982) and/or was reluctant or refused to come again. Others have found that workers who do return only provide sitting services because they lack experience with clients with severe disorders and may not know how to engage them in productive activities despite the parents' suggestions. The parents would like their child to be out walking or engaging in some ordinary community activity, but the worker may be reluctant to leave the security of the home, and so they sit, client and worker, waiting, perhaps anxiously, for the parents' return. The bad effects of this arrangement are that: 1) the parents are supposed to be enjoying their break while they instead worry about their child's boredom or unhappiness and 2) an opportunity to reduce the client's dependency on the parents by the worker taking the client into the community is missed. If the parents are the only ones who can or dare to take their handicapped member outside their home, then the message to the child is, "Only your parents can take care of you." The sitter-companion model, which works well for adolescents and adults with moderate handicaps, could be used more often with persons with more severe disabilities to supplement residential respite care if workers were more competent and confident in working with hard-to-serve clients.

For example, a single mother of a 35-year-old man with autism complained that the only workers available to her were 20-year-old women who came to sit in the home. She wanted a male companion for her son who would engage him in community activities. Although severely handicapped by definition (i.e., autism) her son had functional language and community skills. After a recent hospitalization, she sought residential respite care for her son during her recuperation. She was told that the agency could provide only the same service she had received in the past—a young female sitter—when in fact a residential respite care center willing to accept people with problems similar to her son's was less than 20 miles away. Despite family need, the agency persisted in offering the standard model of care, which in this case resulted in no service.

Home health aides, a popular alternative because of available Medicaid funding, are generally trained to work within the home, but are usually not trained to work with persons who are aggressive or self-abusive. The problems are the same as those as noted with sitter-companions.

More than one parent has been told by respite agencies, "We will fund care for your child, if you can find someone willing to work with him; we have no one on our roster who is capable or willing to do so." Other parents, knowing the extremes of their child's behavior (particularly adolescents and adults) are reluctant to leave their child with only one person to provide care when, in their own experience, there have been times when two people were scarcely able to manage the care. Agencies are reluctant to fund two workers for one client even when appropriate and necessary. The result is often that no respite is provided in some of the most difficult cases.

For all these reasons, parents of persons with severe disabilities reject or are rejected by in-home respite care services. Parents who care for their child day after day have difficulty understanding why there is not someone or someplace that can provide care for their child for a week, weekend, or even a day. They feel the rejection of their children and themselves deeply and personally (Goffman, 1963; Kozloff, 1979; Vine, 1982).

Out-of-Home Models of Care Prevailing out-of-home models fare little better in meeting the needs of severely handicapped clients. A significant minority (40%) of families prefer out-of-home care (Cohen & Warren, 1985). In an effort to develop less restrictive models to meet this demand there has been an overreliance on certain models because they are perceived as less costly and less restrictive. Yet, in the long run, not offering the array of supports families need may prove to be both more costly and more restrictive for persons with severe handicaps (Baroff, 1980; Bruininks et al., 1980; Loop, 1980).

Both individual provider's homes and respite care foster homes face the same difficulties (i.e., caregivers may have little or no experience in dealing with severe behavior problems, and they frequently have no timely support or back-up). Although most foster families have the asset of having two adults available, as compared to the individual in-home worker, in some of them their own children can become a concern should the client begin to act out. Besides being naturally protective of their children, respite providers are also understandably protective of their homes. If the client acts out in ways that threaten the surroundings (e.g., feces smearing) or the members of the provider's family (e.g., severe physical aggression), that behavior can signal the end of the respite relationship. The family may be called to remove the client, or the list of transgressions is presented on their arrival, with the usual implications for future care.

Community residences (group homes) are occasionally used to meet residential respite needs. The program's obligations to its residents must be considered first; it is, after all, the residents' home, and particular consideration must be given when the respite client is a stranger to the residents (Lash, 1983). The group home's primary purpose is to provide a home for its clients, whereas respite care is a primary service for the respite care client. Programs that try to meet two primary needs generally fail to meet either or both. Either the residents' personal lives are disrupted, or the respite client's personal needs may be neglected.

The exception, and one closer to normal living conditions, is to provide a respite stay in a community residence to a known client (classmate or worker) who may be under consideration for a permanent place in the residence. Nonhandicapped people have overnight guests whom they know and value. Similar conditions should exist for people with handicaps. When the respite client is a stranger to the program, his or her needs may not be fully recognized; and the respite experience may be uncomfortable enough to discourage parents using that service again or the program from offering it.

Camp programs can and have provided effective respite for families, especially when parents see the camp as a place that provides the camper with new skills and experiences. However, many camps reject the client with behavioral difficulties or return the client before the promised period is ended, usually for lack of staff, knowledge, or experience with the disability and unrealistic expectations of the client. There need to be more camps with age-appropriate programs for adolescents and adults. Because, for the desperate family a wait of 6 months can seem endless and 12 months may be impossible, spring, fall, and winter camping programs should be developed.

Institutional respite care is not a viable alternative for most families, although some professionals and parents (Aanes & Whitlock, 1975; Fernald, 1984) are looking toward future and/or expanded use of institutions as respite centers. If it were desirable or even acceptable, many families who are struggling daily for survival would have sought permanent institutional placement earlier. A few families in extreme emergencies have been forced to use institutions for respite, but, according to institutional staff, some families who brought their children to the institution ostensibly for respite care refused to pick them up when the respite was formally ended. Thus institutional respite care has been a vehicle for gaining institutional admission by default; and burned-out parents have been forced to dissemble in order to gain permanent "relief."

Additional Service Problems

Two system problems that interfere with the delivery of adequate respite care are *lack of transportation* (Upshur, 1982) and *allocation of service*. Transportation problems affect most strongly poor families of persons with all levels of handicaps, but create more difficulties for those with more severe handicaps. It may be difficult or impossible for a parent to travel on public transportation with his or her handicapped son or daughter. Or there may be few cars in the neighborhood and even fewer offers of help. For families with more moderate incomes, the individual parent may have difficulty transporting the respite client by him- or herself. If the client requires a transportation monitor when going to school or the day program for reasons of safety, it should be obvious that the parent requires that same assistance. Because a client has no means of safe transportation to a respite care program it should not be assumed that the client doesn't need a program or the family is not interested in respite care. Transportation needs must be considered in the planning of respite care.

The second problem is the allocation of amounts of respite service to families of persons with severe handicaps. According to Warren (1983), all states allocate respite care equally, without any significant regard for client or family need. Although this system may reflect a concern for distributing scarce resources, the client at greatest risk of institutionalization, usually the behaviorally disordered adolescent or adult (Lakin, Hill, Hauber, & Bruininks, 1982) is treated at the same level of service as younger, less handicapped, and more easily manageable clients, and then only if willing providers can be found. Individual respite agency administrators will confess that they try to use year-end savings or unused respite care to help their most needy families, but they regret and even resent the circuitous routes they must use to do this when the need is so apparent. Any rational policy for distribution of respite resources must take into account family status and need, as well as client's age and degree of difficulty (Cutler, 1985).

Despite workers' efforts, more public recognition of respite needs, and more funding of respite care, the problems of families for persons with severe handicaps in gaining access to respite care persist. To many of the problems discussed in this section, there are exceptions. When creative solutions to the models' usual failures are working appropriately and well for individuals, these exceptions should be continued and supported. However, it is clear from agency and parent reports that a significant number of families of persons with severe handicaps are being failed by the system. Another model must be developed and supported in the respite system, a model that can provide direct and indirect benefits to those with less severe handicaps, as well as meet the urgent needs of the more disabled population. That model is the small community-based residential respite care center.

MODEL OF RESIDENTIAL RESPITE CARE

Residential respite care is an essential component of the respite care system for meeting the needs of families of persons with severe handicaps. It has been viewed by agencies, providers, and other professionals as costly and restrictive; this perspective has limited and, in many cases, effectively denied the delivery of services to low-incidence, high-risk people and their families (Cutler & Helm, in press). It is time that the advantages of residential respite to the hard-to-serve clients and its benefits to the larger disabled population be recognized.

Residential respite care can serve as the core of a respite system, thus maximizing its training benefits, or it can be a separate component of the system. However, for that group of persons who have not been served by current models, its existence is necessary for their long-term survival in the community and as functioning members of their families.

There are a few community-based residential respite programs throughout the country (Cohen & Warren, 1985; Kenney, 1982; Schmickel, 1981). Most of these programs are small (four beds), and most reserve one bed for emergencies. This discussion is based on a community respite residence that the author was instrumental in developing.

Physical Dimensions

The setting can be a house or apartment(s) in a city/town that serves a larger geographical community from which clients can be drawn and that is within reasonable commuting distance for its clients. It resembles other community dwellings in that it has the kitchen, bathroom, living, and sleeping facilities in the usual arrangements of homes. In serving adolescents and adults, it has been found that single bedrooms are effective in reducing expected behavioral difficulties: 1) Usually the client with a history of acting-out behavior has his or her own room at home, regardless of the arrangements for other children in the family, and 2) if a client is having difficulty, staff can work with that client without disrupting another client in the same room. Furthermore the client benefits from being treated as a person who has achieved adult status. Most nonhandicapped adults without mates have their own rooms. Because four to five bedrooms are needed, a single house or duplex may be used, although two apartments could be combined. Because the setting is home-like, it offers natural opportunities to clients to engage in or learn those activities, self-help skills, and chores common to their homes.

If possible, the respite center should be located near public transportation so that all families can have access to their children staying in the program, even if the client needs special transportation arrangements. Easy access to transportation will allow staff to engage certain clients in a wider range of community activities.

The facility should be known to the local hospital and have made arrangements for any medical emergencies.

Staffing and Training

The basic staffing pattern in this model has been one respite worker to two clients at any given time; thus, for a four-bed respite center with a full-time program director who is on call for emergencies (and other problems that have not yet become emergencies) the ratio is better than 2:1. An assistant director shares the 24-hour responsibility for meeting staff and client needs.

Before accepting clients into the program, all staff receive training in emergency care, first aid, physical intervention techniques, and instructional techniques for a range of ages, disabilities, and degrees of severity. For the first half-year of the program's operation, training should be limited to the center's staff. In the second half of the year, training can be extended to other providers interested in working with hard-to-serve clients. Given the transitory nature of in-home service, it is critical that training and recruitment of providers be tied to a facility-based program so that many workers have the experience of hands-on supervised training. For those workers who intend to meet the needs of the more disabled/behaviorally disordered clients in less supported settings (i.e., the client's or worker's home), direct supervised experience is even more important.

There are some extensive book and lecture training models currently available (ENCOR Respite Provider Training Manual [Cahill & Vohoska, n.d.]; Montana Training Manual [Lukenbill et al., n.d.]; Respite Project of Central New York [Edinger, Schultz, & Morse, 1984]; Temporary Care Services Respite Care Manual [Cobb et al., 1984]; University of Washington In-Home Respite Manuals [Edgar, Kenowitz, & Suizhacher, 1978]), but without exposure to real difficulties (seizures, aggression, etc.) isolated providers can become anxious or frightened the first time that they encounter such behavior in a private home. In the respite center, in addition to having other staff available and client records on hand, staff experience and are supported through such difficulties under the close supervision of a director and other experienced staff. Trained, experienced, and supported, some center workers will also be willing to provide occasional in-home relief to clients they have known in the program, especially if they feel connected to a center on which they can call for advice and back-up. Families who may want or require in-home care from time to time can feel assured that their children will be well cared for because: 1) the respite provider already knows their child and his or her history, 2) the family knows the provider has direct experience in working with the family member and similarly handicapped persons, and 3) they know the center is involved in the placement and will respond to the client's and worker's need for help.

If the residential center is at the core of the respite system, it can become a major training resource for large numbers of respite providers. With adequate training and back-up, even very handicapped people can be provided with occasional or even regular short-term care (day or evening) in the home when doing so meets the families' needs. Moreover, a person trained to work with clients with severe handicaps will also be capable of working with people with less severe handicaps. Finally, staff turnover does not exclude a client from service because the center is in continuous operation and has a core of trained providers to serve the client.

Clients: Setting Priorities

Given the additional expense of operating a continuous residential service and the program's special capacity to serve clients who can not be served or served well in other respite models, it is essential that the center set service priorities to guard against a tendency over time to serve clients with less critical needs who can be better or more appropriately served in other settings.

Working over the past 15 years with parents seeking services, the author has found it helpful to advise parents to ask providers first, "What clients does your agency exclude?" Programs that present themselves as offering service to clients with an array of difficulties and that then during intake tell parents that their clients must be toilet trained, have independent self-help skills, not be disruptive to other clients, and not have any medical needs requiring medication or nursing care, cause still more pain and suffering to parents to have once more invested time and energy in seeking service. Constant rejection drains parents of both the energy and self-esteem they need to survive (Farber, 1979; Goffman, 1963; Kozloff, 1979; Vine, 1982). In the initial contact with families, the agency should state clearly whom it serves and under what conditions (e.g., schedules of client groupings, periods when client use of the program is low so that a hard-to-serve client can be worked in, and availability of additional or specialized staff).

Priorities for service to clients with severe disabilities can be developed in the following order:

1. Clients in medical or other family emergency
2. Clients who have been refused respite care and have no resources beyond their immediate family
3. Clients who have received minimal, marginal, or inappropriate service
4. Clients with less severe handicaps whose families are in crisis and who have no or limited resources at the time of the emergency

Families of persons with severe disabilities may live in a state of continual crisis, dealing day by day with difficulties that would stagger the average person. For example, a state legislator stopped at a home in time to see the behaviorally disordered adolescent son overturn the kitchen table during breakfast. The legislator was overwhelmed. The father told him, "Now you see why we need a break. All I want is to sleep a little later on Saturday morning, and then eat my breakfast and read my paper in peace." A modest request.

There are families who sleep in shifts and/or have locks on doors that are not locked in the average home. For these families the routine of turmoil, disruption, anxiety, and anguish has become their daily life. Only an illness, death, or other act of God is perceived as a "real crisis." These families may need other supports, but first they need planned respite care. Unless providers can prove through the provision of respite care that they are capable of managing the difficult client, they should not offer parent training programs in behavior modification or counseling for family members. If professionals cannot provide care, then what reason have the parents to believe that other offered interventions will be effective, especially when those other interventions make still more demand on the family's dwindling resources?

Although the families who live in routine crisis are second priority, those in the first priority are not likely to fill the four or so beds because their needs depend on "acts of God." Second priority clients will be the most frequent service recipients. The third priority, however, is an important one because, when clients are poorly served, families tend to use that service less. Coming home to find the client unhappy or anxious or the house a shambles does not generate more requests for respite. If parents understand that the worker is not coming back, they may not try to find another because workers are too hard to find, the search itself is an ordeal, and those who are finally located do not stay for long. Families with such experiences will after a time fit into the second priority.

Although it is possible that a parent can return to a center to find an unhappy child and a report of difficulties, it is less likely because staff are supervised, supported, and have extensive client information on hand.

The center should be responsive to less severely impaired clients when their families with limited networks and resources are in crisis states. If these priorities are adhered to, this group of clients will not impede the provision of service to clients with more severe handicaps.

It can be expected that the greatest demand will come from families of adults and adolescents, although there is a real but lesser demand for out-of-home care from parents of young children with severe disabilities. Because of the size of the program, it is possible to accommodate younger children and occasionally less disabled children in family crisis.

Although parents and other family members are clients of the center in that they receive the relief they seek, the disabled family member is the direct recipient of the program's care and thus the focal client in that his or her needs must be well met in order for the family to use and benefit from the service. Therefore, it is incumbent on the program to ensure that the handicapped client is safe, comfortable, and well cared for in ways that families can accept.

Outreach and Intake

To attract appropriate clients for the program, effective outreach to parents is essential. Obviously, as is indicated by the anecdotal material presented throughout this chapter, many families will have difficulty believing that their disabled family member will be accepted into the new respite program and will be kept there for the planned period of time. They need to be reassured that the program believes that they and their children are worthy of service and that the staff can provide the necessary care.

For example, a parent who several years ago sent her adolescent son to a residential respite camp after being assured many times by staff that her son was both appropriate and manageable, was called within 3 days to take her son home. Her son was and is still in a day program, proving that some people were able to work with him. But when the promise was broken, the experience was so painful that the mother, now a widow and relying on her daughter for help, refuses to seek respite care because, "No matter what they say, they won't keep him." Parents with similar experiences will be slow to apply to a new program that claims to serve hard-to-manage clients.

Yet, there are formal and informal ways to coax reluctant and/or rejected parents to a center that will keep its promise. The formal ways include setting up an advisory board that is composed of a majority of parents, including some parents who intend to use the services. Second, wherever possible, the program can hire a qualified parent as a staff member. One respite center has employed a parent experienced in direct care in a combined position of direct service, management, and outreach. In referring a parent to this program, it is more reassuring to a worried parent to say, "When you call the Center, be sure to talk to Roz. She's a parent." At that point there is usually a brightening in the parent's voice and the response, "Then she'll know what I'm talking about."

Informal parent-to-parent connections are also highly effective in reaching parents. The program should build and use its own informal network of parents to find those clients who match its priorities. Parents sharing "war stories" about life at home and the search for respite care can convince unserved and cautious parents that the program is established to meet the needs of families similar to theirs. Parent networks often encourage parents to try out the service; with good experiences, parents will return their sons and daughter for more extended stays. Once the connection is made, program staff must then demonstrate that the program can and will meet the needs of its clients and client-families for competent care and relief.

Intake is more than the usual information processing. Families' concerns, fears, and past experiences in accessing services must be given full consideration and respect (Donnellan & Mirenda, 1984). Although some families will immediately welcome a full week of respite, others will be more cautious and even distrusting. Because no one else could care for their child in the past, why should they expect this program to be any different? These families need to be invited to leave their son or daughter for just a few hours at this first respite. If they are reassured by the first experience, they may ask for a night or a weekend. Families who are allowed to move slowly into the service can become the program's best advocates and will bring other skeptical families in when those families learn that they have the option of gradually introducing their handicapped family member into the program. The gradual introduction is also in the client's best interest because he or she does not have to handle the stress of an extended separation at the outset. With successful service, the families are ready to plan further stays to meet their actual needs. Until parents ask to bring their children back for more and extended respite it is difficult to know if the services are adequate and appropriate to their needs.

Since respite care has become a viable service, the author has heard professionals use terms such as "overprotective," "guilt-ridden," and "you actually have to pry these kids away from their families," (without questioning why these terms might be partially or particularly true) when such statements as "concerned," "fearful," or "alienated" would have been less pejorative and more productive. Asking questions about fears and previous experiences can help the provider assist the parents in taking some first steps toward using a service they desperately need. It is ironic that parents can be seen as a liability in the provision of respite care when these are the people for whom the service was originally designed. Further, they can be a major resource in the provision of competent care, particularly for persons with severe disorders of communication and behavior.

Before the client comes into the program for the first short-term trial, an adequate history must be taken. For the client with severe handicaps, an adequate history must be extensive, especially with regard to that information that only the family can share (Beckman, 1984; Cutler, 1981). For example, in discussing such problems as crying, seizures, self-abuse, self-stimulation, and aggression, parents can be asked these questions: What times are the behaviors likely to occur, what events lead to the problem behaviors, can they tell when a behavior is coming and what are the signs, how long is the behavior likely to last, and what kinds of things do they do to prevent or cope with the problem behavior? The empathic worker can elicit much valuable information from the parents by first accepting information and then probing for more details. Desperate families without support can develop some unusual coping strategies (e.g., "since he likes baths, we give him a bath when he's upset and sometimes he has five baths in one day"; "she screams when the radio or TV is on so we keep them turned off but sometimes after she is finally asleep we sneak them on at a low volume"; or "he threatens to break windows when he doesn't like the food we give him so we give him what he wants"). These strategies may seem like poor or strange ways to live, but families have used them to survive with some success. Their difficulties and successes, however limited, must be acknowledged and respected. Respite care programs are not likely to develop or promote such strategies, but even staff, when they have exhausted their repertoire of methods and are feeling stressed, might say, "Let's give him a bath" or "give him one of those candy bars his mother packed." Without specific and extensive information, staff under pressure might not have these strange but potentially useful last-resort strategies.

Parents want to share the good things their children do, even when those things are done to excess (e.g., "she's wonderful about taking her medication, but of course, she'll swallow anything in sight that resembles a pill"; "he really plays the piano well, but he'll play all day or night so we keep it locked a lot of the time"; or "he can totally dress himself, but he has to do it his own way and you can't rush him"). There will be some surprises: The young man who lacks communication and self-help skills may be an accomplished swimmer. Some of these traits can be useful in identifying potential problems and in planning program activities. Although most of them may in the long run need shaping that is beyond the temporal capabilities of the program, staff can translate or expand them into useful learning activities.

Perhaps most important to the care of clients in the absence of their parents is the information learned from parents about how their children with limited communication skills express their needs or wants. It may be a list of 25 functional signs, or echolalic expressions that the person uses consistently to communicate in a particular context (Prizant, 1983), or physically disruptive behavior that brings the desired item or terminates an unpleasant (to the client) activity (Donnellan, Mirenda, Mesaros, & Fassbender, 1985).

Parents, more than anyone else, have useful and extensive information (Beckman, 1984; Cutler, 1981; Stancin, Reuter, Dunn, & Bickett, 1984; Vincent et al., 1983) if staff will use it or help the parent more clearly articulate it. No one expects the respite center to create exactly the conditions of a home whose members are struggling to survive or to have the same expectations of the client that the parents have, but staff can use the information for scheduling groups of clients, creative planning of activities, and coping with the behaviors that brought the client to the program in the first place.

The center should do more than routine intake; its staff should make a strenuous effort to elicit information from those poeple who are the most knowledgable (i.e., the parents). Information should also be gathered from other sources, including past and current records of service, medical records, and evaluations and assessments. Information should be updated regularly so that staff are aware of recent changes, both desired and undesirable. The reward for this exhaustive intake is that the client may present fewer and/or less severe behavior problems and may more easily engage in more productive activities. Program successes, especially those based on parent information, can be shared with parents: "She wouldn't eat her breakfast until I remembered what you told me about her favorite juice; then she ate everything so she could have the juice," or "he took his bath in a hurry when I told him his favorite TV show was coming on." These are the kinds of reports that make it easier for parents to come back for more respite care.

Primary and Secondary Program Functions

The primary functions of center-based care are to: 1) provide care to priority clients in a setting that is home-like, safe, and staffed by people who are trained and experienced in working with persons with severe disabilities, and that engages clients in activities that are familiar, pleasing, and based on their strengths and needs; and 2) provide other family members with relief that allows them to remain in their own homes if they choose that setting to recover from the demands of full-time care of their handicapped member. Both functions must be equally well served in order to meet the respite needs of families of persons with severe disabilities. If the family is not satisfied with the setting and quality, their respite care may be ineffective and/or they may resist using the service.

The respite center can have a number of secondary functions, depending on its location in the respite system, its support from the community, and the adequacy of its funding.

First, a function of significant benefit to the larger community of clients and respite providers is to provide hands-on supervised training to potential caregivers. For the program, it means additional staff on occasion and a roster of potential providers who can be matched to clients for occasional or even regular in-home relief. For the larger number of less disabled or younger clients, it means that parents, knowing that workers have had direct experience in their training, will be reassured that the respite worker is capable of handling difficulties that may arise (Cohen & Warren, 1985). For the worker, it means that he or she has tested competence, is prepared to deal with difficult situations, and is therefore less intimidated by the threat of predictable problems.

Second, the center can serve an *information and referral* function for families. It can help families find other forms of respite care when the program is filled through its extensive client information system and its knowledge of the wider respite system of providers. Or it can expand this function to provide referral to other services, specialists, and advocates (Downey, Castellani, & Tausig, 1985). Families who have been well served through the center's program will tend to trust and to look to the center staff for advice and direction. However, information and referral to low-incidence clients should include rigorous follow-up (Fearing, 1979). Otherwise the parents may experience the same rejection with which they are so familiar from other agencies.

Third, the center can fill a *coordinating role* in respite service based on its assessment of client and family needs. Staff can assist families in developing Individual Respite Plans to meet their needs. The Individual Respite Plan should be based on actual needs and not on the availibility of funds or staff (Cutler, 1979). Provision of services does of course depend on available resources, but the plan is the guide for meeting family needs. Creative planning can incorporate a combination of respite models: in-home, companion care, and center-based care. A reluctant family may be willing to try other forms of respite with familiar and experienced workers if they know that they are scheduled for regular relief at the center or that they may turn to the center when things are not working out.

These three secondary functions are directly related to the provision of adequate respite services. There are other secondary functions less directly related to respite care that can benefit both the families and the center. These are parent training, advocacy, and mutual support.

Parent training can be offered to families when the program is established and has a proven record of success in dealing with severely handicapped clients. Respite care, however, should not be provided contingent on training; such a condition can add still another burden to already overburdened families. But many parents who see that their children can be well managed, productive and relatively content at the center will be receptive to new educational and behavioral ideas, skills, and principles used successfully in the program with their children (Wikler & Hanusa, 1980); and after some service, they may be interested in training for themselves. Frequently new staff are understandably eager to change clients' behaviors. Given the intermittent short-term nature of the program, it is more beneficial to involve staff in data-based assessments, recording critical incidents, and in incidental teaching than in trying to establish formal programs that they cannot fully implement in the time the client is with them. The exception is when the program can provide an extended stay of several weeks; then a formal program may be undertaken. However most states do not allow such extended service; in those states that do, parents may be reluctant to use their full allocation of service all at one time (for fear of future emergencies) or to have such an extended separation from their son or daughter. Although change is not an intrinsic goal of the program, carefully collected staff observations, data, and anecdotal materials can lead to parents' interest in training and additionally to recommendations for other client services.

Advocacy, within the fiscal and staff constraints of the program, is another ancillary but vital service to families. Because the center provides 24-hour service to its clients, it accumulates extensive information about the clients that can be useful in the development of other service plans, such as IEPs (Individualized Education Plan) and ISPs (Individual Service Plan). If the program has the capacity and financial support, staff can attend meetings of other agencies with parents as family advocates. Staff have the potential for becoming effective advocates in that they know the clients and parents, they probably have little vested interest in the other agency, they are likely to be the professionals most trusted by parents, and they will be available to the parents over time because they will continue to provide an intermittent but regular service to families. Advocacy is not a central function of respite care, but given the center's knowledge and experience, it can provide a vital service to client and family.

Finally, a center that by its very nature provides regular service over time has an opportunity to *bring parents together* for support, information, and for acquiring skills to improve the quality of family life (Intagliata & Doyle,

1984; Pizzo, 1983) and reduce the risk of institutionalization. Parents of persons with severe handicaps have less opportunity to congregate through other services because they represent a low-incidence population. In helping parents form parent groups/networks there is also a direct advantage to the center; parents in contact with each other may become a nucleus of citizen support for the center's continued operation and funding.

Many of the functions described above overlap with case management services. The center can be an appropriate place to assist persons with severe handicaps and their families through case management if there is adequate support and funding. Families will turn to and tend to trust that agency that provides them with an ongoing, vital, and needed service.

PROBLEMS OF CENTER-BASED CARE

There are two major problems in developing community-based residential respite models; these problems derive from current attitudes of those who provide, fund, and promote respite care.

Cost

The first problem revolves around funding. "Money concerns engulf the problem. The state is well aware of the savings that derive from using respite care to encourage families to keep their disabled relatives at home and spare the state the expense of caring for them. Conversely, the state is apprehensive about the cost of paying for respite care. . . ." (*Boston Globe,* June 27, 1985, p. 20).

Residential respite care is seen as too costly and the small community-based center as even more costly. This argument holds only if one ignores client needs and focuses solely on the basic costs of different models of care. In that simple comparison, the maintenance of a center is considerably more expensive than the models that pay individual workers at an hourly rate. The continued maintenance of a facility can require substantial public funding. Yet such a limited view does not take into account other costs incurred when adequate respite care is not provided to families of low-incidence, hard-to-serve clients most at risk of institutionalization. Respite care for such clients in community residential centers is only a fraction of the cost of institutionalization (Loop, 1980) because respite, by definition, is a temporary and intermittent service. Compare 30 days, even 60 days, of residential care per year with the cost of year-round, long-term care at a state or private facility, and the expensive community alternative is clearly a cheaper and more cost-effective model.

The financial and human costs to families who receive marginal respite services or none are hard to measure. Morton (1978) and Bayley (1973) describe lives of restriction and isolation. Any attempt to try to quantify the actual costs of such lives would lead to lists of "might-have-been's," "maybe if's," and "too late's." We act as if we must operate respite care on a triage model, making a high priority of those families who have a high probability of community survival with minimal supports and a low priority of those families with major needs who have a low probability of community survival. Although the purpose in setting up respite care programs is to prevent needless institutionalization, we shrink from serving those who are most likely and soonest to be institutionalized (Suelzle & Keenan, 1981).

Professionals need to look at the reasons for this avoidance. Is it the greater effort demanded, more risk of failure, discomfort with clients with hard-to-manage behavior or their families who have made greater sacrifices than we would have made under the same conditions, or a belief that certain clients really belong in institutions? Cost alone is not sufficient to explain the resistance, lethargy, or disinterest in developing and supporting community-based respite residences. Such respite programs are, as are the clients they try to serve, orphans of the systems. Both are low-incidence entities without the numbers to develop popular support (Cutler, 1983) unless the larger community of parents and professionals recognizes that the needs of more severely handicapped people and their families are an important and legitimate priority and concern.

Institutions provide the most restrictive form of respite care (Salisbury & Griggs, 1983). Those who see the institution as part of a continuum of respite care and who refer clients who do not fit into current models of service to institutional respite should be aware of the costs inherent in legitimizing institutional care for persons who are still community clients, however marginally served. First, such acceptance provides institutions with another reason for their maintenance (i.e., as a last resort for people denied in the community). Second, it delivers the message to families that only the institution can provide care for their handicapped members, thus leading parents to believe that their children can only and must ultimately be served in the institution. This message may have the greatest, most far-reaching cost. Families may institutionalize out of hopelessness generated by community denial of service.

Many persons with severe handicaps are living on borrowed time. Even appropriate respite care programs can not guarantee that all persons with severe handicaps will continue to live outside institutions. But respite care in adequate amounts and appropriate settings can buy time for the families of persons with severe handicaps to find or develop more and better community services to meet the client's long-term needs. Restricting clients with severe disabilities to the institutions is an expensive option that undermines the claims of respite care providers and advocates to prevent institutionalization.

Problem of Restrictiveness

Next to institutions, center-based service is seen as the most restrictive option in the respite system (i.e., more restrictive than community residences, foster homes, and in-home care). However, as described above, the other models are often not available for families of high-risk clients. It is more restrictive to fit clients into programs that do not meet their and their families' needs and in which the client is merely tolerated and no beneficial social experience is provided to the client. Services that are not acceptable or available are the most restrictive "options." For respite care to succeed there must be services for hard-to-serve clients that families want to use.

The size of the community center is a major determinant of its degree of restrictiveness. A large center serving more than six clients at a time can become restrictive. Yet, the center model described in this chapter is smaller than the average group home (Bruininks et al., 1980), and therefore can be described as less restrictive than a community residence. Yet, restrictiveness is determined by more than program size; quality of interactions and activites are equally important determinants. For the hard-to-serve client the quality and effectiveness of the respite intervention may be better met in a small center than in the client's, worker's, or foster family's homes where interactions may be minimal, stressful, and/or counterproductive for the reasons described above. Degrees of restrictiveness are better measured in the context of the clients' and families' needs; the physical dimensions of the setting; adequacy of staffing patterns, skills, support, and supervision; availability of client information; appropriateness of activities for the client; and the feelings of security families have about the program. When both the clients' and families' needs are met, that model of service that meets those needs is the least restrictive.

Communities without residential respite options can begin to test the advantages of community-based residential respite by using a core staff to set up part-time (weekend or seasonal) services in available facilities, such as religious retreat centers or college dormitories. Even part-time centers can offer training and support to develop a cadre of knowledgeable and competent respite workers both for providing center-based care and for increasing more appropriate and beneficial forms of home-based care to supplement the center.

There is a risk to the respite community in ignoring the needs of families of hard-to-serve clients. Their dramatic stories helped move legislators to fund respite care. Yet today legislators are still receiving calls from desperate families who are not being served by the system. Some of them are bewildered; some of them are angry. They thought that the most needy would be served.

Issues of cost and restrictiveness have been raised as obstacles to the development of community-based respite centers. The real obstacles, however, may be the attitudes of the service community that tend to ignore the needs and in effect deny adequate service to low-incidence, high-risk persons and their families. In the words of one middle-level bureaucrat who denied funding to a community respite residence, "Of course, there'll always be people who won't be served." Without funding, without concern, without commitment, he will, of course, be proven right (Cutler, 1983).

CONCLUSION

Because respite care was developed to support families and prevent institutionalization and because popular models of respite services are not meeting the needs of persons with severe handicaps, small community-based residential respite centers should be recognized as an important component of any respite care system. Respite centers can meet the needs of clients with severe behavioral and communication difficulties, a population that to date has been marginally served or not at all.

Benefits to the clients and families include regularly scheduled out-of-home respite, enabling families with little physical, emotional, or financial resources to leave their homes, to use their respite time in their homes if they so choose. Families further benefit from knowing that their handicapped members are in small home-like settings that are well staffed and supervised. As families develop trust in a center's capacity to serve their sons or daughters, they may be referred to or provided with additional basic services, such as parent training, parent support groups, and advocacy. Clients are served in small, controlled settings by staff who are experienced in working with similar clients and are knowledgeable about clients' strengths and needs. They are provided with age-appropriate, meaningful, productive, and pleasing activities during their stays. Clients can return to familiar and comfortable settings for future respite services, and they may be occasionally served in the community by respite workers trained and supported by the centers.

To the wider respite care community, centers offer opportunities for supervised, hands-on training in serving clients with severe disabilities. They also serve as back-up emergency care for less disabled persons whose families have limited resources.

Arguments against the development and funding of community based residential centers usually revolve around issues of cost and restrictiveness. However, these arguments neither stand up against the reality of unmet needs of clients and families nor against the high risk of institutionalization of persons with severe disabilities.

Both community respite facilities and low-incidence, high-risk clients are the orphans of the respite system. In order for poorly-served clients to be served adequately and appropriately, the respite care community must make the small community respite residence a priority of the system.

REFERENCES

Aanes, D., & Whitlock A. (1975). A parental relief program for the mentally retarded. *Mental Retardation, 13*(3), 36–38.

Arizona Division of Developmental Disabilities and Mental Retardation Services. *Family support services: Respite-sitter-in-home program handbook.* Phoenix, AZ.

Apolloni, A., & Trieste, G. (1983). Respite services in California: Status and recommendations for improvement. *Mental Retardation, 21*(6), 240–243.

Baroff, G. (1980). On "size" and the quality of residential care: A second look. *Mental Retardation, 18*(3), 113–118.

Bayley, M. (1973). *Mental handicap and community care: A study of mentally handicapped people in Sheffield.* London: Routledge & Kegan Paul.

Beckman, P. (1984). Perceptions of young children with handicaps: A comparison of mothers and program's staff. *Mental Retardation, 22*(4), 176–181.

Blacher, J. (1984). Sequential stages of parental adjustment. *American Journal of Mental Deficiency, 22*(2), 55–68.

Blacher, J., & Meyers, C. (1983). A review of attachment formation and disorder of handicapped children. *American Journal of Mental Deficiency, 87*(4), 359–371.

Boggs, E. (1979). Economic factors in family care. In R. Bruininks & G. Krantz (Eds.), *Family care of developmentally disabled members: Conference proceedings* (pp. 47–62). Minneapolis: University of Minnesota.

Bruininks, R. (1979). The needs of families. In R. Bruininks & G. Krantz (Eds.), *Family care of developmentally disabled members: Conference proceedings* (pp. 3–12). Minneapolis: University of Minnesota.

Bruininks, R., Hauber, F., & Kudla, M. (1980). National survey of community residential facilities and residents in 1977. *American Journal of Mental Deficiency, 84*(5), 470–478.

Cahill, N., & Vohoska, D. (n.d.). *ENCOR respite provider training manual.* Omaha: Eastern Nebraska Community Office of Retardation.

Cobb, P., Gurry, S., Hall, H., Jones, S., Monnin, D., Weinberger, E., & Williams, G. (1984). *The respite care manual.* Cambridge, MA: Temporary Care Services.

Cohen, S., & Warren, R. (1985). *Respite care: Principles, programs & policies.* Austin, TX: Pro-Ed.

Cutler, B. (1979, June 5). *Keynote address.* Massachusetts Developmental Disabilities Conference on Respite Care, Boston.

Cutler, B. (1981). *Unraveling the special education maze.* Champaign, IL: Research Press.

Cutler, B. (1983). *The erosion of an essential service: Regional respite care.* Paper prepared for the Massachusetts Department of Mental Health. Boston: Autism Services Association.

Cutler, B. (1985, November). *Respite care: An essential community service for families of persons with developmental disabilities.* Presentation to the University Affiliated Facility at the University of Medicine and Dentistry, Rutgers Medical School.

Cutler, B., & Helm, D. (in press). Training parents to access essential services. In

J. Mulick, & R. Antonak, (Eds.), *Transitions in mental retardation.* AAMD Northeast Monograph.

Cutler, B., & Kozloff, N. (in press). Living with autism: Effects on families and family needs. In D. Cohen, A. Donnellan, & R. Paul (Eds.), *Handbook of autism and disorders of atypical development.* New York: John Wiley & Sons.

Donnellan, A., & Mirenda, P. (1984). Issues related to professional involvement with families of individuals with autism and other severe handicaps. *Journal of Association for Persons with Severe Handicaps, 9*(1), 16–25.

Donnellan, A., Mirenda, P., Mesaros, R., & Fassbender, L. (1984). Analyzing the communicative functions of aberrant behavior. *Journal of Association for Persons with Severe Handicaps, 9*(3), 201–212.

Downey, N., Castellani, P., & Tausig, M. (1985). The provision of information & referral services in the community. *Mental Retardation, 23,*(1), 21–25.

Edgar, E., Kenowitz, K., & Suizhacher, S. (1978). *University of Washington in-home respite manuals.* Joint publication of the University of Washington, American Red Cross, and the Division of Developmental Disabilities.

Edinger, B., Schultz, B., & Morse, M. (1984). *Final report.* Syracuse: Respite Project of Central New York.

Editorial: Respite for heroic families. (1985, June 27). *Boston Globe,* p. 20.

Farber, B. (1979). Sociological ambivalence and family care. In R. Bruininks & G. Krantz (Eds.), *Family care of developmentally disabled members: Conference proceedings* (pp. 27–36). Minneapolis: University of Minnesota.

Fearing, F. (1979). Case management/advocacy for the autistic individual. In J. Gilliam (Ed.), *Autism: Diagnosis, instruction, management and research* (pp. 181–204). Austin: University of Texas.

Fernald State School. (1984). *Outwords, 3*(3), 3.

Goffman, E. (1963). *Stigma: Notes on the management of spoiled identity.* Englewood Cliffs, NJ: Prentice-Hall.

Goldenberg, A. (1984). *Respite services for persons with autism.* Paper presented at the 11th annual Northeast Regional Conference on Autism, Lincoln, RI.

Hagen, J., Reasnor, R., & Jensen, S. (1980). *Report on respite care services in Indiana.* South Bend: Northern Indiana Health Systems Agency.

Horejsi, C. (1979). Social and psychological factors. In R. Bruininks & G. Krantz (Eds.), *Family care of developmentally disabled members: Conference proceedings* (pp. 13–26). Minneapolis: University of Minnesota.

Intagliata, J., & Doyle, N. (1984). Enhancing social support for parents of developmentally disabled children: Training in interpersonal problem solving skills. *Mental Retardation. 22*(1), 4–11.

Joyce, K., Singer, M., & Isralowitz. (1983). Impact of respite care on parents' perceptions of quality of life. *Mental Retardation. 21*(4), 153–156.

Kenney, M. (1982). *Giving families a break: Strategies for respite care.* Omaha: University of Nebraska Medical Center.

Kozloff, M. (1979). *A Program for families of children with learning and behavior problems.* New York: John Wiley & Sons.

Lakin, K., Hill, K., Hauber, F., & Bruininks, R. (1982). Changes in age at first admission to residential care for mentally retarded people. *Mental Retardation. 20*(5), 216–225.

Lash, M. (1983). *Respite care: The development of a preventive support service for families under stress.* Boston: Massachusetts Department of Social Services.

Loop, B. (1980). *Family resources services and support services for families with handicapped children*. Omaha: University of Nebraska Medical Center, Meyer Children's Rehabilitation Institute.

Lotter, V. (1978). Follow-up studies. In M. Rutter & E. Schopler (Eds.), *Autism: A reappraisal of concepts and treatment* (pp. 475–495). New York: Plenum Publishing Corp.

Lukenbill, R., Lillie, B., Sanddal, N., Hulme, J., Calkins, C., & McKibben, M. (n.d.). *Respite care training manual*. Helena: Montana Developmental Disabilities Training Institute.

Morton, K. (1978). Identifying the enemy—a parent's complaint. In A. Turnbull & R. Turnbull, III, (Eds.), *Parents speak out* (pp. 142–148). Columbus, OH: Charles E. Merrill Publishing Co.

Oppenheim, J., & Upshur, C. (1978). *Final report of the respite care policy development project*. Boston: Massachusetts Developmental Disabilities Council.

Pizzo, P. (1983). *Parent to parent: Working together for ourselves and our children*. Boston: Beacon Press.

Prizant, B. (1983). *Recent trends on communication research, assessment and intervention*. Paper presented at the annual conference of the National Society for Children and Adults with Autism, Salt Lake City, UT.

Salisbury, C., & Griggs, P. (1983). Developing respite care for families of handicapped persons. *Journal of the Association for Persons with Severe Handicaps*. *8*(1), 50–58.

Schmickel, A. (1981). *Respite Resources, 1*(1).

Stancin, T., Reuter, J., Dunn, V., & Bickett, L. (1984). Validity of caregiver information on the developmental status of severely braindamaged young children. *American Journal of Mental Deficiency, 88*(4), 388–395.

Suelzle, M., & Keenan, V. (1981). Changes in family support networks over the life cycle of mentally retarded persons, *American Journal of Mental Deficiency, 86*(3) 267–274.

Upshur, C. (1982). Respite care for mentally retarded and other disabled populations: program models and family needs. *Mental Retardation, 29*(1), 2–6.

Vincent, L., Brown, P., & Davis, J. (1983, November). *Parents as assessors of their children's developmental status and ongoing progress*. Paper presented at the 10th annual TASH Conference, San Francisco, CA.

Vine, P. (1982). *Families in pain: Children, siblings, spouses and parents of the mentally ill speak out*. New York: Pantheon.

Wikler, L. (1983). Chronic stresses of families of mentally retarded children. In L. Wikler & M. Keenan (Eds.), *Developmental disabilities: No longer a private tragedy*. Joint Publication of National Association of Social Workers and the American Association on Mental Deficiency.

Wikler, L., & Hanusa, D. (1980). *The impact of respite care on stress in families of developmentally disabled children*. Paper presented at the annual meeting of the American Association on Mental Deficiency.

Wikler, L., Wasow, M., & Hatfield, E. (1983). Seeking strengths in families of developmentally disabled children. In Wikler, L. & Keenan, M. (Eds.), *Developmental disabilities: No longer a private tragedy*. Joint Publication of the National Association of Social Workers and the American Association on Mental Deficiency.

Chapter 10

GENERIC COMMUNITY SERVICES AS SOURCES OF RESPITE

Christine L. Salisbury

Community services that provide opportunities for children to participate in activities outside the home serve a respite function by affording parents the time to engage in recreational, vocational, and/or avocational pursuits. The concept of a "secondary respite effect" has been used to refer to this outcome (Cohen, 1982; Salisbury, November, 1983).

The premise of this chapter is that integrated, generic community services can serve as an important source of social support (i.e., respite) to families of children with disabilities. Furthermore, there are compelling reasons why the integration and expansion of generic services should be considered a priority by policymakers, parents, professionals, and community service providers. This chapter departs from most of the literature on integration and mainstreaming by its focus on nonschool settings and the respite outcome that can accrue to the parent when services are provided to the child.

NATURE OF COMMUNITY RESOURCES

Generic Services

Kenowitz, Gallaher, and Edgar (1977) define generic services as typical services that families with nonhandicapped children either receive outright or are able to purchase for a standard price. Given the subsidized or competitive pricing of such services, Kenowitz and colleagues characterize generic services as organized to serve the greatest number of people at the lowest cost.

Communities generally offer the following services to the public: medical, dental, child care, financial, educational, mass transportation, and recreational activities. These services address the common needs of the public and are structured in such a fashion as to serve heterogeneous populations. Why then are many of these services not accessible to children with disabilities and their families? What attempts have been made to integrate nonschool community resources? What are the factors that influence families' access to and use of generic community resources?

Specialized Services

Specialized services are those developed specifically for members of one group, such as children with handicaps, because their needs, or the ways in which their needs can be met, are assumed to be very different from the needs or strategies used by others (Laten, 1981). These specialized services include special diagnostic and medical care, federally subsidized income programs, special education, special transportation systems, camps and scout troups for handicapped children, and specialized sporting events.

The specialized services model carries an implicit assumption that the methodologies and materials used in clinical and educational programs are uniquely suited to those settings and provide the most effective means of facilitating the student's acquisition of skills. This aptitude-treatment-interaction premise lacks both empirical and social support (Lloyd, 1984). Although professionals have developed improved strategies for enhancing the transfer of information from instructional to applied settings, outcomes have been limited to selected types of skills and settings. In addition, there has been little evidence to support the relationship of skills taught in segregated settings to those required and/or expected in complex community environments (Brown, Nietupski, & Hamre-Nietupski, 1976). Process and outcome research in all phases of individualized instruction, transfer of training, and transition is greatly needed to enable us to work better with all children in a variety of school and nonschool settings.

IMPACT OF COMMUNITY RESOURCES

Presence of Resources

Informal networks made up of friends, neighbors, and kin are used more frequently by families with handicapped and nonhandicapped children than are formalized agency services (Gallagher, Cross, & Scharfman, 1981; Unger & Powell, 1980; Venters, 1981). These resources are used for seeking information, providing services, and/or confirming actions of individuals in solving problems. However, it not clear whether the preference of families of disabled children for informal supportive resources has evolved out of choice or because of the lack of other available options.

Community services are part of the family's social network and play a key role in enhancing individual and family adaptation and coping (Geismar,

1971). According to Geismar's conceptualization of community resources, access to and use of such services support the survival and maintenance functions of the family unit (i.e., employment, food, shelter, medical services). Furthermore, community resources can facilitate social participation, social control, mobility, and social and political expression and can enhance the family's living arrangements. These resources are best seen as the social structures and institutions of our society, those that comprise the social context in which the family system operates. Kenowitz et al. (1977) suggest that these community resources are those that "typical families take for granted and consider a necessary part of everyday life" (p. 31). Families with developmentally disabled members cannot rely on the same extrafamilial resources because many of those services are unwilling and/or unable to serve persons with disabilities. This pattern results in a constricture in the social support networks of these families.

Researchers have investigated the size and effectiveness of social networks in families with handicapped children. In general, these families are found to have smaller informal social support systems compared to their nonhandicapped counterparts (Friedrich & Friedrich, 1981; Kazak & Marvin, 1984). However, the effectiveness of these more tightly knit, but smaller networks, is generally found to be unrelated to size or density (Dunst, Trivette, & Cross, 1986; Gallagher et al., 1981; Kazak & Marvin, 1984).

Many families with developmentally disabled children perceive their informal resources as insufficient to mediate the effects of parenting stress (Bristol, in press; Dunst et al., 1986; Gallagher et al., 1981). Stress in these families appears to be related to the chronological age of the child, general parenting issues, and the caregiving demands posed by the child (Bristol, in press; Gallagher, Scharfman, & Bristol, 1984; Kazak & Marvin, 1984; Korn, Chess, & Fernandez, 1978). In this situation, high levels of unresolved stress can create problems on the interpersonal, individual, and family levels (Hill, 1958; Minuchin, 1974). The smaller social support networks of these families may have a "capacity" or "mediational load" that may be exceeded by the demands presented by the child. Enhancing network density and diversity may prove to be a useful strategy for assisting families whose resources are overextended and are no longer effective in mediating stress.

Other families report that they are adjusting and/or are assessed as adapting to parenting stresses, yet stress levels remain high. As several researchers have pointed out, strategies that meet the needs of particular family units should not be labeled as "deviant" or "abnormal" simply because they do not fit the mode (cf. Gallagher et al., 1984; Kazak & Marvin, 1984). What is of concern, however, are the long-term effects of high levels of stress on the individuals within these families. The need-meeting resources of these parents may have reached "mediational load," forcing them to accommodate to a high-stress life-style. These families would seem to be at-risk for physical and/or emotional difficulties over the long run.

Community resources can influence the family's ability to maintain a dependent family member in the natural home (Robinson & Robinson, 1976; Seltzer & Krauss, 1984; Sherman & Coccozza, 1984). Formal and informal family support services can reduce stress by augmenting existing family resources. These services tend to cluster into: 1) services provided to families that are intended to assist them psychologically, instrumentally, or economically and/or 2) services provided to the children to improve their manageability, thereby making them more acceptable to their families (Seltzer & Krauss, 1984).

These "supports" can, however, influence the parents' decision to pursue out-of-home residential placement. As Rowitz (1974) noted,

> the family must be seen as part of a community network made up of other families, schools, churches, businesses, public and private agencies and so on. Each of these community sources may put pressures on a given family to make certain decisions concerning a deviant family member. (p. 411)

Evidence exists to link the child's level of independence/functioning to the type of residential placement. Children who are less dependent on adults for care and supervision are generally placed in community residential facilities where integration in the community is important in making the placement a successful one (Seltzer & Krauss, 1984; Willer & Intagliata, 1985). Preparation for community nonschool social, work, and living environments can be critical for the long-term welfare of both the child and his or her family.

There is some indication that using generic services can be more stressful for parents than using specialized resources. The impact of integration on the child into nonschool community activities is as yet unknown. However, mainstreaming is one example of a generic service where the daily reminders of the discrepancy between the handicapped child's abilities and those of his or her nonhandicapped peers can be difficult for the parents, despite the service's educational advantages for the child (Winton & Turnbull, 1981). Kenowitz et al. (1977) provide evidence of potential financial stress that can be posed by generic transportation and dental services that are presumably available to handicapped children and adults. Prohibitive fees or stringent eligibility guidelines preclude many families from using "available" generic community services. Thus, barriers exist in many communities to the use of potentially supportive resources by families with handicapped children. Although the nature of these barriers is not clearly documented, general themes from the literature are examined in a subsequent section of this chapter.

Absence of Resources

The absence of services, as well as their use, can be stressful for parents. Bristol and Schopler (1984) specifically identified "the lack of trained babysitters as a source of stress . . . reported by parents of children of all ages" (p. 114). Babysitters and other community child care services are only one of several types of generic resources that are generally not available to parents of disabled children. Other services that have been known to serve disabled children and their families differentially include medical, dental, insurance, religion, restaurants, transportation, social, and beauty/barber (Kenowitz et al., 1977).

One outcome of community resource deprivation for both parents and children is dependency. Children who are not, for example, taught the skills necessary to secure community employment or function in the YMCA recreation program remain dependent on the family unit for maintenance and socialization. Although any family serves maintenance and support functions for its members, the chronicity of the child's dependence for more needs, for far longer periods of time creates additional stress on the family unit (Turnbull, Brotherson, & Summers, 1983). Without the mediating role of social supports, there is a higher probability that family functioning will be negatively affected.

Parents whose children cannot be served in appropriate day programs (e.g., child care, work, activity programs) are often precluded from employment and social opportunities (Boggs, 1979; Bristol & Schopler, 1984; Kenowitz et al., 1977; Seltzer & Krauss, 1984). The absence of economic and social opportunities can influence marital satisfaction, psychological well-being, and family integration (Friedrich & Friedrich, 1981; Hoffman & Manis, 1978). The availability and use of appropriate community resources can, however, mediate the effects of stressor events and enhance the economic self-sufficiency and resilience of the family unit (McCubbin et al., 1980; Unger & Powell, 1980).

CURRENT PRACTICES

A gap between what is philosophically or educationally desirable and actual practice exists in many communities. Kenowitz et al. (1977) described the discrepancy between the ideal, as elaborated above, and reality in many communities. They observed that "it is paradoxical to train the handicapped to use public transportation if they are denied access to or face obstacles in using such services" (p. 31). They go on to discuss a range of generic services that were not available to children with handicaps in several communities in the Northwest (e.g., child care, insurance, religion, transportation, recreation). However, Kenowitz and colleagues do not argue for the proliferation of specialized services as a response to diminished generic service opportunities. Rather, they suggest that the margin between availability and use of existing generic services can be reduced by emphasizing the community's responsibility to persons with developmental disabilities and the obligation of the educational system to prepare these individuals appropriately for life in the community. However, specialized services must still exist to serve the unique needs of handicapped children and their families.

A generally accepted premise of educational and habilitative services in communities across this country is that, within the context of specialized settings, handicapped children should be taught the skills necessary to enable them to function effectively in a broad range of community settings. The strategies chosen to teach the skills inherent in this goal vary across agencies and communities, as do the criteria used to evaluate the outcomes of program efforts. Two dominant approaches have emerged in recent years that serve as both philosophical and instructional referents for designing, developing, and evaluating community-based services for handicapped children and their families.

The principle of normalization (Wolfensberger, 1972) suggests that, to the extent possible: 1) individuals with developmental disabilities be taught to function in normalized settings, 2) that the content of what is taught be that which nonhandicapped individuals are expected to perform, and 3) that the community be required to make typical services and opportunities available to persons with disabilities.

The criterion of ultimate functioning (Brown et al., 1976) and the criterion of the next environment (Vincent et al., 1980) suggest that educational programs must focus their efforts on preparing students to function effectively in subsequent school and nonschool environments. These criteria imply that the content of instruction will necessarily be based on an assessment of expectations and performance competencies in the natural environment. Further, they presume that instruction in nonschool settings is important to ensuring student success in the community. Logically, the execution of these principles is predicated on the availability of training opportunities and support within the community sector.

Recently, there has been growing concern among professionals that specialized recreational programs and events may accentuate the disabilities of the participants, rather than emphasizing the abilities and similarities of these persons to their nonhandicapped peers (Orelove, Wehman, & Wood, 1982; Polloway & Smith, 1978). In addition, opportunities to interact with nonhandicapped individuals are minimized in such events. Orelove et al. (1982) point out that the obvious (although not necessarily simple) solution is to provide handicapped children and youth with the opportunity to participate in community recreation programs. Such programs include church and community center dances, Little League events, 4-H groups, and community swimming classes. (p. 328)

Reports of actual intervention efforts in this area are lacking.

Regarding the educational arena, Stainback and Stainback (1984) reinforce the need to acknowledge the spectrum of individual differences that exist among all children and to minimize costly and largely unfounded practices of dual service delivery systems. They suggest that a "dual system creates artificial barriers between people and divides resources, personnel, and advocacy potential" (p. 105). Many of the arguments and constructs made by Stainback and Stainback apply to the integration of generic community resources as well. They conclude their position paper by stating that "it is time to stop developing criteria for who does or does not belong in the mainstream and instead turn the spotlight to increasing the capabilities of the . . . mainstream to meet the needs of *all* students" (p. 110). Clearly, the integration of generic nonschool services can and should be subjected to the same scrutiny as that applied to public school services and afforded the same opportunities for enhancement.

TOWARD MUTUAL LEARNING OPPORTUNITIES

At issue is not whether generic *or* specialized community services are needed to support persons with developmental disabilities and their families. The position advocated here is that elements from both service delivery systems must be merged to develop integrated programs that are capable of meeting the needs of all persons in the community. A range of fully integrated community programs should be available in every community. There are at least four reasons why integrated generic services should be developed as social supports to families in the community.

First, development and support of specialized community programs are costly (Stainback & Stainback, 1984). The economic impact of developing programs that are used by only a small proportion of the population is, for many communities, a negative one. Given that all families contribute to publicly funded services (e.g., recreation programs, transit, schools, camps) and many others that are subsidized by contributions, it seems reasonable to expect that access to such programs would be viewed as a right, rather than an imposition. In addition, the quality of low-use programs is frequently not comparable or appropriate when compared to "equivalent" programs in the general sector. The integration of existing services appears to be more cost-effective than the development of low-use, high-cost alternatives and clearly offers a more normalized social opportunity for all participants.

Second, other populations (e.g., the elderly, sensory impaired, physically disabled) are already accommodated in many community services. Clearly, the capability of community vendors to modify existing services has been demonstrated. Efforts could be directed at expanding these inroads and developing others that would benefit the developmentally disabled population.

Third, the long-term social costs to the population of persons with disabilities appears far greater when only specialized services are available. Such services emphasize differences among children and perpetuate the notion that segregated services are singularly beneficial and preferable to other models of service. Specialized services are typically not integrated and, consequently, do not offer nonhandicapped persons and their parents the opportunity to interact with and learn from children with handicapping conditions. The cost, here, is a social one that has both long- and short-term consequences for all members of the community.

Finally, provision of integrated generic services serves to broaden the social support network options of *all* families in the community. Consequently, opportunities for leisure, vocational, and educational pursuits are enhanced by the secondary respite effects generated by the presence of such additional services. This concept is particularly critical for families with dependent children. Families of children with handicaps may experience lost opportunities (i.e., jobs or promotions) because of the increased demands made by the child on time and energy and/or of the unavailability of appropriate child care services (Boggs, 1979).

Need for Collaboration

Special education services personnel play a key role in preparing students to move along the continuum of specialized to generic community service options. Their training and expertise are uniquely suited to the task of individualized instruction. Personnel from generic programs are typically not trained to adapt materials and activities to meet diverse individual physical, intellectual, and psychological needs. Yet, their knowledge and skill in the content and processes of the service at-hand (e.g., recreation, dance, child care, dentistry) provide information that is critical to the success of any integrative effort. Thus, both sectors must collaborate to ensure that modifications made in the integration process preserve the integrity of the generic service while simultaneously creating viable opportunities for meaningful participation by persons with developmental disabilities.

The blending of specialized and generic resources has most recently been found in federal, state, and local programs that have focused on the transition of handicapped students from school to community environments. Exemplary programs have demonstrated effective strategies to prepare students to function in community work, residential, and educational settings (Carden-Smith & Fowler, 1983; Gaylord-Ross & Peck, 1985; Sailor & Guess, 1983; Snell, 1983; Wehman, 1981). These projects utilize specialized resources to teach handicapped persons and community providers the skills necessary to facilitate the movement of students into community environments. Specialized instructional settings can effectively enhance the developmentally disabled person's acquisition of critical skills before, during, and after the transition and integration process. However, to ensure that the outcomes of their efforts are socially valid, collaboration with generic service providers must occur.

Kenowitz and colleagues (1977) point out that "there is a disparity between provision for and delivery of services" (p. 34). In order to rectify this disparity, generic services (e.g., recreational, transportation, church, day care) can be adapted to serve individuals with handicapping conditions. Similarly, handicapped children can be taught to utilize the services as they are presently delivered in the community. The enabling mechanisms for either approach require the expertise of special services personnel and emanate from a belief that there is merit in an integrated services model.

RESEARCH ON INTEGRATION

School and Child Focus

One is struck by the almost myopic focus of the integration literature on classroom settings and child outcomes. Reports of efforts at integrating handicapped children into nonschool generic services have been extremely limited, as is research on the impact of integration practices on parents. The vast majority of research on integration has focused on classroom-based settings (Apolloni & Cooke, 1978; Bricker, 1978; Brown et al., 1983; Fowler, 1982; Gaylord-Ross & Peck, 1985; Guralnick, 1978; Hamre-Nietupski & Nietupski, 1981; Snyder, Apolloni, & Cooke, 1977; Stainback, Stainback, & Jaben, 1981; Strain & Cordisco, in press; Taylor, 1981; Wilcox & Sailor, 1980; Ziegler & Hambleton, 1978).

Although a variety of intervention tactics have been used successfully by the preceding authors to positively influence the social interaction of handicapped and nonhandicapped children in mainstreamed settings, structured contact appears to be a key element to their success in tutorial, small group, and large group intervention strategies. Whether the methodologies and results garnered from these settings can be generalized to nonschool environments is not clear. Although the integration of handicapped and nonhandicapped children has been termed "best educational practice" (Vincent, Brown,

& Getz-Sheftel, 1981, p. 18), it is equally appropriate to view it as an accepted matter of public policy (albeit not one of fact) (Strain & Cordisco, in press) that constitutes "best societal practice."

There has been an almost universal emphasis on child outcomes as a dependent variable of the integration process. If one assumes that there is a transactional relationship among child, family, and community activities and interactions, then it is also reasonable to assume that the child's involvement in an integrated program would have repercussions for the parents at points of decision, entry, and participation. This supposition has been supported by preliminary data on the effects of mainstreaming on parents (Winton & Turnbull, 1981), yet it is an area that requires considerably more investigation.

Nonschool Settings

Although persons of normal intelligence with severe physical disabilities have been integrated into community college environments (Heliotis & Edgar, 1980), reports of nonschool integration activities for developmentally disabled persons have generally been restricted to preschool situations or integrated work settings.

Galloway and Chandler (1978) contend that adherence to the principle of normalization (Wolfensberger, 1972) clearly dictates that services to handicapped children must be normalized, individualized, continuous, and integrated if these children are to be provided the best, rather than better, services. They argue that integration will influence how: 1) the handicapped child is perceived by others, 2) specialized settings prepare students for transition, and 3) learning opportunities are afforded to both handicapped and nonhandicapped children. Although their research was classroom-based, the principles espoused in their work can be extended to nonschool integration activities as well.

Fredericks et al. (1978) reported on their efforts to mainstream moderately and severely handicapped preschool children into a normal day care setting. Language and social behavior were designated as outcome measures and served as targets for facilitation by staff members in the integrated setting. Results of their study indicated that moderately and severely handicapped children increase their social and verbal interactions when provided with structured activities. However, these improvements did not result from "typical" staffing patterns or procedures. On the contrary, the handicapped children were not able to keep pace with routine day care center activities without special help. The feasibility of using detailed, time-consuming intervention procedures in a normal day care setting emerged as the major question of this study. The amount of time expended and the level of staff training required to duplicate these results must be balanced against the goals of intervention and the extent to which the outcomes reflect a "normalized" situation.

Smith and Greenberg (1981) conducted a systematic integration study using four preschool children with social, emotional, and cognitive delays. These children were gradually integrated into a normal day care center over the course of a 9-month period. Time sampling and incidence data on the social and verbal behavior of all of the children were collected at three points. Results revealed significant increases in interaction behavior for some children and withdrawals for others. The mainstreamed children did not display the same rate of developmental progress as did handicapped children who were not integrated and who remained in the treatment settings. It is important to note that there are acknowledged limitations to this report. First, the small sample size limits appropriate interpretation of the results. Second, because no provision was made to facilitate interactions systematically among the children, the authors observed that "merely placing handicapped children with nonhandicapped children is not sufficient to bring about meaningful integration. Some plan to increase beneficial interaction must be part of any mainstreaming project" (p. 100). Finally, the gradual integration strategy likely contributed to the lack of interaction between the children. Smith and Greenberg stated that "if anything, the . . . children's perception of being different was developed and sharpened. In retrospect, we realize that this may have been the result of the initial plan to 'gradually' integrate the handicapped children" (p. 100).

Results of these investigations suggest that strategies for integrating children with moderate and severe disabilities into normal child care settings must continue to be refined. Although using strategies found to be effective in classroom settings may be one means of enhancing the probability of successful integration in a child care setting, there are inherent restrictions in using normalized generic settings. Fredericks et al. (1978) point out that "the children will benefit if the environment has been adequately prepared . . . (yet) whether or not it is feasible to adequately train staff and conduct the programming necessary . . . is a serious concern" (p. 205). Appropriate training continues to be a major factor affecting the facilitation and provision of integration experiences.

Examination of classroom-based integration strategies may provide critical prescriptive information that can be used to teach, support, and remediate in both specialized and generic settings. Extrapolating from these data bases, integration of individuals with developmental disabilities into generic nonschool activities will likely meet with greater initial success when child, staff, and parent variables are addressed before, during, and after the integration process (Fowler, 1982; Strain & Cordisco, in press).

Barriers to Integration

Given that social, educational, legal, and interpersonal justifications have been cogently forwarded in support of integrated community services (Bricker, 1978; Guralnick, 1978; Strain & Cordisco, in press; Taylor, 1981; Vincent, Brown, & Getz-Scheftel, 1981), why then do parents of handicapped children experience difficulties obtaining generic nonschool services for their child? Although there have been no specific investigations to identify expressed barriers to integration efforts in nonschool environments, there appear to be at least five types of problems facing parents who seek integrated nonschool resources for their developmentally disabled son or daughter.

Diversity of Services Many parents voice problems with the range of nonschool community options available to their child. In many communities, integrated resources are limited to public services (e.g., restaurants, theaters, transportation, and library). By their very nature, these programs require adult supervision if the child is young and at least indirect monitoring if the individual is a young adult. The interaction of inadequately prepared children and the dearth of trained generic service providers create a situation wherein parents of developmentally disabled children are usually expected to or "get saddled with" the responsibility of direct supervision. Parents of nonhandicapped children, on the other hand, are likely to be more confident about their child's level of independence and the ability of the service providers to address the needs of their child so that there is less need for direct supervision. The paradox in these cases is evident; such services have the potential to provide relief (i.e., respite) to the parents, yet the parents of handicapped children themselves often become directly involved in the activity. Data on the needs of families suggest that services that provide secondary respite benefits are, in many cases, perceived as more needed than primary respite care services.

Salisbury (1983, May) investigated parental needs for social support. Parents of developmentally disabled children ranging from preschool age to adulthood listed what they perceived to be their most pressing needs regarding their child or family situation. Statements were independently transcribed and sorted into nondesignated categories by two raters. These categories were then sorted into theoretically based dimensions of intraindividual, intrafamilial, and extrafamilial social support needs. Figure 1 depicts the distribution of parental needs across the three types of support resources. For this particular sample of parents, external support in the form of community services (e.g., child care, recreation) that could provide secondary respite effects was perceived as most needed.

When the descriptive statements were reclustered into primary versus secondary respite categories across preschool, school-age, and post-school-age groups, the need for secondary respite became even more evident. Figure 2 reveals this relationship. Not surprisingly, parents of school-age handicapped children expressed the least need for secondary respite services. Consistent with other research, school was apparently meeting the families' need for relief from caregiving, serving both a primary and a secondary respite

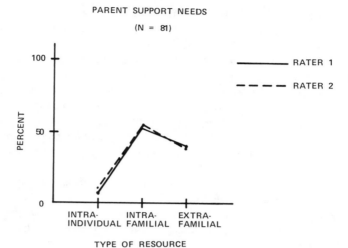

Figure 1. Parent support needs (categorical sort by two independent raters of 126 parent statements).

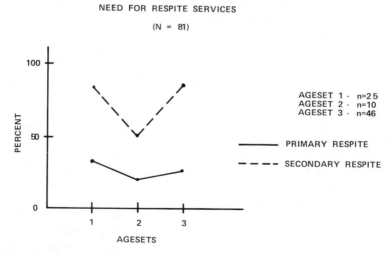

Figure 2. Need for respite services. (*Note:* Not all parents chose to respond to this item.)

function (Blacher, Chapter 11). Parents of preschool and adult developmentally disabled children, however, indicated a strong desire for community services designed to serve their child appropriately.

Although the number of organizations interested in serving persons with developmental disabilities is increasing (e.g., church groups, scouts, swimming, teen programs, day camps, child care, and dance), their intent is frequently to serve only handicapped children. Clearly, expressions of interest are a necessary step toward developing positive attitudes and productive programs. Efforts are needed to adapt the delivery of existing generic services to achieve a proportional balance between generic and segregated programs in the community. Diversity of need-meeting resources may be a particularly critical variable in mediating the effects of parenting stresses in families with developmentally disabled children.

Quantity of Services   Communities often develop one integrated program as a prototype and revel at the great number of persons using the service (e.g., Saturday recreation). Yet, rather than develop more of the same, they establish waiting lists. Equally often, they limit the number of special needs children, using either "normal population proportions" or "ability to handle" as exclusionary justifications. This latter criterion is one that typically excludes persons with significant medical, physical, behavioral, and/or intellectual difficulties. Thus, services are not always matched to the families in greatest need, nor are they equally available to all families in a given geographic region. Location of services is a particularly salient issue for families in sparsely populated areas where distance and critical mass often determine whether a service will be used or even developed. Efforts are needed to expand the number of programs willing and able to accommodate children with special needs so that the size of the potential social support base available to parents is increased.

Access to Services   This problem is inextricably linked to the others. Here, attitudes, preconceptions, eligibility requirements, and other exclusionary tactics effectively reduce the probability that handicapped children and their families would want or be able to use needed nonschool, generic support services. In addition, even if children with developmental disabilities were permitted access by the provider, the probability of maintaining enrollment in the program would likely be low because of concerns about competencies of the provider, negative attitudes toward the disabled child, and/or ability of the provider to meet individual needs appropriately. Lack of accurate information about children with handicapping conditions (Galloway & Chandler, 1978; Thurman & Lewis, 1979) and insufficient training of providers (Fredericks et al., 1978; Galloway & Chandler, 1978) have been identified as significant factors that can influence the relative success of an integration experience.

Blacher-Dixon, Leonard, and Turnbull (1981) point out that teacher/provider competence, pedagogical approaches, and parent participation are also relevant variables that influence the outcome of mainstreaming (integration) experiences. Clearly, accessibility studies are needed to ascertain how child, family, and resource characteristics interact with the process of integration in nonschool settings.

Content/Quality of Services   Within the population of parents of children with developmental disabilities, there are different opinions about what expectations are reasonable for providers of community-based services. On the one hand, many parents are so grateful that their child has something to do or somewhere to go that they are rather nonjudgmental about the content and quality of the services rendered. This is particularly true for parents of older developmentally disabled individuals (Salisbury, 1984, November; Salisbury, Weed, Brown, & Evans, 1984). On the other hand, parents of younger handicapped children have more stringent expectations about the appropriateness of what is offered and the relationship of this material to their child's long-term growth and development (Salisbury, 1984, November; Salisbury et al., 1984). In the area of respite services, the most frequently voiced concern is that related to the capabilities of the provider to meet the needs of their child appropriately (McGee, Smith, & Kenney, 1982; Salisbury & Griggs, 1983; Upshur, 1982a; Webb, Shaw, & Hawes, 1984). The modification and support of community-based programs must include input from parents if we expect services to address the needs of their child and the family as well. Without such involvement, one runs the risk of developing a service that may not match or fulfill the needs of the consumers it had hoped to serve.

Cost of Services   With the notable exception of the report by Kenowitz et al. (1977), there have been no data presented on the cost of generic services as a deterent to their use. However, data from respite care service projects provide some insight into the potential for cost to be a viable issue, particularly when the move is made from special to generic services. Respite programs have reported cost to be a deterrent (Upshur, 1982a; Webb et al., 1984) and that family subsidies are often required to offset the high costs associated with highly trained personnel for both in- and out-of-home services (Moore, Hamerlynck, Barsh, Spieker, & Jones, 1982; Upshur, 1982b; Webb et al., 1984; Zimmerman, 1984). One must realistically acknowledge the financial implications of integration. If we expect community providers to adapt materials and undergo extensive training, then this investment will likely be recovered in additional costs to the consumer. The nature and extent of adaptations required of community providers must be closely examined throughout the integration process to minimize escalation of costs and prohibit the subsequent exclusion of parents and children in need.

RECOMMENDATIONS FOR CHANGE

Establishing parity between the community resources available to families of handicapped and nonhandicapped children is an important task. The position espoused here is that many existing generic programs can be adapted to include developmentally disabled persons. Greater community opportunities will be reflected in a broader social support base to families, which can subsequently be used to mediate the effects of parenting stressors. Bolstering the diversity and quality of informal social supports must, however, be complemented by the addition of formalized services. These latter resources are valuable in teaching parents specific interpersonal problem-solving skills (Intagliata & Doyle, 1984; Wikler, 1981) that can subsequently enable them to use more effectively informal social supports and deal with the structural fluctuations that accompany out-of-home services. Acknowledging and planning for this latter dynamic may prevent the potential deleterious effects that can accompany the provision of isolated, nonsupported informal resources (Rodgers, 1983; Wikler, 1981). Clearly, research and community development efforts are needed to translate theoretical suppositions into practice, the outcome of which are services that are functional for community providers, developmentally disabled persons and their families, and the general community at large.

Facilitating Integration

Recent attempts at integrating generic nonschool services have utilized the structured contact approach. This approach incorporates many specific tactics that have as their focus changing peer-peer interaction patterns in the mainstreamed situation. Strain and Cordisco (in press) have identified the following strategies as effective in facilitating social competency and social interaction skills in handicapped children (p. 20):

1. Reinforcement of play or prosocial behavior using contingent praise and attention
2. Use of play materials that require interaction
3. Peer modeling
4. Peer-mediated social skills training
5. Direct training in sociodramatic play

Yet, addressing only the skill deficiencies of the handicapped child ignores other variables that ultimately influence the success of the integration effort. As Strain and Cordisco (in press) point out,

> It (skill training) is a necessary, but not sufficient means for achieving successful mainstreaming. While there is reason to believe the social isolation and rejection experienced by some handicapped children is based, in

part, on their lack of skill, it is also true that peers' perception of and behaviors towards handicapped children significantly influence social integration. (p. 8)

Thus, it is equally important to address the cognitive/attitudinal variables that can influence the nature of social interactions among handicapped and nonhandicapped persons.

Thurman and Lewis (1979) suggest that one reason handicapped children are singled out as different is that integration has occurred only at the behavioral level and has failed to address the nonhandicapped child's cognitive understanding of what makes these children different. Information (i.e., addressing integration at the cognitive level) appears to be one key element in maximizing the probability of social interaction.

Clearly, adults, as well as children, can benefit from informational intervention and training in specific skill areas. Yet, specific strategies for accomplishing integration in nonschool settings are limited. To be maximally effective, providers, handicapped and nonhandicapped children, and their parents must be included in planning, intervention, and evaluation activities to ensure that the goals, strategies, and outcomes of what is done meet the needs and expectations of all participants.

CONCLUSION

This chapter addressed the integration of generic community services as a critical area where out-of-home programs can provide respite to families with developmentally disabled children. It was argued that the development and expansion of integrated community services should be a priority area in communities. The dearth of information on how to accomplish this objective and to provide the necessary outcome data that will produce a flow of resources to generic, as well as specialized, services provides rich ground for future research and community development efforts.

REFERENCES

Apolloni, T., & Cooke, T. P. (1978). Integrated programming at the infant, toddler and preschool age levels. In M. Guralnick (Ed.), *Early intervention and the integration of handicapped and nonhandicapped children* (pp. 147–165). Baltimore: University Park Press.

Blacher-Dixon, J., Leonard, J., & Turnbull, A. P. (1981). Mainstreaming at the early childhood level: Current and future perspectives. *Mental Retardation, 19*(5), 235–241.

Boggs, E. (1979). Allocation of resources for family care. In R. H. Bruininks & G. C. Krantz (Eds.), *Family care of developmentally disabled members: Conference proceedings*. Minneapolis: University of Minnesota.

Bricker, D. D. (1978). A rationale for the integration of handicapped and nonhandicapped preschool children. In M. Guralnick (Ed.), *Early intervention and the integration of handicapped and nonhandicapped children* (pp. 3–26). Baltimore: University Park Press.

Bristol, M. M. (in press). The home care of developmentally disabled children: Some empirical support for a conceptual model of successful coping with family stress. In S. Landesman-Dwyer & P. Vietze (Eds.), *Environments for developmentally disabled persons*. Baltimore: University Park Press.

Bristol, M. M., & Schopler, E. (1984). A developmental perspective on stress and coping in families of autistic children. In J. Blacher (Ed.), *Severely handicapped young children and their families: Research in review* (pp. 91–141). New York: Academic Press.

Bronfenbrenner, V. (1976). The experimental ecology of education. *Educational Research, 5,* 5–15.

Brown, L., Ford, A., Nisbet, J., Sweet, M., Donnellan, A., & Gruenewald, L. (1983). Opportunities available when severely handicapped students attend chronological age appropriate regular schools. *Journal of the Association for the Severely Handicapped, 8*(1), 16–24.

Brown, L., Nietupski, J., & Hamre-Nietupski, S. (1976). Criterion of ultimate functioning. In M. A. Thomas (Ed.), *Hey. Don't forget about me! Education's investment in the severely, profoundly and multiply handicapped* (pp. 2–15). Reston, VA: Council for Exceptional Children.

Carden-Smith, L., & Fowler, S. A. (1983). An assessment of student and teacher behavior in treatment and mainstreamed classes for preschool and kindergarten. *Analysis and Intervention in Developmental Disabilities, 3,* 35–37.

Cohen, S. (1982). Supporting families through respite care. *Rehabilitation Literature, 43*(1–2), 7–11.

Dunst, C., Trivette, C. M., & Cross, A. H. (1986). Mediating influence of social support: Personal, family and child outcomes. *American Journal of Mental Deficiency, 90*(4), 403–417.

Fowler, S. A. (1982). Transition from preschool to kindergarten for children with special needs. In K. E. Allen & E. M. Goetz (Eds.), *Early childhood education: Special problems, special solutions* (pp. 309–334). Rockville, MD: Aspen Systems Corporation.

Fredericks, H. D. B., Baldwin, V., Grove, D., Moore, W., Riggs, C., & Lyons, B. (1978). Integrating the severely and moderately handicapped preschool child into a normal daycare setting. In M. J. Guralnick (Ed.), *Early intervention and the integration of handicapped and nonhandicapped children* (pp. 191–206). Baltimore: University Park Press.

Friedrich, W., & Friedrich, N. (1981). Psychosocial assets of parents of handicapped and nonhandicapped children. *American Journal of Mental Deficiency, 85,* 551–553.

Gallagher, J. J., Cross, A., & Scharfman, W. (1981). Parental adaptation to a young handicapped child: The father's role. *Journal of the Division for Early Childhood, 3,* 3–14.

Gallagher, J. J., Scharfman, W., & Bristol, M. (1984). The division of responsibilities in families with preschool handicapped and nonhandicapped children. *Journal of the Division for Early Childhood, 8*(1), 3–12.

Galloway, C., & Chandler, P. (1978). The marriage of special and generic early education services. In M. Guralnick (Ed.), *Early intervention and the integration of handicapped and nonhandicapped children* (pp. 261–287). Baltimore: University Park Press.

Gaylord-Ross, R., & Peck, C. A. (1985). Integration efforts for students with severe mental retardation. In D. Bricker & J. Filler (Eds.), *Severe mental retardation: From theory to practice* (pp. 185–207). Lancaster, PA: Lancaster Press.

Geismar, L. (1971). *Family and community functioning: A manual of measurement for social work practice and policy.* Metuchen, NJ: Scarecrow Press.

Guralnick, M. (1978). Integrated preschools as educational and therapeutic environments: Concepts, design and analysis. In M. Guralnick (Ed.), *Early intervention and the integration of handicapped and nonhandicapped children* (pp. 115–145). Baltimore: University Park Press.

Hamre-Nietupski, S., & Nietupski, J. (1981). Integral involvement of severely handicapped students within regular public schools. *Journal of the Association for the Severely Handicapped, 6*(2), 30–39.

Heliotis, J., & Edgar, E. (1980). Issues in mainstreaming students with cerebral palsy in a community college. *Journal of The Association for the Severely Handicapped, 5*(1), 86–99.

Hill, R. (1958). Generic features of families under stress. *Social Casework, 39,* 139–150.

Hoffman, L. W., & Manis, J. D. (1978). Influences of children on marital interactions and parental satisfactions and dissatisfactions. In R. M. Lerner & G. B. Spanier (Eds.), *Child influences on marital and family interaction: A life span perspective* (pp. 165–213). New York: Academic Press.

Intagliata, J., & Doyle, N. (1984). Enhancing social support for parents of developmentally disabled children: Training in interpersonal problem solving skills. *Mental Retardation, 22*(1), 4–11.

Kazak, A. E., & Marvin, R. S. (1984). Differences, difficulties and adaptation: Stress and social networks in families with a handicapped child. *Family Relations, 33*(1), 67–78.

Kenowitz, L. A., Gallaher, J., & Edgar, E. (1977). Generic services for the severely handicapped and their families: What's available. In E. Sontag & J. Smith (Eds.), *Educational programming for the severely/profoundly handicapped* (pp. 31–39). Reston, VA: Council for Exceptional Children.

Korn, S. J., Chess, S., & Fernandez, P. (1978). The impact of children's physical handicaps on marital and family interaction. In R. M. Lerner & G. B. Spanier (Eds.), *Child influences on marital and family interaction— A life span perspective* (pp. 299–326). New York: Academic Press.

Laten, S. (1981). *Mothers of young handicapped children: Their emotional responses and their perceptions of needs and resources.* Unpublished doctoral dissertation, University of Wisconsin, Madison.

Lloyd, J. (1984). How shall we individualize instruction—Or should we? *Remedial and Special Education, 5,* 7–15.

McCubbin, H., Joy, C., Cauble, A., Comeau, J. K., Patterson, J. M., & Needles, R. H. (1980). Family stress and coping: A decade review. *Journal of Marriage and the Family, 42,* 865–870.

McGee, J. J., Smith, P. M., & Kenney, M. (1982). *Giving families a break: Strategies for respite care.* Omaha, NE: Media Resource Center, Meyer Children's Rehabilitation Institute.

Minuchin, S. (1974). *Families and family therapy.* Cambridge, MA: Harvard University Press.

Moore, J. A., Hamerlynck, L. A., Barsh, E. T., Spieker, S., & Jones, R. R. (1982). *Extending family resources.* Seattle, WA: Children's Clinic and Preschool, Spastic Aid Council, Inc.

Orelove, F., Wehman, P., & Wood, J. (1982). An evaluative review of Special Olympics: Implications for community integration. *Education and Training of the Mentally Retarded, 17*(4), 325–329.

Polloway, E. A., & Smith, J. D. (1978). Special Olympics: A second look. *Education and Training of the Mentally Retarded, 13,* 432–433.

Robinson, N. M., & Robinson, H. B. (1976). *The mentally retarded child: A psychological approach* (2nd ed.). New York: McGraw-Hill Book Co.

Rodgers, J. (November, 1983). *Respite care for families with deaf-blind children.* Paper presented at the annual convention of the Association for the Severely Handicapped, San Francisco, CA.

Rowitz, L. (1974). Social factors in mental retardation. *Social Science and Medicine, 8,* 405–412.

Sailor, W., & Guess, D. (1983). *Severely handicapped students: An instruction design.* Boston: Houghton Mifflin Co.

Salisbury, C. (1983, May). *The respite care network: Requisite factors in model development.* Paper presented at the annual convention of the American Association on Mental Deficiency, Dallas, TX.

Salisbury, C. (1983, November). *Research and training issues in the provision of respite care services.* Paper presented at the annual convention of the Association for the Severely Handicapped, San Francisco, CA.

Salisbury, C. (1984, May). *The respite function and its relationship to generic community resources.* Paper presented at the annual convention of the American Association on Mental Deficiency, Minneapolis, MN.

Salisbury, C. (1984, November). *Parent judgments of educational outcomes: A cross-sectional comparison.* Paper presented at the annual convention of The Association for Persons with Severe Handicaps, Chicago, IL.

Salisbury, C. (1984, December). *Outcome evaluation of social support services.* Invited paper presented at the Governor's Conference on Family Supports. Albany, NY.

Salisbury, C., & Griggs, P. (1983). Developing respite care services for families of handicapped persons. *Journal of The Association for Persons with Severe Handicaps, 8*(1), 50–57.

Salisbury, C., Weed, K., Brown, F., & Evans, I. (1984). *Parent perceptions of education outcomes: A comparison of regular and special education services* (Tech. Rep. No. 5, Project SPAN). Binghamton, NY: University Center, Department of Psychology.

Seltzer, M. M., & Krauss, M. W. (1984). Placement alternatives for mentally retarded children and their families. In J. Blacher (Ed.), *Severely handicapped young children and their families: Research in review.* New York: Academic Press.

Sherman, B., & Cocozza, J. J. (1984). Stress in families of the developmentally disabled: A literature review of factors affecting the decision to seek out of home placements. *Family Relations, 33,* 95–103.

Smith, C., & Greenberg, M. (1981). Step by step integration of handicapped preschool children in a day care center for nonhandicapped children. *Journal of the Division for Early Childhood, 2,* 96–101.

Snell, M. (1983). *Systematic instruction of the moderately and severely handicapped.* Columbus OH: Merrill Publishing Co.

Snyder, L., Apolloni, T., & Cooke, T. P. (1977). Integrated settings at the early childhood level: The role of nonretarded peers. *Exceptional Children, 43*(5), 262–266.

Stainback, W., & Stainback, S. (1984). A rationale for the merger of special and regular education. *Exceptional Children, 51*(2), 102–111.

Stainback, W., Stainback, S., & Jaben, T. (1981). Providing opportunities for interaction between severely handicapped and nonhandicapped students. *Teaching Exceptional Children, 13*, 72–75.

Strain, P., & Cordisco, L. K. (in press). Child characteristics and outcomes related to mainstreaming. In J. Anderson & T. Black (Eds.), *Issues in preschool mainstreaming.*

Taylor, S. J. (1981). From segregation to integration: Strategies for integrating severely handicapped students in normal school and community settings. *Journal of the Association for the Severely Handicapped, 7*(3), 42–49.

Thurman, S. K., & Lewis, M. (1979). Children's response to differences: Some possible implications for mainstreaming. *Exceptional Children, 45*, 468–469.

Turnbull, A. P., Brotherson, M. J., & Summers, J. A. (1983). *Family life cycle: Theoretical and empirical implications and future directions for families with mentally retarded members.* Paper presented at NICHD conference on "Research on Families with Retarded Children."

Unger, D., & Powell, D. (1980). Supporting families under stress: The role of social networks. *Family Relations, 29*, 566–574.

Upshur, C. (1982a). Respite care for mentally retarded and other disabled populations: Program models and family needs. *Mental Retardation, 20*, 2–6.

Upshur, C. (1982b). An evaluation of home-based respite care. *Mental Retardation, 20*, 58–62.

Venters, M. (1981). Familial coping with chronic illness: The case of cystic fibrosis. *Social Science and Medicine, 15*, 289–297.

Vincent, L., Brown, L., & Getz-Sheftel, M. (1981). Integrating handicapped and typical children during the preschool years: The definition of best educational practice. *Topics in Early Childhood Special Education, 1*(1), 45–56.

Vincent, L. J., Salisbury, C., Walter, G., Brown, P., Gruenewald, L. J., & Powers, M. (1980). Program evaluation and curriculum development in early childhood/special education. *Criteria of the next environment.* In W. Sailor, B. Wilcox, & L. Brown (Eds.), *Methods of instruction for severely handicapped students* (pp. 303–328). Baltimore: Paul H. Brookes Publishing Co.

Webb, A. Y., Shaw, H., & Hawes, B. A. (1984). *Respite services for developmentally disabled individuals in New York State.* Albany, NY: Office of Mental Retardation Developmental Disabilities.

Wehman, P. (1981). *Competitive employment: New horizons for severely disabled individuals.* Baltimore: Paul H. Brookes Publishing Co.

Wikler, L. (1981). Stress in families of mentally retarded children. *Family Relations, 30*, 281–288.

Wilcox, B., & Sailor, W. (1980). Service delivery issues: Integrated educational systems. In B. Wilcox & R. York (Eds.), *Quality education for the severely handicapped: The federal investment* (pp. 277–304). Washington, DC: U.S. Department of Education.

Willer, B., & Intagliata, J. (1984). *Promises and realities for mentally retarded persons: Life in the community.* Baltimore: University Park Press.

Winton, P., & Turnbull, A. P. (1981). Parent involvement as viewed by parents of preschool handicapped children. *Topics in Early Childhood Special Education, 1*(3), 11–19.

Wolfensberger, W. (1972). *The principle of normalization in human services.* Toronto: National Institute on Mental Retardation.

Ziegler, S., & Hambleton, D. (1978). Integration of young TMR children into a regular elementary school. *Exceptional Children, 42*(8), 459–461.

Zimmerman, S. (1984). The mental retardation family subsidy program: Its effects on families with a mentally handicapped child. *Family Relations, 33*(1), 105–118.

Chapter 11

THE SCHOOL AS RESPITE FOR PARENTS OF CHILDREN WITH SEVERE HANDICAPS

Jan Blacher and Phyllis Prado

> . . . The only thing that got me through the year Joey turned 3 was knowing each day would come to an end. Right about that time we got the respite care. And then school . . . it was so much easier to take care of him once school started.
>
> —Mother of boy with severe handicaps,
> from Meyers & Blacher (1985b)

T his chapter provides a historical perspective on public schooling and families. It is shown in the first section that schooling today provides respite for all families, with or without a handicapped child. That schooling is even *more* important for parents of children with severe handicaps is emphasized in the second section of this chapter, where the context of respite is reviewed. Of course, schooling serves other functions, not the least of which are educational programming and teaching. In the third section, data on parents' perceptions of schooling, its benefits, and respite effects are presented. The fourth section discusses issues and dilemmas for parents provoked by publicly mandated schooling and parent involvement activities. The chapter concludes with policy implications affecting severely handicapped children and their parents.

Preparation of this manuscript was supported in part by grant no. RO1 HD14680 from the National Institute for Child Health and Human Development.

PUBLIC SCHOOLING AND FAMILIES: HISTORICAL PERSPECTIVE

In our eagerness to study the impact of schooling on families with handicapped children, it is easy to overlook the impact that public schooling in America has had on the functioning of *all* families. During much of the 19th century many Americans pursued their education within families and churches and through other informal means. By the late 1880s, schooling began to alter traditional family functioning (Keniston, 1977). It changed the role of the family three ways. First, consider that at that time many American families lived on farms where children were part of the family productive unit. Sending children to school meant that they would no longer be available to help out on the family farms. To accommodate families needing extra help during the summer, the peak farm season, the now traditional long summer vacation was established. Note that the year-round schooling schedule thus brought about a change in family functioning by decreasing the economic value of children (i.e., they were no longer producers for most of the year) and increasing their economic dependency on parents.

A second change in family functioning catalyzed by public schooling was the removal of education from the family. Earlier, most education was conducted at home through reading the Scriptures or learning a trade. The major responsibility for this education fell on parents, with school having a lesser role. Today the average American child spends the better part of his or her weekdays *not* in the presence of the family, but in the presence of teachers, day care workers, or peers—undeniably a striking change in family functioning over time. The family role as primary teacher has faded dramatically.

A third change in family functioning is almost a by-product of schooling. Writes Keniston (1977), ''Schooling thus permits mothers to enter the paid labor force by indirectly providing the equivalent of 'free' baby-sitting making working possible without expensive child-care arrangements'' (p. 20). In today's complex society, all parents seem to need additional help to balance work and the raising of children. It appears that, for many families, schooling serves this function very early on, when their children are quite young.

Thus, by the end of the 19th century, there were a number of positive changes in the role and function of school. Public schooling at that time was still optional for some children; for others it was imposed by parents whose social circumstances (i.e., need for work) caused them to send their children to school (Cremin, 1980). The purpose of the school was to prepare youngsters for adulthood and to ease their way into the world of work, with valued lessons on punctuality, adherence to rules and procedures, and literacy. The progressive education movement fueled the broadening of school functions to include concern for health, vocation, and quality of family and community life (Cremin, 1961). This movement also advocated a kind of individualizing of education, tailoring instruction to different kinds and classes of children.

These early historical works on schooling in America do not speak directly to the educational needs of handicapped children; however, three aspects of this early schooling had implications for the education of handicapped children: 1) attempts to individualize instruction, 2) concern for both family and school life, and 3) the use of public schooling as respite for parents. It is this latter, rather implicit, function of schooling that is addressed by the remainder of this chapter.

PUBLIC SCHOOLING AND FAMILIES OF
SEVERELY HANDICAPPED CHILDREN: THE CONTEXT OF RESPITE

All parents need respite from time to time. Indeed, most parents have access to respite (e.g., neighborhood babysitters, grandparents to fill in when Mom and Dad go away, friends who have children the same age) when they need it. Ironically, parents who really do need respite—those with young severely handicapped children, particularly with behavioral problems—do not usually have a cadre of friends and neighbors on hand to help out. Moreover, they may even be excluded from some respite care programs because of the severity of their child's handicap (Cohen & Warren, 1985; Rimstidt, 1983)!

The meaning of respite or relief is likely to be very different for families with severely handicapped children, as opposed to families with only nonhandicapped children. One might expect the frequency with which relief is needed, the form that relief takes, and the reasons given for needing respite to be quite different. This section discusses the context of respite for families of very impaired children.

Daily Care Burden on Families

> "I get so tired of saying, 'Ralphy, NO!' "
>
> —Mother of child with severe handicaps,
> from Meyers & Blacher (1985b)

Sometimes the day-to-day care and management of young children with severe handicaps is relentless, with a constant need to sing out the phrases learned in those behavior management programs for parents: "Hands down," "good boy." In addition to the constant need to manage the behavior of a young child with severe handicaps, there are other complicating factors in the daily care of such a child:

> Why is this so difficult a task? There are several reasons. The first is that many severely disabled individuals can do so little for themselves. They need to be fed, dressed, toileted, bathed, and sometimes carried. Parents do this for all their children, but they do these things for 2 or 3 years. They do

it for children who weigh 20 or 25 pounds. What makes doing these things particularly difficult is doing them year after year, for a child who is 8 or 12 years old instead of 1 or 2, for a child who weighs 70 or 80 pounds instead of 20, for a child who menstruates; and for a child who is turning into a woman or a man. (Cohen & Warren, 1985, p. 4)

What is clear is that the caregiving role for parents of very impaired children disrupts the development of the normal family life cycle (Farber, 1979; Skrtic, Summers, Brotherson, & Turnbull, 1984). The period of childhood dependency is extended, and parents may never witness the blossoming of full independence in their child. The emergence of self-help skills and other mileposts of independence in children are themselves forms of respite for parents of nonhandicapped children that parents of severely handicapped children may never experience.

An additional care burden derives from the time parents, especially mothers, spend as therapist, teacher, trainer, and transporter of their severely handicapped child. As Keniston (1977) pointed out, parents of nonhandicapped school children have been freed of this role historically, allowing them time to devote to jobs or more family-oriented activities. These extra roles for mothers of handicapped children often result in the mother-handicapped child pair splitting off from the rest of the family for large amounts of time. These additional responsibilities interfere with other work opportunities and often create a sense of (if not actual) isolation for mothers (Wahler, 1980).

In short, respite is not a luxury for families that they could easily live without. As Cohen and Warren (1985) aptly point out, many families would "collapse" under the pressures, stress, and exhaustion caused by never having a break from caregiving.

What Respite Is . . . And What It Is Not

Various models of respite service are delineated throughout Part II of this book. Here, the intent is to highlight the relationship between school services and functions of respite.

Current definitions of respite care emphasize its function as "temporary relief" to parents from caregiving responsibilities associated with having a disabled child (Salisbury & Griggs, 1983). Respite also refers to temporary care provided to a developmentally disabled or otherwise dependent individual for the purpose of providing relief to his or her primary caregivers. The notion of temporary does not usually exceed 30 continuous days, but it may extend up to 90 days under special circumstances (Cohen & Warren, 1985).

There are two major functions of respite care described by Salisbury and Griggs (1983) that contribute to our understanding of how the school may also serve as respite. First, respite can consist of short-term, out-of-home residential placement for the handicapped child. Examples of this function include overnight stays with relatives or trained respite workers. Second, respite can serve the same relief function through short-term, in-home care that provides immediate relief for other family members. Services provided by home teachers, parent trainers, and respite day workers fulfill this function. Some community-based services, on the other hand, provide respite as a by-product (Cohen, 1982), often called secondary respite. This type of secondary respite is provided by summer camp, day care, and, of course, the school. In all these services, the handicapped child is receiving direct care, instruction, or entertainment of some sort; the result for the parents is a form of respite during the hours that the activity or service is being provided.

The significance of secondary respite in providing relief to families can be profound. In a study of respite care utilization and its relationship to other variables, such as family characteristics, family functioning, and likelihood of long-term out-of-home placement, it was noted that the one service found to be significantly more effective than others offered was a 30-hour-a-week preschool program (cited in Cohen & Warren, 1985).

Hypothesized Relationships Between Respite, Social Network Supports, and Coping with Stress

There are other resources available to families that may buffer the demands of a severely handicapped child. These include money, skills in negotiating the service delivery system, good mental and physical health, a support network of family and friends, a strong marriage, and healthy family interaction patterns (Cohen & Warren, 1985). McCubbin et al. (1980) cite the following dimensions as facilitators of family coping: 1) personal resources of individual family members (economic or physical well-being, problem-solving ability, self-esteem); 2) internal family resources (family environment dimensions, cohesiveness, adaptability); and 3) social support (belonging to a network made up of family and friends.) The latter dimension—use of social support networks—is "unquestionably crucial" (Schilling & Schinke, 1983, p. 384) to the quality of life of the disabled individual and family.

Members of one's social support network often provide respite for families with handicapped children. The network can include more than one friend in addition to a spouse and is defined by Garbarino (1983) as a set of interconnected relationships that endure across many forms and provide mutual reinforcement. Social support networks, sometimes also referred to as family or personal social networks (Powell, 1980), can grow out of other preexisting groups (e.g., when co-workers become a resource for each other). They may also be created deliberately (e.g., groups formed by and for parents of handicapped children).

Social support networks are but one of several systems now believed to mediate family functioning and the stress presumably associated with having a retarded child. In their recent review of issues concerning the adaptation of families with mentally retarded children, Crnic, Friedrich, and Greenberg (1983) mention other systems in the ecology of the family that also serve this function—the home environment, workplace, neighborhood, social agencies, school, and the interrelationships among these systems.

The Respite Function of School

Mandated public schooling for severely handicapped children is a relatively new phenomenon. Before the passage of Public Law 94-142, the Education for All Handicapped Children Act, many severely impaired children received no, or inadequate, educational services. Today there is a tremendous growth of new programs for severely handicapped infants and preschoolers. Families now interact more frequently with a host of school-related individuals from whom they may receive social support or respite. Furthermore, parents have reported that school or day care teachers were an important source of information about child development, child rearing, or behavior management (Meyers & Blacher, 1985a; Powell, 1980). Public school programs alone remove the burden of care from parents for 25 to 30 hours a week, if not longer. Extension of the school year from 10 to 12 months also provides relief during the summer (Stotland & Mancuso, 1981).

To summarize, respite can refer to either a direct service (as in respite care) or an end result (as in the sense of relief provided by the service.) It can help families cope with both daily stresses and emergency situations (Upshur, 1983), it can have a positive impact on family relations and social activities (Joyce, Singer, & Isralowitz, 1983), and it has been shown to be satisfying for parents (Ptacek et al., 1982).

Respite is *not,* however, a cure-all for families with young severely handicapped children. It is, as pointed out by Elsie Helsel (1985), "a service whose time has come" (p. x). There are other services and rights for handicapped children that parents have deemed necessary, for which parents have fought long and hard (Turnbull & Winton, 1984)—education, treatment, and even citizenship. Formal respite services are also not universally available to families; such services vary within and across states. An exception to this is the secondary effect of public schooling for all handicapped children.

PARENTS' PERCEPTION OF SCHOOLING: DATA FROM A LONGITUDINAL STUDY

Today the political and social *zeitgeist* reflects strong preference for home placement of most handicapped children. Living at home today, in the post–Public Law 94-142 era, means that one way or another parents will be keenly aware of and frequently involved in their child's schooling. This section reviews how current legislation can affect parents and then presents data from a study of parents' perceptions of schooling under this new legislation.

Two major components of the Education for All Handicapped Children Act directly affect parents and families. One, the provision of free appropriate education, results in the handicapped child being gone for 6 hours or so each day. Hence, the secondary respite effect of schooling mentioned earlier. The other component, mandated parental participation in schooling, provides a number of new roles and responsibilities for parents. These range from a minimal awareness of their child's actual school program as described in the individualized education program (IEP) to maximum involvement as teachers, advocates, and decision makers (Baker, 1984; Turnbull & Winton, 1984). Thus, the law has an explicit effect on handicapped children, the provision of a free, appropriate education, and an implicit effect on parents— the provision of respite and the opportunity for involvement. Ironically, school-provided respite and school participation may have opposite effects on families. The first provides relief by removing the child from the family setting, and the second may produce stress by removing the parent (usually the mother) from the rest of the family.

The extant literature contains no reports of systematic attempts to determine whether or how the public school serves as a form of respite. However, there have been attempts to measure the extent of parent involvement following implementation of the law. Most studies have examined the extent of parental participation in the development of their child's IEP (Baker & Brightman, 1984); no studies reported to date have focused exclusively on parents of severely handicapped children. For example, one recent study that attempted to assess parent participation using an instrument developed for this purpose (Cone, Delawyer, & Wolfe, 1985) obtained data from families of children varying widely in age and level of handicap.

In the special case of families with severely impaired children, the mandated role of parent participation in schooling is bound to affect not only the school process itself but also parent-child dynamics. Presumably, schooling will help modulate the impact of the severely handicapped child on the family. This, in fact, is the topic of a 3-year longitudinal study, the UCLA Project for Severely Impaired Children and their Families (Meyers & Blacher, 1985b). The purpose of this project is to assess the impact of schooling on: 1) family adjustment to a severely impaired child, 2) parental involvement and participation in educating their child, and 3) the development of extrafamily social supports and networks. Data presented here are delimited to the second focus above; namely, parents' perception of schooling.

Participants and Procedures

One hundred families were secured through developmental disabilities service centers. These agencies mailed invitations to parents of children labeled "severely handicapped" within the age range of 3 and 8 years. Subject families were those that responded positively to the invitation.

Ninety families reported the mother as principal caregiver. In two families, the father was the principal care provider, and in eight more the father shared the role equally with the mother. The predominant ethnic group was Anglo-white, with Hispanic and black families second and third in frequency; there were few families of mixed or Asian ethnicity. Education levels of parents ranged from incompleted elementary school through graduate school, with 30% of mothers and 46% of fathers having completed college. Occupation levels ranged from unskilled to professional/managerial categories. Most fathers were employed; 33% of mothers were employed, whereas 52% of mothers regarded themselves as housewives. Eighty-eight percent of the informants were married or living together and considered their families intact. The data indicate that families were somewhat above average in terms of employment, education, and marital intactness, but the sample had a broad range in all characteristics.

At initial contact, children were all between the ages of 28 and 99 months (mean = 66); 66 were male and 34 female. Their adaptive behavior was consistent with the profound to severe levels of mental retardation (Grossman, 1983). Ratings given by mothers as informants on selected items of the Adaptive Behavior Scale (Nihira, Foster, Shellhaas, & Leland, 1974) showed that most of these children were incapable of self-feeding, toileting, dressing, and language. Most, however, had adequate vision and hearing.

The information on which this report is based was derived from an interview with parents that was conducted yearly as part of a longitudinal study. Complete interviews lasted from 2 to 6 hours and were audiotaped to permit reliable coding of certain responses. Parents responded to questions about the child's effect on the family and the school placement. The interviews included structured and unstructured formats. Portions of the interview, focusing on mother-child interactions, were videotaped.

The interview protocol, "Parents' Perception of School and Their Relation to It," contained a number of open-ended questions regarding the child's school placement. Audiotapes made during the 2- to 6-hour interview were transcribed verbatim. These were carefully studied by project staff, and responses were assigned numerical codes according to four major dimensions of interest: 1) parents' satisfaction with the school program, 2) benefits derived from schooling, 3) parents' involvement in the school program, and 4) parent-school communication. Two independent raters coded these transcripts with an interrater agreement of .96. Scales (with high item-to-total correlations) were constructed for each of the four dimensions.

This report focuses on parents' responses about the school placement as a form of respite care for the primary caregiver (usually mother). During the second year of this 3-year project, in the course of a discussion about the benefits of schooling for themselves and their families, mothers were asked,

"Do you see the school as respite?" Subsequent coding and interpretation of their responses follow.

Results and Interpretation

Five different types of parental responses were identified. These categories were: 1) parent views the school mainly as providing respite care for primary caretaker, but not necessarily as having educational value for child; 2) school is viewed as providing both respite for parent and educational value for child; 3) school is identified as having educational value, but not as providing respite; 4) school is sometimes viewed as respite care for parent, sometimes as education for child, but never both; 5) school is neither viewed as respite care nor as having educational value.

A Category I ($N = 43$) parent is one who considers school a blessing in helping her cope with her handicapped child. Most of the Category I parents (78%) depend on school for respite care in order to attend to other obligations in their lives. Twenty-one percent stated that they would "go crazy" if their child were not in school, whereas others simply could not fathom having their child home continuously. About half (42%) ot the parents in this category viewed the school as giving Mom and child a "break" from each other, the result being that mother developed a more positive attitude toward and increased tolerance for her child. Parents in Category I could recognize that "the indirect respite care [of school] is invaluable." Eleven percent (about five parents) stated that they would institutionalize their child if there were no public schooling.

A Category II ($N = 43$) parent believes the school has respite value for herself, but also great educational value for her child. Many parents in Category II simply feel that an education for their severely handicapped child is just as important as an education for their other nonhandicapped child or children; 62% stated that they would still manage to provide an education somehow, if there were no public schooling available. Parents in Category II tend to see the respite value of school as less profound than the educational value; 58% acknowledged the relief in responsibility for promoting development of their child. These parents recognized that it was "important that their child always be in an educational situation."

The Category III ($N = 9$) parent is not too dissimilar from the Category II parent, with both viewing the school as educational for their child. Unlike the Category II parent, however, the Category III parent does not acknowledge the school as having any respite value. Instead, approximately 70% of these parents express the need to provide the best possible education for their child. Overall, these parents hold strong convictions about the value of education and what should be provided for their child.

Category IV ($N = 3$) parents, though small in numbers, view the school alternatively as respite for themselves and as education for their child. For these few parents, school is always viewed as a benefit regardless of the situation; they just do not seem to recognize both aspects of the school at once. They recognized that "the benefits [of school] value both parent and child."

Category V comprises only 2% of our sample—those parents who view school as having neither respite nor educational value. One of these families reported unhappiness with the school program and receiving no benefits from schooling; justifiably, this parent found no value to the child's school placement. The other family saw the school placement as necessary for socialization purposes only; the mother, by her own choice, attended school with the child all day and was neither seeking nor found respite value in that situation.

It is striking that, within these 5 categories of parental responses, 98% of our parents view public schooling as beneficial for either child or parent; 89% mentioned respite as a benefit of schooling (categories I, II, IV). In 43% of the families schooling apparently benefits both the child and parent. The number of parents finding no value to schooling whatsoever is inconsequential (although the reasons for their dissatisfaction are not, and are definitely worth pursuing.)

Exactly *why* some parents view school as respite and some do not is not clear at this time. In both Categories I and II, for example, about 30% of mothers worked; some of these working mothers viewed their own jobs as "respite," not as economic necessity. Of the other mothers in these categories, a majority felt that having their child in school would allow them to consider having a job if the need arose. It is not surprising that mothers at home, as housewives, find respite value in the school and appreciate the educational gains for their child.

A review of child and parent characteristics reveals a few major differences between respite categories I and II. (See Table 1 for the means and *t* tests for selected characteristics.) Category II mothers, those who saw the school as respite *and* as having great educational value, are significantly older than mothers in Category I; there were no differences, however, in mothers' educational levels or marital adjustment. Children of Category II mothers are significantly higher in overall adaptive behavior, particularly in cognitive-linguistic ability and walking/running skills. Overall maladaptive behavior, the occurrence of specific stereotypical behavior, and chronological age did not differentiate the two groups.

Clearly, the mothers in our sample whose children are somewhat higher in adaptive behavior have greater expectations for schooling and for their children's progress. These mothers also tend to be slightly older than the mothers who see school more as respite than as education; the older mothers

Table 1.   Means and summary of *t* tests by respite category group

Variable	Category I (N = 43)		Category II (N = 43)		t	p<
	M	SD	M	SD		
Child characteristics[a]						
Adaptive behavior	24.4	13.7	30.5	12.9	2.10	.04
Cognitive-linguistic ability	9.6	4.7	12.0	6.3	1.96	.05
Ambulation	1.3	1.8	2.3	2.0	2.33	.02
Maladaptive behavior	12.0	8.4	12.1	8.7	0.05	NS
Stereotypical behavior	1.2	1.5	1.5	1.7	0.78	NS
Age (Mos.)	63.2	20.0	68.2	18.2	1.22	NS
Parent Characteristics						
Mother's age[b]	31.5	5.5	34.7	5.9	2.59	.01
Mother's education[c]	5.3	1.4	5.4	1.3	0.62	NS
Marital adjustment[d]	114.8	17.4	105.6	25.4	1.81	NS

[a]Scores on child characteristics not available for 2 children, Category I.
[b]Mother's age unavailable for 1 parent, Category II.
[c]Mother's education as follows: 1 = Grade 1–6; 2 = Grade 7–8; 3 = Grade 9–10; 4 = Grade 11–12; 5 = some college or trade school; 6 = junior college; 7 = completed college or beyond
[d]Marital adjustment scores from Locke & Wallace (1959) are based on N = 36 Category I, N = 37, Category II.

are likely to have reared children longer and thus also to have experienced relief from schooling; now they acknowledge the educational benefit as well.

From the parents' perception of school interview were obtained total scores on parental satisfaction with their child's education and parental involvement in this education for 99 families (one family did not yet have their child in school at the time the study began). The satisfaction score refers to the parents' satisfaction with their child's teacher, therapists, overall attitude of the school toward them as parents, and the benefits the parent perceives from schooling. Parent involvement is also a composite variable, including involvement in child assessments, IEP development, parent-groups, home teaching, behavior management at home, and the like.

These scores, reported here for the first year of the study, reveal some interesting findings. First, the majority of parents were highly satisfied with their child's schooling; of a total possible score of 25 on the satisfaction scale, the mean was 17 (range=3–24). Only 15 parents did not attain a score of at least 12, the minimum needed for interviewers to determine a rating of very satisfied. Second, the group as a whole was highly involved in their child's education; of a possible total of 17 points for parent involvement, the mean was 11 (range = 1–17). Only 37 of our parents received a score of less than 11 and were thus considered not highly involved. Only 5 were both dissatisfied and uninvolved.

The high level of involvement among parents, who for the most part found the school to be a source of respite, is very surprising. It also raises a number of issues and dilemmas for parents of very handicapped young children. This chapter concludes with a brief discussion of these issues.

INVOLVEMENT VERSUS RESPITE: DILEMMAS FOR PARENTS

It is paradoxical that, although parents of severely handicapped young children acknowledge and indeed enjoy the respite provided by public schooling, they find themselves very involved in it. The real dilemma is as follows: Can parents feel relieved of responsibility, yet at the same time accept additional responsibilities? Public schooling frees them of child caregiving during the day, but can shoulder them with several additional burdens, including mandatory attendance at IEP meetings, parent-teacher conferences, daily communication with teachers or other school personnel, and home teaching. Eighty-six percent of the parents in the Meyers and Blacher (1985a) study identified the school as a definite source of respite for them. Most also indicated a high level of involvement in their child's school program, which included participation in such activities as assessment, IEP development, therapy, and a variety of forms of daily communication with teachers. Most also are highly satisfied with their child's school program and their involvement in it.

Some parents feel reluctant to report the respite value of schooling, for fear that the actual educational provisions of Public Law 94-142 and the more recent Education of the Handicapped Amendments Act of 1983 may be cut. Many of these parents live in constant fear that the reduction of educational services from the full day school program to a few hours of day-care-type service is possible. The guaranteed educational program under the current law also guarantees year round respite.

There are still other benefits of schooling for parents and siblings of handicapped children. These are summarized in Table 2. Although all these benefits were mentioned by 100 parents in the study reviewed above, many have also been indicated in research with parents reported elsewhere (see, for example, Blacher, 1984). The interactions between parents and teachers, as well as between parents and other parents of handicapped children, provide both a source of social or emotional support and a source of teaching or training tips for use at home. Parents of severely handicapped children have reported increased gains in child development knowledge and skill acquisition, as well as gains in their own confidence in the care and management of a

Table 2. Summary of benefits of public schooling for parents of severely handicapped children

1. School provides respite for mother, father, and siblings.
2. Interaction with other parents and teachers provides social support to parents.
3. Parents learn skills/techniques to use at home with their handicapped child.
4. Increases in skill training and behavior management lead to improvements in parental confidence in the care and development of their child.
5. Gains in child development/progress due to schooling can improve parent-child interaction and subsequent attachment to child.
6. It helps parents think more productively and realistically about the future for their child.

very impaired child. The emphasis on individualized education, undergirded by the IEP with its goals and objectives for progress, helps parents think more productively and realistically about the future of their child. These points are highlighted here in order to emphasize the positive role that public schooling has in the lives of many families with severely handicapped children. Even a remote hint of cutbacks to services creates alarm, for the respite function of schooling alleviates what McCubbin and colleagues (McCubbin et al., 1982) refer to as a ''pile-up'' of family events and strains.

Temporary Respite versus Permanent Placement

Respite often helps families avoid painful placement decisions. Helsel (1985) hails respite as a societal need if handicapped children are to be kept at home and fully integrated into society. Most retarded individuals have historically and still do reside in heir own homes (Meyers & Blacher, in press.)

Temporary respite, even if not available on a regular basis, can help reduce stress and strain for families with severely handicapped children. The literature suggests, in fact, that the presence of such a child can predispose a parent toward abuse (Frodi, 1981; Meier & Sloan, 1984).

The use of respite can ironically better prepare some families for a more permanent placement decision. For example, Ackerman (1985) notes ''Friends and family need to find ways to help parents stay involved in mainstream and adult life while they are raising their handicapped children, so that adjustment to life-after-placement is not so severe.'' (p. 151) Time provided to parents by temporary respite care can enable them to build up personal social networks, to establish friendships and supports that will remain after the handicapped child is placed.

As with other types of formal or informal sources of respite, the provision of public schooling may also affect placement decisions. In her writing about issues related to institutionalization and deinstitutionalization, Avis (1985) states:

> In my recent experience the need for placing young children out of their own homes to receive training has been reduced by mandated school programs. If outside placement is needed for other reasons, placements are preferably made in a community training home where the education and family-like relationships continue. Even this option is offered only when direct assistance to the whole family has been insufficient. (p. 194)

The UCLA Project for Severely Impaired Children and Their Families (Meyers & Blacher, 1985) studied parents' perceptions of schooling as one of several key dimensions that may affect their decision to keep or place their severely handicapped child. It also examines factors related to family adjustment (marital harmony, sibling adjustment, the quality of the family environment and child rearing, coping ability and so forth), social support networks (sources of formal and informal support and respite), and child characteristics (adaptive and maladaptive behavior, temperament, attachment, responsivity, and the like). The ultimate aim is to determine, using a prospective research design, which factors dispose a family to place their child and which dispose the family to keep the child at home. It was hypothesized that public schooling would have a tremendous impact on families' decision to keep such a child. After 3 years of study, only seven families have placed their child, and two more are in the process of placement. As more children reach puberty, placement grows more likely (Meyers, Borthwick, & Eyman, 1985), and it should be possible to monitor further the role of schooling and other forms of respite in family decision making.

Future Research on Respite

Descriptions of types and forms of respite are currently available (Cohen & Warren, 1985; Salisbury & Griggs, 1983; this text); we know families need respite, but it is difficult to predict how much respite individual families need at what point in their family life cycle. Ongoing investigations, such as the UCLA Project, can determine the role that primary respite services, as well as secondary respite provided by the public school, play in family decision making regarding a severely handicapped child. A research program is needed that could: 1) identify the stressors confronting families of severely handicapped children, 2) identify sources of respite or relief available to ease these stressors, and 3) relate patterns of stress and respite service utilization patterns to family characteristics.

As pointed out by Yando and Zigler (1984), no further research is needed to show that various respite services and facilities *should be* available for families; the issue is to design such services with flexible programming to enable families to utilize them. For example, these authors propose a model of services within a state or region that includes multiple local programs for preschool and school-age children, all integrated into the public school system. In addition to providing coordinated parent training and clinical services, districts or regions could also share a residential facility offering respite care. Through creative public-private cooperation, funding for such programs may become feasible (Zigler & Finn, 1981). Clearly, we have neither exhausted the possibilities for providing respite nor for evaluating the effectiveness of such services for families.

IMPLICATIONS FOR POLICY

There is an ongoing need for public advocates and policies that address future, as well as present, needs of families. With continued emphasis on normalization, mainstreaming, and deinstitutionalization, more handicapped individuals will remain at home, and more families will need access to respite services. Writes Keniston (1977):

> Indeed, in our complex, fragmented, often overwhelming society, parents can be driven to institutionalize a child by the sheer lack of resources and support in training of a kind and intensity that a normal parent with limited resources cannot always give. The failure of most of our communities to provide homemaking or babysitting services, respite care, special education, or daytime programs for handicapped children has been documented at length. (p. 193)

Public schooling has been and will continue to be a paramount need. It is one of the oldest and best established "family services" in this country (Keniston, 1977). As pointed out by Weicker (1985), there is still the need to train parents to participate in their children's special education, particularly as they deal with the critical transition of their child from school to some kind of employment activity.

Although a number of studies note that parents find a variety of respite services highly satisfying (Joyce et al., 1983; Ptacek et al., 1982; Seltzer & Krauss, 1984), such services are either not universally available, or they are available only on a limited basis. Informal supports to families might include help from friends and family, whereas formal support includes clinical services, financial incentives, parent training, and respite services. Furthermore, studies reviewed by Seltzer and Krauss (1984) indicate that the extent of formal support provided to severely retarded persons who live at home and to their families is considerably less than that provided to persons in out-of-home placements. Given these findings, one has to question policy and service system priorities for maintaining severely handicapped persons in their own homes.

CONCLUSION

Let us return to the historical role of schooling highlighted by Keniston (1977). He noted that schooling originally: 1) freed parents to work, 2) decreased family responsibility for teaching their children, and 3) decreased the economic value of children.

Increased schooling for handicapped children parallels the first of these roles—freeing parents to work, spend time with their nonhandicapped children, or pursue other activities. Yet, the parallel ends here. Families' responsibility for teaching is in some ways increased by the provisions of Public Law 94-142, and the economic value of children is implicitly increased by providing training for children who were formerly ignored. The overall impact of public schooling for the overwhelming majority of families with severely handicapped children appears to be positive.

REFERENCES

Ackerman, J. (1985). Preparing for separation. In H. R. Turnbull & A. P. Turnbull (Eds.), *Parents speak out: Then and now* (pp. 149–156). Columbus, OH: Charles E. Merrill Publishing Co.

Avis, D. W. (1985). Deinstitutionalization jet lag. In H. R. Turnbull & A. P. Turnbull (Eds.), *Parents speak out: Then and now* (pp. 193–199). Columbus, OH: Charles E. Merrill Publishing Co.

Baker, B. L. (1984). Intervention with families with young, severely handicapped children. In J. Blacher (Ed.), *Severely handicapped young children and their families: Research in review* (pp. 319–375). Orlando, FL: Academic Press.

Baker, B. L., & Brightman, H. P. (1984). Access of handicapped children to educational services. In N. D. Reppucci, L. A. Weithorn, E. P. Mulvey, & J. Monahan (Eds.), *Children, mental health, and the law* (Vol. 4, pp. 289–307). Beverly Hills, CA: Sage Publications.

Blacher, J. (1984). *Severely handicapped young children and their families: Research in review*. Orlando, FL: Academic Press.

Cohen, S. (1982). Supporting families through respite care. *Rehabilitation Literature, 43*, 7–11.

Cohen, S., & Warren, R. D. (1985). *Respite care: Principles, programs, and policies*. Austin, TX: Pro-Ed.

Cone, J. D., Delawyer, D. D., & Wolfe, V. V. (1985). Assessing parent participation: The parent/family involvement index. *Exceptional Children, 51*, 417–424.

Cremin, L. A. (1961). *The transformation of the school. Progressivism in American education. 1876–1957*. New York: Vintage Books.

Cremin, L. A. (1980). *American education. The national experience. 1783–1876*. New York: Harper & Row.

Crnic, K. A., Friedrich, W. N., & Greenberg, M. T. (1983). Adaptation of families with mentally retarded children: A model of stress, coping, and family ecology. *American Journal of Mental Deficiency, 88*, 125–138.

Farber, B. (1979). Sociological ambivalence and family care. In R. H. Bruininks & G. C. Krantz (Eds.), *Family care of developmentally disabled members: Conference proceedings* (pp. 27–36). Minneapolis: University of Minnesota.

Federal Register. (1977, August 23). Washington, DC: U. S. Government Printing Office.

Frodi, A. M. (1981). Contribution of infant characteristics to child abuse. *American Journal of Mental Deficiency, 85,* 341–349.

Garbarino, J. (1983). Social support networks: Treatment for the helping professionals. In J. K. Whittaker, J. Garbarino, & Associates (Eds.), *Social support networks: Informal helping in the human services.* New York: Aldine Publishing Company.

Grossman, H. J. (Ed.). (1983). *Classification in mental retardation.* Washington, DC: American Association on Mental Deficiency.

Helsel, E. D. (1985). Foreword. In S. Cohen & R. D. Warren, *Respite care. Principles, programs, & policies* (pp. ix–x). Austin, TX: Pro-Ed.

Joyce, K., Singer, M., & Isralowitz, R. (1983). Impact of respite care on parents' perceptions of quality of life. *Mental Retardation, 21*(4), 153–156.

Keniston, K., & The Carnegie Council on Children. (1977). *All our children: The American family under pressure.* New York: Harcourt Brace Jovanovich.

Locke, H. J., & Wallace, K. M. (1959). Short marital-adjustment and prediction tests: Their reliability and validity. *Journal of Marriage and Family Living, 21,* 251–255.

McCubbin, H. I., Joy, C. B., Cauble, A. E., Comeau, J. K., Patterson, J. M., & Needle, R. H. (1980). Family stress and coping: A decade review. *Journal of Marriage and the Family, 42,* 855–871.

McCubbin, H. I., Nevin, R. S., Cauble, A. E., Larsen, A., Comeau, J. K., & Patterson, J. M. (1982). Family coping with chronic illness: The case of cerebral palsy. In H. I. McCubbin, A. E. Cauble, & J. M. Patterson (Eds.), *Family stress, coping, and social support* (pp. 169–188). Springfield, IL: Charles C Thomas.

Meier, J. H., & Sloan, M. P. (1984). The severely handicapped and child abuse. In J. Blacher (Ed.), *Severely handicapped young children and their families. Research in review* (pp. 247–272). Orlando, FL: Academic Press.

Meyers, C. E., & Blacher, J. (1985a). *Parents' perception of schooling for their severely handicapped child.* Unpublished manuscript, UCLA Project for Severely Impaired Children and Their Families, UCLA-NPI Mental Retardation Research Center, Los Angeles.

Meyers, C. E., & Blacher, J. (1985b). *The effect of schooling on severely impaired children and their families.* NICHD Grant No. R01HD14680, UCLA School of Medicine, NPI-Mental Retardation Research Center, Lanterman State Hospital Research Group.

Meyers, C. E., & Blacher, J. (in press). Historical determinants of residential care for mentally retarded people. In S. Landesman & P. Vietze (Eds.), *Living with retarded persons,* washington, DC: American Association on Mental Deficiency.

Meyers, C. E., Borthwick, S. A., & Eyman, H. K. (1985). Place of residence by age, ethnicity, and level of the mentally retarded/developmentally disabled population of California. *American Journal of Mental Deficiency, 90*(3), 366–370.

Nihira, K., Foster, R., Shellhaas, M., & Leland, H. (1974). *AAMD Adaptive Behavior Scale.* Washington, DC: American Association on Mental Deficiency.

Powell, D. R. (1980). Personal social networks as a focus for primary prevention of child mistreatment. *Infant Mental Health Journal, 1,* 232–239.

Ptacek, L. J., Sommers, P. A., Graves, J., Lukowicz, P., Keena, E., Haglund, J., & Nycz, G. R. (1982). Respite care for families of children with severe handicaps: An evaluation study of parent satisfaction. *Journal of Community Psychology, 10,* 222–227.

Rimstidt, S. (1983). When respite care does not exist. *The Exceptional Parent, 13*(6), 45–48.

Salisbury, C., & Griggs, P. (1983). Developing respite care services for families of handicapped persons. *TASH Journal, 8,* 50–57.

Schilling, R. F., & Schinke, S. P. (1983). Social support networks in developmental disabilities. In J. K. Whittaker, J. Garbarino, & Associates (Eds.), *Social support networks: Informal helping in the human services.* New York: Aldine Publishing Company.

Seltzer, M. M., & Krauss, M. W. (1984). Placement alternatives for mentally retarded children and their families. In J. Blacher (Ed.), *Severely handicapped young children and their families. Research in review* (pp. 143–175). Orlando, FL: Academic Press.

Skrtic, T. M., Summers, J. A., Brotherson, M. J., & Turnbull, A. P. (1984). Severely handicapped children and their brothers and sisters. In J. Blacher (Ed.), *Severely handicapped young children and their families: Research in review* (pp. 215–246). Orlando, FL: Academic Press.

Stotland, J. F., & Mancuso, E. (1981). U. S. Court of Appeals decision regarding *Armstrong v. Kline:* The 180 day rule. *Exceptional Children, 47*(4), 266–270.

Turnbull, A. P., & Winton, P. J. (1984). Parent involvement policy and practice: Current research and implications for families of young, severely handicapped children. In J. Blacher (Ed.), *Severely handicapped young children and their families: Research in review* (pp. 377–397). Orlando, FL: Academic Press.

Upshur, C.C. (1983). Developing respite care: A support service for families with disabled members. *Family Relations, 32,* 13–20.

Wahler, R. G. (1980). The insular mother: Her problems in parent-child treatment. *Journal of Applied Behavior Analysis, 13,* 207–219.

Weicker, L., Jr. (1985). Sonny and public policy. In H. R. Turnbull & A. P. Turnbull (Eds.), *Parents speak out: Then and now* (pp. 281–287). Columbus, OH: Charles E. Merrill Publishing Co.

Werner, E. E., & Smith, R. S. (1982). *Vulnerable but invincible: A study of resilient children.* New York: McGraw-Hill Book Co.

Willer, B., Intagliata, J., & Wicks, N. (1981). Return of retarded adults to natural families: Issues and results. In R. H. Bruininks, D. E. Meyers, B. B. Sigford, & K. C. Lakin (Eds.), *Deinstitutionalization and community adjustment of mentally retarded people* (pp. 207–216). Washington, DC: American Association on Mental Deficiency.

Yando, R., & Zigler, E. (1984). Severely handicapped children and their families: A synthesis. In J. Blacher (Ed.), *Severely handicapped young children and their families. Research in review* (pp. 401–416). Orlando, FL: Academic Press.

Zigler, E., & Finn, M. (1981). From problem to solution: Changing public policy as it affects children and families. *Young Children, 36*(4), 31–32, 55–58.

Chapter 12

PARENTS' PERSPECTIVES
FOCUS ON PROVIDERS

Noreen Quinn Curran

The two kinds of respite care we have always preferred are in-home respite for an overnight or weekend and out-of-home respite at Christine's camp setting, not a respite facility. In-home respite seems to be the most preferred respite by many parents of children with mild to moderate delays, for the obvious reasons that there is less disruption of family life and the environment remains fairly consistent for the individual with developmental delays. Presently existing respite facilities seem to be more appropriate for the severely handicapped, although in a world with more options for parents, a respite facility designed for the person with mild to moderate disabilities should be available.

Summer camp for Christine has proven to be a very normalized respite for us, as well as a constructive, highly mainstreamed activity for Christine. Now, at 17, having 10 years behind her at her same regular girls' summer camp, she is in the counselor-in-training program, assisting on the waterfront and with other camp activities. What a boost to her self-esteem! What peace of mind and pride this brings to us! Unfortunately, it has been difficult to get some respite agencies to consider this kind of camping experience as a legitimate use of respite monies, especially when used to support funding for an integrated camp.

Recreation programs are another form of short-term respite for families that, in my opinion, should be vastly expanded. In my past work with parents in the urban Boston school system, many parents of adolescents with mild/moderate developmental delays chose, in an assessment of needs, after-school recreational programs as their first, and often only, choice of respite programs. It is crucial that, for parents to take advantage of respite, the services must be designed to meet their needs and be sensitive to cultural/ethnic preferences.

AVAILABILITY

We have experienced increased success with respite care services over the past 10 years. Our experiences with public agencies (Department of Social Services and Department of Mental Health) continue to be very positive ones. Our daughter enjoys the experience, and the workers seem to enjoy her. My requests for services are handled courteously and efficiently, with minimum hassle to me, which, as a broker in the world of my daughter's special services, I appreciate.

The kind of people we—my daughter and I—have come to prefer are young female college students. These women are now seen as Christine's companions. When Christine was younger, we preferred to use our regular babysitter, who eventually came to be called a "kidsitter." I urge agencies to be more open to the person of the parents' choice (e.g., the regular babysitter) as this person knows the child well, knows the parents' expectations and routines, and there is less adjustment for the young child to make to a new person in the home, as well as less stress for the parents. A respite is supposed to provide a break, not another reason for the parents to worry.

A SIMPLE PROCESS

The process of obtaining respite care is as follows:

1. A telephone call is placed requesting service, usually with 2 weeks advance notice.
2. Two to three days later, the agency calls me with an identified person who can accept the assignment.
3. This person calls me, and we have a brief chat about Christine and her needs.
4. When Christine was younger, if the person was new to us, I would ask that she come to visit for a half-hour or so and charge that time, including travel time, to our respite hours. Now, I feel comfortable enough with the women the agency sends, as well as with my daughter's ability to adapt, to talk only briefly over the telephone and then observe the person for a few minutes with Christine. This affords me an opportunity to make any necessary comments.

Our criteria has become simpler over the years; we ask for someone who likes children, particularly teenagers, and who is reasonably responsible.

TRAINING

All the respite workers appear to have had some training. Their transition into our home and with Christine is quite smooth, and everyone seems to enjoy the experience.

Some training components I would suggest be included before placement with a family would cover these areas:

1. An overview of handicapping conditions and their effect on the child and his or her family
2. A clear description of what is expected at the placement
3. A discussion of the agency's guidelines for the kind of activities in which the respite worker can participate (e.g., taking the child in his or her own car, taking care of other siblings). (One worker would not accept responsibility for Christine's brother, then age 10 or 11. We had to decline the respite, because we had no family member at the time to whom we could send our son.)
4. Some "suggested activities" to do with children or young adults with disabilities

The informal "training" I give consists of the following:

1. A brief overview of my expectations: 1) that Christine enjoy the respite and 2) that regular routines be followed (e.g., limit setting on eating, television, and bedtime)
2. A review of Christine's usual planned activities and a discussion of new possible activities mutually worked out between her parents, Christine, and the respite worker
3. A list of emergency numbers to call (e.g., doctors, friends, neighbors, relatives)
4. A discussion of information resources that are readily available (i.e., Christine's brother and Christine herself). Drawing attention to Christine by indicating her competency gives her an important boost in her self-esteem and seems to enhance her perception of the respite worker as a companion/friend.

COSTS

We have never been charged for respite care services. We use the time we need, not necessarily what the agency (Department of Social Services) has established for us. The time allotted by this agency is the same for all families; therefore, not needing as much time as some other families, we generally use less than half of our allotted time in a year.

I firmly believe that families with children or adults who are handicapped should be legally entitled to services at government expense, just as a child who is handicapped is entitled to a free appropriate education at public expense under PL 94-142. If children and young adults with handicaps are to remain at home in a positive environment, then the government must provide funds to support families in this important yet tiring endeavor. The total cost of quality services (i.e., education, recreation, vocational training, and adequate respite) in 1 year cannot compare with the exorbitant cost of institutionalization for an adolescent with developmental disabilities for the same period of time.

Harriet Horowitz Bongiorno

Fifteen years ago when our need for respite care was at its zenith, respite care as we know it today was unavailable in our community. Today, thankfully, this situation is beginning, albeit slowly, to change. The local developmental center will offer up to 30 days respite care for those parents whose children are enrolled in nonresidential services offered by the center. This service is based on the availability of space on a suitable unit. It is offered to a limited number of families who feel the need to be relieved of the burden of caring for their severely handicapped child, as well as to families who are considering placing their child in a developmental center. The local developmental center is also in the process of initiating a home health care/homemaker service to provide limited respite in the home. Although progress is being made, only a minute number of families are being served.

TRAINING OF PROVIDERS

It is my feeling that the nurses' aides, therapy aides, and nurses at the developmental center appear to be well trained for their respective positions. An extensive mandated inservice program must be completed as a condition for continued employment. It would be my hope and/or recommendation that part of the curriculum include seminar courses in family counseling, care of the developmentally handicapped, family crisis intervention, pharmacology, and sensitivity training in the awareness of the special needs and pressures of parents who have handicapped children.

I believe that respite care services should be provided to the parents of handicapped children at no cost to the family. Most of the affected families would probably be single-income families with other dependents who are already overburdened by unusual expenses for medications, special equipment, medical bills, and dietary supplements. Current financial statistics indicate that the cost of maintaining a child at a developmental facility is approximately $60,000 per year. If one were to consider only the economics of this situation it should seem readily apparent that many children/families could be afforded home respite aide for the same dollar-for-dollar cost of maintaining one child in a facility. The cost of respite care should be underwritten by the state, federal, or local government and not by the families because most families lack the resources for such an undertaking.

Providing in-home respite services to families of handicapped children would not only alleviate some of the tremendous burden experienced by the families but would also allow the members of the family to share their love and lives with each other . . . at home.

Part III

EVALUATING
RESPITE SERVICES

Chapter 13

HOME-BASED RESPITE CARE, THE CHILD WITH DEVELOPMENTAL DISABILITIES, AND FAMILY STRESS

SOME THEORETICAL AND PRAGMATIC ASPECTS OF PROCESS EVALUATION

Lynn McDonald Wikler,
Darald Hanusa, and Judy Stoycheff

W hen families with children who are developmentally disabled are asked to name services that would be helpful to them, respite care is usually mentioned first. Respite care programs often claim one of their articulated goals to be the reduction in stress in the families of the person with developmental disabilities (Cannon, 1978; Hitzling, Loop, Lyons-Ross, & Miller, 1976; Moore & Seachore, 1977; Warner, 1978). The assumption is made that respite care reduces family stress because it relieves the family's relatively uninterrupted caregiving responsibility for the child's extraordinary needs. Parental responses to survey questionnaires administered after the provision of respite care services have supported this perspective (Upshur, 1983). However, there has been no systematic study of the impact of respite care on family stress nor any careful discussion of the ways in which the process might be quantitatively evaluated.

This chapter summarizes some of the literature on family stress, indicates ways in which respite care may function to affect those stresses, and illustrates these topics by describing the evaluative process of two prevention-oriented respite care projects conducted by the authors.

In both these pilot projects, process data were collected at regular intervals over time. In contrast to simply taking pre/post-measures, process evaluation was able to describe more fully some features of interventional respite care for individual families. The projects were similar in that each provided a nonnegotiable, noncontingent 6 hours-per-week minimum of respite care. The training of the respite care workers was also similar. However, the two projects had distinctly different goals. The first project provided respite care to five families of children with developmental disabilities who had recently been discharged to the community and remained at risk for reinstitutionalization because of chronic severe behavioral problems. Respite care was begun as an intervention to avoid placement. The focus of evaluation was on regular monitoring of the behavioral problems of the handicapped child as the producer of family stress.

In the second project, families with developmentally disabled children in the community who were committed to keeping their child at home volunteered to receive respite care. The evaluative focus was on monitoring the stress levels of each family throughout the provision of the respite care services.

Process data collected during the administration of both respite care projects showed a reduction in the targeted problem areas. Parents reported high satisfaction with the projects; quantitative outcome data were also collected. However, each of the fifteen families also varied widely in their responses on attitudes and stress levels; some benefited more than others from the receipt of respite care.

The final section of this chapter discusses the theory of respite care, and, using a family stress model, considers the theoretical impact of respite care on a family's functioning. Recommendations for future research are then presented.

BACKGROUND

Families with developmentally disabled children are reported to experience several unique, chronic stresses over the life cycle of the child. Among these is the extraordinary burden of care that is both prolonged and continuous (Wikler, 1981). Management problems related to the specific handicapping condition of the child, such as hyperactivity in a nonverbal child or spasticity and lack of bowel control in a teenager, are physically exhausting to the primary caregiver. As the child grows larger, these extraordinary needs become more burdensome (Berger & Foster, 1976; Holt, 1958). Added to these physical burdens is the psychological stress of the prolongation of these children's dependency needs far beyond the period of preschool, during which all parents expect the extensive dependency needs of their children. Mothers of developmentally delayed children cannot look forward to engaging in activities in which parents of normal children moving toward adulthood can participate (Birenbaum, 1971; Farber, 1976). Finally, the prolonged and extraordinary burden of care is likely to be continuous; there are few breaks available to the caregiver from the constant demands. This burden of care may be related to the increased social isolation reported by these families (Barsch, 1968; Farber, 1959, 1960, 1968; Holt, 1958; Jacobs, 1974; Levinson, 1975; Stone, 1965) and the significantly fewer social contacts of families of mentally retarded children as contrasted with families of normal children (Davis & MacKay, 1973; McAllister, Butler, & Lei, 1973).

One family resource or community support for parents of normal children has always been babysitters, teenage neighbors or relatives who provide brief periods of child care enabling the parents to conduct a normal social life. Families of the mentally retarded child, however, are less likely to procure this resource. Because one coping behavior that has been identified as related to family adaptation is the procuring of community and social supports (Mc-Cubbin & Patterson, 1983), one question is whether the families themselves are maladaptive in this way, or whether the community and societal stigma inhibits the success of such transactions.

Respite care has emerged as an institutional response to this support deficit to assist families in their care for their handicapped offspring. Defined as temporary relief from the continuous burden of care, respite care is offered in several forms, including in-home services (sitter/companion and companion services) and out-of-home services (planned and emergency weekend/2-week respite care provided in foster homes, group homes, nursing homes, homes of other parents of developmentally disabled children, and institutions). The respite care programs offer substitute care to families for periods of time ranging from several hours to days or weeks. These can be pre-scheduled or in response to emergencies (Warren, 1981). Thus, there is variability in frequency, duration, spontaneity, and continuity.

In general, service providers, rather than the families themselves, have been responsible for determining which type of service will be most likely to achieve the goals of supporting the family as a whole, reducing family stress, and improving the behavior of the child in question within the home.

FIRST PROJECT DESCRIPTION

Five developmentally disabled children at severe risk for reinstitutionalization were targeted in a small prevention-oriented respite care project (Wikler & Stoycheff, 1975). Each had been hospitalized for management of severe behavioral problems, during which time careful inpatient behavior management programs had been developed and implemented. At discharge the professional staff was concerned about the transition period of returning home:

Would the families be able to maintain these programs at home? The stresses that led to hospitalization, in addition to the parents' reported difficulty in engaging babysitters, were thought to jeopardize (at minimum) the consistent enforcement of the behavioral programs at home. To require that the mothers take on the continuous, uninterrupted burden of extraordinary care subsequent to the hospitalization period could also increase the potential of parental burnout for several reasons. First, the mothers had grown accustomed to time without the child. In addition, there was the potential for the deterioration of the behavioral gains the child had made in the hospital setting, and finally, there was the risk of the family's placing the child outside the home a second time, but this time permanently.

Over a 4-month transition period, a respite care project was developed that provided in-home respite care for 6 hours a week per family by students trained in behavior management techniques. The project was described to the parents as a routine part of the program: the transition phase. Five college students were selected and trained to provide in-home respite care. These students were among 15 who responded to a description of the project as a student employment service. The selection criteria were: 1) interest in learning about mental retardation and behavior modification; 2) minimum of a sophomore standing in college, with a major related to handicapped children; 3) previous experience with children, preferably with handicapped children; and 4) willingness to commit 6 months to the project.

Procedure

The students participated in six weekly 2-hour seminars and three 2-hour practicums with mentally retarded children in an inpatient setting. The seminars covered: 1) information on mental retardation and the characteristic problems of working with mentally retarded children; 2) principles of behavior modification with children, such as defining, observing, and charting behaviors and consistent carrying out of contingent reinforcement and time-out behavior interventions; and 3) assignments of reading and practice exercises between sessions to promote understanding and discussion.

The practicum was designed to expose the trainees to mentally retarded children with severe behavioral problems and to the professional staff's methods of handling those problems. The first session was spent observing the staff interact with the patients in the inpatient setting; the second included recording data on a specified behavior of a child and playing with that child; and the third session was spent implementing behavioral intervention while playing with the child. A nurse trained in behavioral techniques supervised the students' experiences by observing them and discussing their performance. No more than two students had a practicum at any one time.

The five trained respite care workers were then matched as closely as possible to five families of discharged patients who were interested in the respite care project. The matching was done on the basis of the child's problems, the student's skills, and location. The students then met individually with the project coordinators to become familiar with the particular assigned child and family. Student and parents agreed to the prescribed minimum involvement of 6 hours per week for sixteen consecutive weeks at a cost to the families of $1.50 per hour. The students decided with the parents which behaviors should be targeted. Specific behavioral programs were developed with the supervisor, weekly data on changes in the child's target behavior were kept, and regular supervisory meetings were required of the respite care workers. Supervision entailed weekly supportive phone calls from the nurse, monthly workshop discussions to review the behavioral programs and share experiences with one another, and two final sessions to compile the data and evaluate the project.

Case Descriptions

Case A was a 3½-year-old boy with borderline intelligence and autistic behaviors. The respite caretaker was able during daily, hour-long sessions using immediate candy reinforcers to increase the child's obedience of commands from 18% to 100%, given a constant number of commands. The student also noticed an increase in the child's verbalizations and worked to shape them with positive reinforcement (candy and praise) into frequent full sentences (see Figure 1).

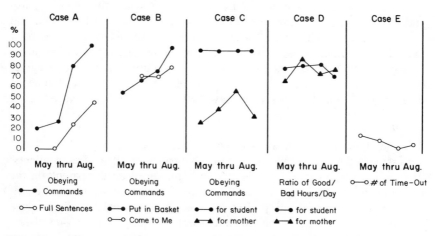

Figure 1.   Target behaviors of five children with developmental disabilities over a 4-month intervention period in the home. (Observations made by trained respite caregivers and parents.)

Case B was a 4½-year-old severely mentally retarded and autistic girl. She had been treated both as an inpatient and an outpatient to reduce her destructive behavior and increase her attention span. The mother could find no one to manage the child whom she could trust. The respite caregiver spent her time focusing on two specific commands, while using candy reinforcers and praise. Improvement was slow, but steady.

Case C is a mildly retarded 7½-year-old boy with behavior problems of aggression, withdrawal, and encopresis. The family has been involved with both the outpatient and inpatient services at the Neuropsychiatric Institute for 2 years. The child would respond in an appropriate way to the professional after treatment, but not to his mother. Extensive counseling and training still left the mother's behavior inconsistent with her son. This inconsistency maintained itself throughout the project. Although the student-therapist tried to support the mother in being consistent, the student had no problems with the boy's following commands and spent time playing positively with him.

Case D was a 4-year-old boy with severe aggressive and destructive behavioral problems. The goal of the respite caregiver was to maintain the positive ratio of "good" hours per day (i.e., without temper tantrums or destroying things) to "bad" hours per day. The parents kept a star chart during each week that they reviewed with the student, who used the same one when he babysat. This child was given time-out on a chair for 5 minutes after aggressive behavior and was rewarded with stars, play activities, and praise for a certain number of good hours. The child maintained an acceptable level of behavior over the 4-month period.

Case E was a 7-year-old mildly retarded boy with mild cerebral palsy and manipulating behavior. He would throw things, scream for hours, and vomit in order to get his way. The student-therapist was able to gain control of the child's manipulative temper tantrums, which never entirely disappeared, by consistently using a contingent time-out procedure. The respite caregiver developed such a positive relationship with the boy that the parents left her to care for him while they took a long-awaited two-week summer vacation.

Evaluation

The underlying goals of this respite care project were: 1) to avoid behavioral regression and maintain behavioral gains that had been attained as inpatients, 2) to reduce the extraordinary burden of care placed on the parents in the transition following hospitalization, and 3) to avoid reinstitutionalization.

The evaluation of this project included observational data on selected behaviors of the mentally retarded child over time, questionnaires on satisfaction with the respite care services, and pre/post measures of parental attitudes toward their mentally retarded child.

Table 1. Changes in family functioning of nine families receiving respite care over a 2-month period

Perception of changes	Functioning of developmentally disabled child	Functioning of mother	Marital relations	Social relations
Positively perceived changes	20.5%	17.6%	14.3%	53.5%
Mixed perception of changes	2.5	3.1	20.0	2.3
Negatively perceived changes	5.1	7.9	8.5	2.3
No reported changes	71.8	71.4	57.2	41.9
	100.0%	100.0%	100.0%	100.0%

Children's Behavior   There was no increase in maladaptive behaviors and no deterioration for any of the five children shown in the charting over a 4-month transition period (Table 1). Instead, maintenance or improvement of selected behaviors charted by the respite care workers was evident in each case. This data were also consistent with the informal reports of overall behaviors given by both the respite care workers and the parents.

Respite for the Parents   The parents unanimously expressed satisfaction and relief at having a consistent, reliable, and trained person to share their responsibilities of child care. In the postproject questionnaire, they reported an increase of times per month they had gone out. Each family found its own way of using this opportunity.

Placement   Parental response to an open-ended question in the informal evaluative questionnaire reflected an increase in positive attitudes toward their child. A simple five-point scale was used to test parents both before and after the project in order to measure quantitatively changes in parental feelings about their mentally retarded child. Although there were some changes, there were no consistent patterns in either direction on this scale, in contrast to what was evident in the answers to the open-ended question. None of the families requested readmission of their child over the critical 4-month transition period.

Discussion

In the process of evaluation, an important point emerged. Concern about readmission due to the behavioral problems of this target population resulted in a direct focus by the respite care workers with the parent on the use of behavioral techniques to avoid behavioral regression. The collaborative emphasis on the child's behavior seemed to function to shield the parents from the actual goal of the enterprise, which was to provide relief to them in their caregiving role. The parents were often hesitant to express openly their need to "take a break." It was as though a "good" mother should never complain about her own exhaustion or frustrations. By portraying the respite program as a benefit to the child, the respite care workers entered into a face-saving process, which then enhanced the likelihood of the program being effectively used. When the parent returned refreshed, worker and parent discussed the child's progress, rather than overtly acknowledging that this refreshment was the project's goal. In addition, the special training of the respite case worker seemed to support the notion that the child was difficult to manage and that the mother did have an extraordinary burden of care. The affirmation of the complexities of the tasks faced by the mother seemed to restore her perception of herself as a competent parent facing a difficult challenge.

SECOND PROJECT DESCRIPTION

In contrast to the first project in which short-term institutionalization had already taken place, the target population in the second project consisted of families in the community who had kept their developmentally disabled child at home and who volunteered for the respite care project (Wikler & Hanusa, 1980).

Rather than focusing on the developmentally disabled child's behavior, the overt goal was to provide relief to the parent as primary caregiver of the continuous care. Stresses experienced by families of the child with developmental disabilities were routinely monitored as they received respite care by one assigned, trained respite caretaker over a 2-month period. The intervention was basically the same as in the first project, with a non-negotiable *6-hours-per-week* respite care in the home, scheduled according to the needs of the family and the availability of the caregiver. Respite care was provided at no cost to the family by trained graduate students. However, no specific behavioral program was developed.

Families with developmentally disabled children living at home were made aware of the project through fliers posted at parent associations, preschools, churches, and clinics. Eighteen such families responded, and 14 completed the preliminary assessment forms. Of these, 10 were randomly selected to fill the 10 slots in the respite care project.

The parents varied widely in regard to demographic variables. Seven were married, two were divorced, and one was a foster parent (mother). Four families earned over $18,000 year, four between $9,600 and $18,000, and two under $9,600. Eighty-eight percent of all the parents had an advanced education, 6% had a high school diploma, and the remaining 6% had education at the elementary level.

There were six male and four female developmentally disabled children, with ages ranging from 2 to 20 years. With the exception of one severely mentally retarded individual, all were functioning in the moderately mentally retarded range. They had various other handicaps, including cerebral palsy, Down syndrome, autism, microcephaly, and deafness.

Before the project, the ten families had used babysitters between zero and two times per week, averaging 1.85 hours per week. Three families reported using no babysitters at all. This project would therefore be tripling the amount of respite care they were receiving. In order to participate in the project, the parents agreed to use 6 hours of respite care per week. The parents' average rating of satisfaction with their current use of babysitting-respite care services was 1.88 on a scale of 1 through 6 (6 being highly satisfied).

Case Descriptions

Case 1 was a mentally retarded 12-year-old boy who was the elder of two brothers. He was attending a small class for children with autistic-type behavior. The cause of his multiple problems was not known; however, he required constant supervision. Before the onset of this program, respite was provided by a relative who cared for the boy for a couple of hours once a week. However, this break was only reluctantly used.

Both before and after participation in the respite care project, the family reported stress in several areas: 1) they had financial difficulties, 2) the mother was depressed, and 3) the second child was manifesting problems at school.

Despite hesitation and even initial suspicion, this family reported enormous benefit from the respite worker. The mother noted an improvement in her general ability to cope. Her attitude toward the mentally retarded child became more positive, and the parents were able to give their other child more attention. For the first time ever, the mother reported feeling comfortable leaving her child with a nonrelative. The parents expressed their complete satisfaction and positive benefits from respite care.

Although it is clear that the problems in this family were considerable, particularly for the mother, the impact of respite care was positive. She reported that the change of routine alone helped her gain some perspective on her own feelings, which in turn improved her relationship with her mentally retarded child. In her own words, "Worry free fun temporarily made me feel less stressed and able to face the world every day without becoming bogged down in grief."

Case 2 was a 21-year-old female who lived with her parents at home. She was both profoundly deaf and severely mentally retarded. Although she could do many things for herself, such as dressing and eating, she required much attention. On weekdays she attended a program for retarded adults who could not attend sheltered workshops. She spent the rest of the time with her mother at home.

A major obstacle to this family's having time to themselves was the absence of suitable respite care; this was due in part to their social isolation, but mainly because of their daughter's difficult behavior. Before the respite care program, they perceived no available alternatives; supervising the daughter was a continuous and overwhelming task, because she could not be left alone at home.

The family reported a considerable decrease in stress after provision of respite care and expressed an increased ability to cope. They also wanted respite care to continue. The mother reported an improved relationship with the mentally retarded child, and the latter's behavior was markedly better. The entire family reported benefiting from the brief intervention.

Evaluation

The formal assessment of this project included four components: 1) subjective process evaluation of the familial stress level taken by the respite caregiver following each visit, 2) a Family Changes Questionnaire administered at the end of the project by the student assigned to that family, 3) pre/post intervention scores on a standardized questionnaire on family stress (Holroyd, 1974), and 4) parental evaluation of the program submitted anonymously by mail after the last formal contact. The results are summarized below.

Process Evaluation of Family Stress Levels   After each visit, the respite caregivers rated the familial stress level on a scale of 1 (none) to 6 (extreme stress); the results are shown in Figure 2. There may have been a bias in the ratings given by the committed caregivers who were hoping to see change. However, because they were familiar with the families, they may have been better able to make valid assessments. The individual families' stress assessments over time were graphed. At the outset of the program, these assessments were averaged at 4.0 and decreased to an average of 1.8 during the final home assessment, a reduction of more than half.

Family Changes Questionnaire   This questionnaire, administered by the respite caregivers to the mother at the end of the project, identifies areas of family functioning in which behaviorally specific changes assumed to reflect stress have occurred. These include the developmentally disabled child, 6 items; socializing patterns of the family members, 5 items; marital relationship, 5 items; and mother's functioning, 7 items. For each reported

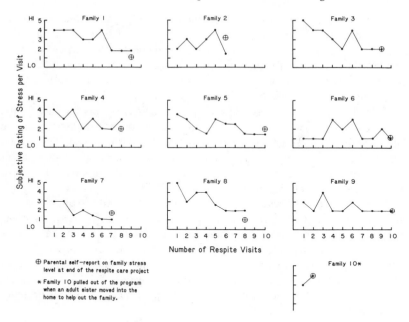

Figure 2. Stress levels of families with children with developmental disabilities over 10 weeks of in-home respite care. (Observations made by trained respite caregivers and parents.)

change, the respondent was asked to state if she thought there had been a change and, if so, whether it was positive, negative, or mixed.

Grouped data reported in percentages showed positively perceived, negatively perceived, and mixed perception changes in each area of family functioning. Although there were more positively perceived changes than negatively perceived changes reported in each category, the greatest amount of positive change was in social relations (see Table 1).

Pre/Post Scores on Standardized Questionnaire The Questionnaire on Resources and Stress (QRS, Holroyd, 1974) is a tool for evaluating the extent and types of stress experienced by the family as it cares for the handicapped child. It is an objective, multidimensional, self-administered test. The test includes 285 items representing family and respondent difficulties in coping, as well as items reflecting actual handicap or dependency in the index case. The items are arranged into 15 nonoverlapping scales: 1) poor health/mood, 2) excess time demands, 3) negative attitude toward the index case, 4) over-protection/dependency, 5) lack of social support, 6) overcommitment/martyrdom, 7) pessimism, 8) lack of family integration, 9) limits on family opportunity, 10) financial problems, 11) physical incapacitation, 12) lack of activities for index case, 13) occupational limitations for index case, 14) social obtrusiveness, and 15) difficult personality characteristics. The QRS has successfully discriminated between stresses in families with children of varying handicapping conditions (Beckman, 1983; Friedrich, 1979; Holroyd & Guthrie, 1979; Holroyd & McArthur, 1980).

Tests for differences between pre- and poststress ratings for each of the 15 Holroyd scales were computed using Wilcoxon's T Statistic for the Matched Pairs Signed Rank Test (Wilcoxon & Wilcoxon, 1964). There were significant decreases (p < .05) in both the negative attitudes of the mother toward the child with developmental disabilities and in the reported number of difficult personality characteristics.

Postrespite Care Evaluations These evaluations were solicited at the end of the project. On anonymously returned evaluation forms, the parents rated their own estimate of reduction of family stress due to respite care. They assessed their own overall stress reduction as 4.00 out of a possible 5. In addition, they rated their overall satisfaction with the respite care project; on a scale of 1 (low) through 5 (high) they rated the project as 4.88. At the outset, one should recall that their satisfaction with previously available arrangements was 1.88.

Discussion

Because the amount of respite care offered per week was not considered negotiable, the question of when parents ask for respite did not arise. However, it did seem that these mothers probably would not have requested this much respite time at the outset of the program. (This was different from the first project in which each of those children had recently been discharged from inpatient care). These women seemed so entrenched in their daily routines of essentially uninterrupted caregiving that they lost their initiative in self-care and lowered their expectations of breaks for themselves. Again, there seemed to be a belief that the "good" mother concerns herself first, and possibly only, with the needs of others. This myth can present problems of several kinds. First, the mother may not be easily able to monitor her own exhaustion level and so may become suddenly surprised at finding herself emotionally depleted. Second, the mother may be seriously inhibited in requesting respite care because she assumes that she would be judged as an inadequate mother by others, as well as by herself. However, such potential problems were avoided by predetermining the amount of respite care, so that the mothers did not have to request the amount.

Whereas in the first project, the respite care workers had collaborated with the parents around a specific focus—activities with the child with developmental disabilities—in the second project extensive discussion revolved around ways in which the parents could use the 6 hours per week of newly available time. The respite care workers discovered that mothers had difficulty planning for free time. Under supervision, the students worked with the mothers to devise creative and inexpensive activities that would be satisfying to them.

The discussions with these mothers made clear that the theory of providing a respite to the caregiver of a person with developmental disabilities differs from the practice. What is respite to one person may not be respite for the next. For one mother, respite care meant 2 weeks of vacationing with no responsibilities for child care. For another, respite meant working in her garden for 3 hours without interruption while listening to the contented sounds of her child being entertained in the house. Another mother needed ideas on how to use respite care. Eventually, she went to three dress stores, tried on dresses in each one, and did not buy anything. The luxury of shopping without a specific purchase in mind was meaningful to her. One mother needed someone to drive her wheelchair-bound son to and from an activity as her respite. The variability of people's needs reflects the diversity of people's life-styles, and respite for families should be responsive to the uniqueness of each family's circumstances. In this case the only restraints were time. The parent and the respite care worker negotiated openly to find the most suitable arrangement for each individual mother.

Perhaps the most notable trait brought out by the process evaluation was the variability over time of the family stress levels. There was no single profile that could characterize these families. Although overall the stress levels were reduced by more than half, each family had a unique pattern of recorded stress levels.

This finding confirms the understanding that each family has not only its own definition of respite but also its own specific context. And as the family processes the contextual information from schools, from work, and from friends, relatives, and neighbors, it responds. If the external or internal information is problematic, the observed family stress levels increase. Many of these stresses will be unrelated to the handicap of the child and yet are cumulative in effect, and so they co-exist with the chronic stresses of the child's disability.

Because there were no requests made for respite, it is unclear whether requests would have been made when excessive multiple stresses occurred in families. However, it seems safe to conjecture that the parent would often allow the family stress levels to rise significantly before turning to outside sources for help.

Yet, if respite could exist as a preventive service, it could function as a buffer for these families. Respite provided automatically, as it was in these projects, could offer an additional consistent family resource. Respite could be an antidote to chronic family stress and could increase family resilience in coping with the additional acute stresses of normal family life.

SPECULATIONS

Why, in theory, would respite care effect a reduction in reports of family stress? Family stress theorists propose two factors that can buffer the impact of hardship on a family and help avoid a family crisis: the family resources available for handling the hardships and the perception the family holds about the hardships (Hill, 1958; McCubbin et al., 1980).

In the two projects described here, the provision of respite care on a regular basis by one person in the home clearly functioned to reduce the hardship itself (i.e., the burden of care for the primary caregiver). Improving the behavior of the child reduced the extraordinary caregiving needs of the child with developmental disabilities, whereas provision of respite care interrupted the continuous demands on the mother.

Respite care additionally may have had an impact on both of the buffering factors discussed by Hill (1958). The family's resources were expanded simply by having another person available to participate in the caregiving activities of the child with developmental disabilities. In addition, because of the respite care for the primary caregiver, more of her time and energy was available for making social contacts outside the home. For example, of the four dimensions of family functioning in which the mother reported change over the respite care period, the most dramatic change was in the increase of social relations. Reducing the social isolation of the family by the provision of regular respite care may also function to increase the resilience of the mother. Both socializing and having an alternative caregiver may increase the family resources available for managing the hardship of the burden of care.

The perception held by the primary caregiver about the continuous burden of care seems also to have been altered and improved by the provision of respite care. Negative attitudes toward the child may build up in part due to the physical and emotional drain on the family. This perception could be altered by respite care as provided in these projects. These parents had an opportunity to observe the respite care worker's attitude, skills, and knowledge as he or she interacted in the family's own home with their child. Through such modeling, parents may come to change their attitude toward the child. For example, on the QRS scales scores, significant change was observed in the negative attitudes toward the child with developmental disabilities. Observing their child interacting pleasantly with another adult, as well as seeing another person manage the youngster's difficult behaviors, may alter their own attitudes and energy in subsequent interactions with that child.

Boggs, a long-time advocate and lobbyist for developmentally disabled children, recommends that in-home supports for families of young developmentally disabled children should be made available with an emphasis on frequency, demand responsiveness, and reliability (1979). She supports a more proactive service, one that might offer, for example, a minimum of a set number of hours per week of in-home respite services.

RECOMMENDATIONS FOR FURTHER RESEARCH

In order to support the idea that respite care can indeed effect behavioral improvements of the child with developmental disabilities and reduce stress in the families, an experimental design should be developed that avoids threats to internal validity and external validity. For example, such a study might contrast two randomly assigned groups: a control group and a group that received this special form of prevention-oriented respite care. Having a control group would test the possibility that naturally occurring changes over time explained the results. The passage of 2 months and 4 months in the two respite care projects, for example, could account for changes that occurred in the families.

Second, the two groups should be randomly drawn from a population of families with developmentally disabled children. These groups could be compared to determine whether they were similar in various characteristics that may play a role in the families' responsiveness to the respite care; doing so could determine variations of respite programs that might best serve a more diverse population.

Further careful study could help answer the following questions. Does respite care effect a reduction in stress in families of the developmentally disabled and an improvement in the social and behavioral competence of the developmentally disabled child? Is the prevention-oriented type of in-home respite care being proposed in this chapter more effective than respite care as currently available in the community? Some of the families were more affected by the respite care intervention than were others; another study could begin to determine why the variable effect occurred.

Third, an independent interviewer who is unaware of the family's treatment status should administer the various assessments of familial stress and of the developmentally disabled children's behavior. Doing so would avoid the obviously confounding effect of having the assessments conducted by the respite caregivers who had a relationship with the family and an awareness of the goals of the project. It would also reduce the parental awareness of the impact of their responses on their respite caregiver. The problem of the parents being recipients of a highly valued service could be managed by using an objective assessor.

Another plausible explanation for the positive family changes resulting from respite care projects could be the social contact alone, rather than the respite care. An often-documented stress of families with developmentally disabled children is their relative social isolation. If another treatment group were established in which a person regularly visited the families, this intervening variable could be held constant.

The respite care projects described here had a preventive orientation in that they provided a set amount of respite care that was not contingent on requests for services. They aimed at reducing the stress of the extraordinarily continuous burden of care, and as a consequence, they supported the integrity of the family as a unit. A related benefit of these respite care programs was an improvement in the behaviors manifested by the developmentally disabled child. The interaction between stress experienced by the primary caregiver and difficult behaviors exhibited by the child should be further explored.

Finally, both of these respite care projects were conducted with a very small number of middle-class, white families. Larger numbers of families with more variability in social class and ethnic backgrounds should be included in the next study in order to determine variations of respite care services that might best serve a diverse population.

The goals of respite care are: 1) to provide refreshing, energizing breaks that will increase the family's ability to carry out home care while decreasing the emotional costs to its members; 2) to maintain the optimism and loving that the family member as caregiver can best provide; and 3) to avoid burnout that might precipitate neglect, major family disruptions, or placement. Yet, each mother has a unique constellation of personality features, support networks, additional responsibilities, caregiving histories, and social class and ethnic background that will affect her choice of respite care, as well as her satisfaction with it. These differences should be incorporated into evaluations of respite care services.

If respite is truly the goal, each family served should be interviewed about their unique circumstances and wishes, rather than having only one form of respite care available. Researchers should obtain the answer to this question: What supports could you imagine needing if you were to keep Johnny home for the next 5 years? Or, what is the type of problem that most makes you contemplate placement outside the home? This information increases the potential of delivering a true match to each family's situation. Then, as the care is provided, workers must monitor the family's satisfaction and intervene to alter the service if there are problems or concerns.

Outcome evaluations provide quantitative data about many families and indicate failure or success. They are useful for reporting purposes. However, outcome evaluation glosses over the nuances of each family's personal experiences. If the goal of evaluation includes the need to understand how and why respite care is effective, it requires careful observation of intimate accounts of the family's use and perception of the services over time. It is process evaluation that gives us the information needed for improving a program, for altering the services being provided, and for enhancing the fit between the respite caregiver and the family.

REFERENCES

Arnold, I. L., & Goodman, L. (1975). Homemaker services to families with young retarded children. In J. Dempsey (Ed.), *Community services for retarded children.* Baltimore: University Park Press.

Barsch, H. (1968). *Parents of the handicapped.* Springfield: Charles C Thomas.

Beckman, P. (1983). Influence of selected child characteristics on stress in families of handicapped infants. *American Journal of Mental Deficiency, 88* (2), 150–156.

Berger, M., & Foster, M. (1976). Family level interventions for retarded children: A multivariate approach to issues and strategies. *Multivariate Experimental Clinical Research, 2,* 1–21.

Birenbaum, A. (1971). The mentally retarded child in the home and the family cycle. *Journal of Health and Social Behavior, 12,* 55–65.

Boggs, E. M. (1979). Economic factors in family care. In R. H. Bruininks & G. C. Krantz (Eds.), *Family care of developmentally disabled members: Conference proceedings* (pp. 47–76). Minneapolis: University of Minnesota.

Cannon, G. (1978). *Annual report Archdiocese of Denver respite service project.* (Project No. 77-018a). Denver, CO.

Cook, J. J. (1963). Dimensional analysis of child-rearing attitudes of parents of handicapped children. *American Journal of Mental Deficiency, 68,* 354–361.

Crnic, K. A., Friedrich, W. N., & Greenberg, M. T. (1983). Adaptation of families of mentally retarded children: A model of stress, coping, and family ecology. *American Journal of Mental Deficiency, 88*(2), 125–138.

Cummings, S. T., Bayley, H. C., & Rie, H. E. (1966). Effect of the child's deficiency on the mother: A study of mothers of mentally retarded, chronically ill, and neurotic children. *American Journal of Orthopsychiatry, 36,* 595–608.

Davis, M., & MacKay, D. (1973). Mentally subnormal children and their families. *The Lancet,* October 27, p. 5.

Erickson, M. T. (1968). MMPI comparisons between parents of young emotionally disturbed children and mentally retarded children. *Journal of Consulting Clinical Psychology, 32,* 701–706.

Farber, B. (1959). Effects of a severely mentally retarded child on family integration. *Monographs of the Society for Research in Child Development, 24* (Serial No. 71).

Farber, B. (1960). Family organization and crisis: Maintenance of integration in families with severely retarded children, *Monographs of the Society for Research in Child Development, 25* (Serial No. 75).

Farber, B. (1968). *Mental retardation: Its social context and social consequences.* Boston: Houghton Mifflin Co.

Farber, B. (1975). Family adaptations to severely mentally retarded children. In M. Begab & S. Richardson (Eds.), *The mentally retarded and society: A social science perspective.* Baltimore: University Park Press.

Fotheringham, J. B. (1970). Retardation, family adequacy and institutionalization. *Canada's Mental Health. 18*(1), 15–18.

Friedrich, W. N. (1979). Predictors of the coping behavior of mothers of handicapped children. *Journal of Consulting and Clinical Psychology, 47,* 1140–1141.

Graliker, B. V., Koch, R., & Henderson, R. A. (1969). A study of factors influencing placement of retarded children in a state residential institution. *American Journal of Mental Deficiency, 74,* 50–56.

Hill, R. (1958). Generic feature of families under stress. *Social Casework, 39,* 3–9.

Hitzling, W., Loop, B., Lyons-Ross, K., & Miller, H. (1976). *Respite Services Community Development Project, Project Description.* Omaha, NE: Center for the Development of Community Alternative Service Systems.

Holroyd, J. (1974). The Questionnaire on Resources and Stress: An instrument to measure family response to a handicapped member. *Journal of Community Psychology, 2*(1), 92–94.

Holroyd, J. & Guthrie, D. (1979). Stress in families with neuromuscular disease. *Journal of Clinical Psychology, 35,* 734–739.

Holroyd, J., & McArthur, D. (1976). Mental retardation and stress of the parents: A contrast between Down's Syndrome and childhood autism. *American Journal of Mental Deficiency, 80*(4), 431–436.

Holt, K. S. (1958). The home care of severely retarded children. *Pediatrics, 22,* 746–755.

Jacobs, J. (1974). *The search for help: A study of the retarded child in the community.* New York: Brunner/Mazel.

Joyce, K., Singer, M., & Isralowitz, O. (1983). Impact of respite care on parent's perception of quality of life. *Mental Retardation, 21*(4), 153–156.

Kerschner, J. R. (1970). Intellectual and social development in relation to family functioning: A longitudinal comparison of home vs institutional effects, *American Journal of Mental Deficiency, 75,* 276–284.

Levinson, R. M. (1975). *Family crisis and adaptation: Coping with a mentally retarded child.* Unpublished doctoral dissertation, University of Wisconsin-Madison Department of Sociology.

McAllister, R., Butler, E., & Lei, T. (1973). Patterns of social interaction among families of behaviorally retarded children. *Journal of Marriage and the Family, 35,* 93–100.

McCubbin, H., Joy, C., Cauble, E., Comeau, J., Patterson, J., & Needle, R. (1980). Family stress and coping: A decade review. *Journal of Marriage and the Family, 42*(4), 855–870.

McCubbin, H., & Patterson, J. (1983). Family stress adaptation to crises: A double ABCX model of family behavior. In H. McCubbin, M. Sussman, & J. Patterson (Eds.), *Social stresses and the family: Advances and developments in family stress theory and research* (pp. 39–60). New York: Haworth Press.

Mederer, H., & Hill, R. (1983). Critical transitions over the family life span: Theory and research. In H. McCubbin, M. Sussman, & J. Patterson (Eds.), *Social stress and the family* (pp. 39–60). New York: Haworth Press.

Menolascino, F. J. (1977). *Challenges in mental retardation: Progressive ideology and services.* New York: Human Sciences Press.

Mercer, J. R. (1966). Patterns of family crisis related to reacceptance of the retardate. *American Journal of Mental Deficiency, 71,* 19–32.

Moore, C., & Seachore, C. (1977). *Why do families need respite care? Building a support system.* (Report prepared for the Montgomery County Respite Care Coalition and the Maryland State Planning Council on Developmental Disabilities.)

Moroney, R. (1980). *Social services and social policy: The issue of shared responsi-*

bility (DHHS Pub. No. ADM 80–846). Washington, DC: U.S. Government Printing Office.

Salisbury, C., & Griggs, P. (1983). Developing respite care services for families of handicapped persons. *Journal of the Association for the Severely Handicapped, 8*(1).

Stone, N. D. (1965). Family factors in willingness to place the Mongoloid child. *American Journal of Mental Deficiency, 72,* 16–20.

Townsend, P. W., & Flanagan, J. J. (1976). Experimental pre-admission program to encourage home care for severely and profoundly retarded children. *American Journal of Mental Deficiency, 80,* 562–569.

Upshur, C. C. (1983). Developing respite care: A support service for families with disabled members. *Family Relations, 32,* 13–20.

Warner, P. (1978). *Respite care: A family resource service.* (Report prepared for the State of Wisconsin, Division of Policy and Budget, Division of Health and Social Services.)

Warren, R. C. (1981). *For this respite, much thanks . . . Concepts, guidelines and issues in the development of community respite care services.* New York: United Cerebral Palsy Association.

Wikler, L. (1981). Chronic stresses in families of mentally retarded children. *Family Relations, 30,* 281–288.

Wikler, L. (1986). Periodic stresses in families of older children with developmental disabilities. *American Journal of Mental Deficiency,* May.

Wikler, L., & Hanusa, D. (1980). *The impact of respite care on stress in families of mentally retarded children.* Paper presented at the American Association for Mental Deficiency Annual Convention, San Francisco.

Wikler, L., & Stoycheff, J. (1975). Babysitters as community resources used to maintain retarded children in the home, *Exchange, 3*(1), 24–48.

Wikler, L., Wasow, M., & Hatfield, E. (1981). Chronic sorrow revisited: Parent vs. professionals depiction of the adjustment of parents of mentally retarded children. *American Journal of Orthopsychiatry, 51*(1), 63–70.

Wilcoxon, F., & Wilcoxon, R. A. (1964). *Some rapid statistical procedures.* New York: American Cyanamic Co.

Wolfensberger, W. (1967). Counseling the parents of the retarded. In A. A. Baumeister (Ed.), *Mental retardation: Appraisal, education and rehabilitation* (pp. 329–400). Chicago: Aldine Publishing Co.

Chapter 14

Assessing the Impact
of Respite Care Services
A REVIEW OF
OUTCOME EVALUATION STUDIES

James Intagliata

Evaluation and research data have played an important, if not essential, role in the development and survival of many human services programs. In the field of developmental disabilities in particular, outcome evaluation studies have provided information that has shaped and given continued life to such key programmatic initiatives as deinstitutionalization and mainstreaming. Unfortunately, although respite care services are widely believed to provide a crucial support to both individuals with developmental disabilities and their families, the evaluation data that could substantiate the beneficial impacts of respite care, enhance its effectiveness, and be used to justify its continued existence and expansion are extremely limited both in amount and sophistication (Cohen & Warren, 1985; Slater [Chapter 4]; Wikler, Hanusa, & Stoycheff [Chapter 13]).

This chapter has three main objectives. The first is to provide a conceptual framework within which outcome evaluation questions regarding respite care services can be systematically formulated and interrelated. The second is to identify where those evaluation studies that have been conducted to date fit within this framework and to assess the nature and quality of the evaluative information they have generated. The third and final objective of the chapter is to identify the crucial gaps that currently exist in our evaluation data base on respite care and to describe the types of studies that are needed to fill these gaps.

THE EVALUATION CONTEXT

According to Knutson (1969), evaluation efforts may be undertaken for a variety of reasons, including:

1. To determine whether or not a program is developing in the right direction
2. To determine whether a program is meeting the needs for which it was designed
3. To obtain evidence that might help in demonstrating the effectiveness of a program
4. To compare different program methods or approaches in terms of their relative impact
5. To justify past or projected expenditures
6. To gain support for program expansion

As is probably apparent from the wording of several of these possible motivations for conducting evaluation efforts (e.g., numbers 3, 5, and 6) evaluators are sometimes firmly committed to a program and personally convinced of its value and effectiveness before ever systematically examining it. This is a common reality of the political context of many evaluation and research efforts. In those situations where the individuals evaluating the program also happen to be carrying it out or are otherwise clearly advocates for it, it is particularly important that the evaluation be conducted in an objective fashion that does not predetermine its outcome. This is essential if the results are to be viewed as credible by the intended audiences of the evaluation effort. This objectivity is also crucial if the results obtained from the evaluation are to be genuinely constructive in helping those delivering the program or service to do so more effectively or efficiently. The same points apply with equal weight in those cases where an external party is conducting the evaluation of a program, especially if that party is perceived to have already decided that the program's funding should be reduced or discontinued before the data are gathered.

In keeping with the objective of setting an even-handed context within which to conduct an evaluation effort, the author would identify an additional reason for doing an evaluation in addition to the six already described above. This is:

7. To identify those factors both internal and external to the program or service that facilitate or inhibit it in making its intended impacts

This motive for conducting an evaluation has several important characteristics. First, rather than presupposing that the given program or service is effective or ineffective from the start, it presupposes only that there is a legitimate need for the program and that those providing the service are attempting to meet this need. Second, it is oriented to generating new information that will help program providers understand what is occurring. If the program is working well it will help identify those factors that are most responsible for this success. Alternatively, if the program is ineffective it will attempt to identify what is impeding its success. Finally, because the focus is on generating an understanding of *how* the program is working, rather than merely labeling it a success or failure, this approach is developmental in nature and can greatly assist its providers in reshaping or strengthening the program so that it meets its objectives more effectively.

AN EVALUATION FRAMEWORK

The conceptual framework that is used in this chapter to discuss outcome evaluation of respite care services in the developmental disabilities field has three major components:

1. *Independent variables* that include those factors that are clearly under the control of program providers and that define the respite intervention itself (e.g., amount and frequency of respite, in-home versus out-of-home models)
2. *Intervening variables* that are contextual in nature and that moderate or influence the nature and degree of the program's effects on those receiving it (e.g., the availability of other out-of-home services for clients, the family's own natural support system)
3. *Outcome variables* that include intermediate outcomes (e.g., reduced numbers of hours that parents must care for their developmentally disabled child), as well as ultimate outcomes (e.g., reduced levels of stress, improved family functioning)

Salisbury (Chapter 10) addresses many of these factors and their potential relationship to the integration of persons with disabilities into generic community services. Attainment of primary and secondary respite program objectives can be evaluated using the three component model.

Figure 1 graphically portrays this conceptual framework and identifies the variables that will be considered in this chapter.

Independent Variables

There are a variety of variables that can be used to describe and characterize respite care services. Each of these variables represents an important dimension on which programs vary one from another. To the extent that these variables are under the control of the individuals administering or evaluating the respite care program, they can be viewed as independent variables. The

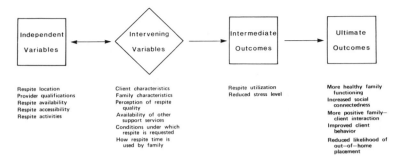

Figure 1.   Respite care evaluation framework.

clearest case for treating them as independent variables would be in evaluation studies where they are purposefully manipulated to assess how such variation influences program outcomes. Regardless of whether or not they are intentionally manipulated, it is important that these variables be considered when conducting an evaluation. If for no other reason than to provide an accurate description of the respite program, data on the following independent variables ought to be gathered as part of any evaluation effort:

1. The location in which respite is provided
2. The qualifications of the respite care providers
3. The availability of the respite care to families
4. The accessibility of the respite care to families
5. What activities take place between the respite care provider and client during respite

Each of these variables is discussed in relation to findings in the current evaluation literature, as well as with regard to their place within any evaluation of respite care services.

Location   Much attention has been paid in the respite care literature to the first variable to be considered; namely, the location in which respite care is provided. Respite care services have been and continue to be provided in a wide array of different settings. In general, these settings fall into two categories, in-home and out-of-home respite care. In-home care involves an individual coming into the residence where the client and family currently live and supervising or serving as a companion to the developmentally disabled individual. Out-of-home respite care may take place in a variety of different settings, including the homes of respite care workers, foster care homes, group homes, nursing homes, and institutions.

The location in which respite care is made available is an important program characteristic to consider when evaluating respite care services. One example of how the location variable can influence the outcome of a respite program is suggested by the fact that parents of persons with developmental disabilities generally prefer to use in-home rather than out-of-home respite care services (Brickey, 1982; Cohen, 1980; Hagen, Reasnor, & Jensen, 1980; Upshur, 1982). Given that such a preference exists, one would expect that the location in which respite services are made available would strongly affect the degree to which a program's services are utilized. Further, to the extent that location affects the level of participant utilization, it may in turn also affect the amount of overall program impact.

It should be noted that there are certainly circumstances in which the characteristics of the clients, the families being served, or the purpose for which the respite care is being sought would result in parents preferring out-of-home rather than in-home respite. Which of the two location alternatives is, in fact, preferred is not so much the issue here. Rather, the main point is that families do have preferences regarding respite care location and that these preferences will affect levels of respite utilization. Consequently, the service location(s) that any respite program offers is an important program characteristic that must be taken into account when conducting evaluations.

Provider Qualifications A second group of independent variables that characterize the nature of the respite services being offered and that need to be considered in evaluating respite care programs relate to the qualifications of the individuals who are providing the respite care that families are utilizing. According to a nationwide survey of respite care programs conducted by the Association of Retarded Citizens (1982), 80% of programs require providers to take part in training programs before being approved or certified to deliver respite care. These training programs vary widely in length and in topics covered, but participants are typically given information regarding the causes and consequences of developmental disabilities, meeting basic care needs of clients, responding to safety needs and emergency situations, and the use of general principles of behavior management.

The matter of a provider's qualifications is an important factor to consider in evaluating respite care programs for two major reasons: 1) These qualifications can influence a family's perception of the quality of the respite care offered, which can in turn influence the likelihood of using respite, and 2) these qualifications are likely to influence the nature and quality of interaction that takes place between the provider and the developmentally disabled person during respite. The relevance of this latter point is made clear in an evaluation study described by Wikler, Hanusa, and Stoycheff (Chapter 13). They evaluated a respite care program that required providers to receive specialized training in behavior modification techniques and principles. This type of training was essential because: 1) the program offered respite specifically to families whose developmentally disabled child had significant behavioral problems and 2) the respite time was used by the care provider to work with the client in pretargeted behavioral areas. In this case, the qualifications of the providers not only made the parents more amenable to trusting the providers with their children but also made it more likely that the clients would directly benefit from respite care time. Clearly provider qualifications can be a potent variable to consider when evaluating respite care programs.

Availability A third group of independent variables to consider in evaluating respite care programs relates to the availability of the respite care services offered. There are several aspects of availability. Perhaps the aspect most commonly thought of is the amount of respite that a family is allowed to use over a certain period of time. In the cases where already established respite programs are being evaluated, families usually have an upper limit on the number of hours that they can use, especially if the cost of respite is subsidized. However, families participating in such programs typically use widely varying amounts, anywhere from no time up to the maximum allowed by the program. In other situations where the respite care program is established as part of a systematic research effort, the number of respite hours that are used may be set at a fixed level to which families agree as part of their participation (e.g., see both studies described by Wikler et al. in Chapter 13). This latter approach is particularly useful for learning how respite care works because it can assess the impact of respite: 1) provided at a level that researchers believe significant enough to be likely to have its intended effects, or 2) provided at two different levels that vary widely enough to show correspondingly different levels of impact.

A second aspect of availability relates to the reasons for which the participating families can legitimately request respite. These reasons may be specifically defined in given programs. For example, some programs may provide respite only in situations judged to be emergencies, whereas others may exclude the use of respite in order to allow a parent to work outside the home. Clearly, the reasons for which respite is allowed to be used (if, in fact, they are defined by a program) will likely influence utilization of the service and the type of impact it can potentially make. As noted by Cohen and Warren (1985), the specific limitations imposed by respite care programs on the use of respite by participants may result in some programs being capable of preventing stress, whereas others will be relegated to serving only a crisis intervention function.

A final aspect of availability relates to the times of day, days of the week, or duration that respite care is made available. Some programs, for example, provide all types of respite care, including on weekday days or evenings, weekend days or evenings, and in any amounts ranging from merely an hour or two up to several weeks. This aspect of availability, as with the others already described, can influence not only levels of respite utilization but also the types of functions that respite serves and the effects it can have.

Accessibility   A fourth set of independent variables that need to be considered when evaluating respite services relate to accessibility. As with availability, accessibility has multiple aspects. These include location, cost, and immediacy of response. Regarding location, the distance in time and/or miles between the family and respite is likely to affect the level of respite use. Cost too can be a major factor that makes respite care more accessible to one family than to another (Hagen et al., 1980). As noted by Cohen and Warren (1985), the Developmental Disabilities Council of Louisiana reported in 1978 that 41% of respondents indicated that, if they had to pay anything for respite care services, they would have difficulty using them.

A final aspect of accessibility to be considered is the responsiveness of a respite program to the needs of families. Some respite programs require families to preschedule respite care, giving providers considerable lead time to make arrangements. Other programs have considerably more flexibility and are able to respond quickly to family emergencies. The degree of responsiveness of individual respite programs is a variable that can significantly influence the level of participant utilization, as well as the nature of impacts that the respite care can have (Hagen et al., 1980; Chapter 13).

Respite Activity   A final independent variable to consider when evaluating respite care programs relates to what actually takes place between the respite care provider and the client during respite care periods. Interestingly enough, many respite care program descriptions or evaluation reports do not even address this variable. One guess as to why this is so is that most program providers seem to view respite primarily as a service for the parents. Thus, if any attention is given to the matter of what takes place during respite, it more typically is focused on how the parents or other family members make use of their relief time. Although this is an important consideration that is discussed in the next section of this chapter, what takes place between the provider and the person with developmental disabilities is also a key feature that defines the nature of the respite care service being offered.

What takes place during respite is a relevant variable for two primary reasons. First, it can influence parents' perceptions of the quality and value of respite care and thus affect their likelihood of utilizing it. Second, if client-related outcomes are a concern of the program, what takes place between provider and clients during respite is crucial.

One approach to characterizing the respite activity is simply to let the time be relatively or totally unstructured with the client simply having his or her needs met by the provider in a reactive, responsive manner. This approach would result in great variability between what takes place during one respite visit and another. Other approaches might utilize the time that respite care providers and clients spend together in order to accomplish specific client-related objectives. One example of such an approach was described by Wikler and her colleagues in Chapter 13 this book. Their project used respite care time to have a provider systematically work with a client who had significant behavioral problems in order to improve the client's behavioral control.

Respite care time could just as easily be used to accomplish a variety of other behavorial growth objectives with clients, provided that those giving the respite care are trained appropriately in instructional techniques. The notion of utilizing respite care time to engage the client in either structured programming or in special recreational activities is an alternative that appeals to a number of families (California Institute on Human Services, 1982). The appeal of this approach to respite would be even stronger in those locales where the general availability of out-of-home programming for clients is limited.

Intervening Variables

Intervening variables are those that are generally not under the direct control of program providers and evaluators but that nevertheless can have a profound influence on the degree of impact, if any, that respite care services have on developmentally disabled persons and their families. Although in some cases, certain of these variables may be controllable by program providers and thus became independent in nature, the following list provides examples of variables that are typically intervening in nature and that need to be considered when evaluating respite care programs:

1. The demographic and functional characteristics of the developmentally disabled person served
2. The demographic and functional characteristics of the families served
3. The family's perception of the quality of respite care being offered
4. The availability of other programs and support services needed by client and family
5. The conditions under which family members request respite
6. How family members use their time when receiving respite

Client Characteristics   The client characteristics that have most frequently been reported as influencing the provision of respite care include age, the degree of physical or medical handicap, and the severity of behavioral problems. Findings regarding the influence of these client characteristics have not generally been related directly to the outcome or impact of respite services. Instead, these client characteristics have more often been discussed only to the degree that they affect the availability of respite care for families and the level of its utilization. Results of studies to date have indicated that the provision of respite care is often limited and, in many areas, nonexistent for families whose developmentally disabled son or daughter has serious physical handicaps, serious medical needs, and/or serious emotional or behavioral problems (Apolloni & Triest, 1983; Association for Retarded Citizens, 1982). Despite the relatively more limited availability of respite programs to serve more difficult client populations, there have been a number of demonstrations that programs can be designed to serve these individuals effectively using in-home models of respite care (e.g., Upshur, 1982; Chapter 13).

The other finding related to the influence that client characteristics can have on respite care programs is that, when respite is made available to a general population of families, those whose sons or daughters are more se-verely retarded, more dependent in functioning, more multihandicapped, or who have the most severe behavioral problems are likely to be the heaviest users of these services (Cohen, 1980; Halpern, 1982). Although this is not a particularly surprising finding, it is important to keep it in mind when trying to assess the outcomes associated with any given respite program's serving a sample of families. The reason is that levels of utilization of respite within any given sample of families are likely to be skewed toward those with more difficult clients, unless the level of utilization is fixed at a specific level for all families as part of a program's operating principles. If families with the most difficult clients are trying to cope with the highest levels of stress, the most positive outcomes revealed in an assessment of impact may not occur with those individuals who are using the most respite.

Family Characteristics A second set of variables that may intervene to influence the type or degree of impact that a respite care program has relate to the families being served. These include such variables as the families': 1) demographic characteristics, 2) initial levels of stress, 3) initial levels and styles of function/dysfunction, and 4) degree of available natural support.

Regarding demographic characteristics, findings have indicated that 1) families in which the mother was older tended to make greater use of services (Cohen, 1980) and 2) families living in rural areas are less likely than those in urban areas to be interested in receiving respite care services and are more likely to prefer and request hands-on specialized services for their chil-dren with developmental disabilities (Brickey, 1982; Home Aid Resources Program, 1978, cited in Slater [Chapter 4]).

For a number of reasons, the initial level and sources of family stress are also important intervening variables to consider when evaluating the impact of respite care programs. First, if a significant reduction of family stress is an intended outcome of a respite program, this effect may be relatively more difficult to demonstrate if the initial levels of stress in the families being served are relatively low. Second, although there is evidence that families with high levels of initial stress are likely to be the heaviest users of respite services offered by a program (Cohen, 1980; Halpern, 1982) their stress level may be so high that the provision of respite alone may not be a powerful enough intervention to improve the situation significantly. This is particularly likely to be the case for those families whose sources of stress are multiple and include factors that are independent of the level of burden associated with caring for the developmentally disabled child. Additional significant stresses that may be totally uninfluenced by the provision of respite care include a family income that is below the poverty level, the presence of a number of other siblings who also require significant levels of care, and other assorted stressful life events that may impinge on a family. It may be unrealistic to expect that respite care, even in significant amounts, could counteract such a variety of stressors.

Another important set of intervening family variables relates to the initial levels and styles of function or dysfunction that are present in the families being served. Families, as a result of their levels and styles of functioning, are differentially disposed to experience the potentially positive impacts of using respite care. As noted by Cohen and Warren (1985), some long-term family adjustment patterns may be not only dysfunctional but also largely intractable. If these functioning patterns are impervious to the impact of respite care services and are a major source of stress and dysfunction in the family, respite services are highly unlikely to have any dramatic ameliorative impact.

The final group of family characteristics that may function as intervening variables influencing the outcome of providing respite care relates to the amount and types of support that are already being provided to families by their natural social networks. The availability of natural support to a family can be influential in at least two major ways. First, there is good evidence that those families with relatively larger and stronger support networks are less likely to use the services of a respite care program that employs providers with whom the family does not already have a personal relationship (Brickey, 1982; Halpern, 1982). Second, those families who already use a significant amount of support from an existing natural network and who, in addition, have the support of a formal respite care program to supplement as needed may be more likely to reach a noticeable level of stress relief than those families who must rely solely on a formal respite service system.

It is particularly relevant to consider the evidence and arguments made by Slater in Chapter 4 in discussing the relationship between family support networks and respite care programs. Families, and not just those in rural areas, prefer to use family network members to provide respite care, rather than agency-trained respite care workers. She also suggests that family support initiatives may be most effective when they enable families to meet their daily concerns in as normalized a fashion as possible by helping families to develop or build on already existing natural support networks to meet their needs.

In this regard, it is relevant to note the model of respite care developed by the University Affiliated Facility (UAF) for Developmental Disabilities based at the University of Missouri at Kansas City. This model (C. Calkins, personal communication, March, 1985) is based on family members identifying individuals whom they already know (relatives, neighbors), recruiting them to be trained and certified as respite care providers, and then providing the families with subsidies to assist them in reimbursing these providers for the respite care they provide. Thus, the respite program builds on, rather than usurps, the role of families' natural support networks as a resource in helping them meet their needs.

Perception of Quality   Another key intervening variable that is likely to affect or influence outcomes associated with respite care services is the families' perception of the quality of respite care being offered. This variable has its primary impact by influencing the degree to which families actually make use of the respite care services that are available, with services perceived as higher quality being utilized more frequently (Hagen et al., 1980; Halpern, 1982; Upshur, 1982).

The factors that are likely to influence this perception of quality include the training and experience of respite care workers, their personality traits, and the degree to which there is a good match between the style and values of respite care workers and the particular families served. According to a study conducted by Cohen (1980), behavioral characteristics that differentiated significantly between respite care workers who had been rated at the top versus the bottom of the group by their supervisors included dependability, outlook, judgment, consideration, stability, flexibility, cooperation, supportive communication with clients, client assistance skills, household management skills, and routine medical management skills.

Although this list of characteristics is useful information, it cannot be assumed that respite care supervisors and parents share the same perspective or set of values when rating respite care workers. Further, the issue of match between respite worker and the particular client and family he or she is serving is crucial. In this regard it is relevant to once again point to the respite care model developed by the UAF at the University of Missouri at Kansas City. In this model, respite care workers go through their training along with the parents and clients to be served. Parents are able to actually see the skills and styles of the various respite care workers who will be available before they utilize their services formally. Thus, parents, clients, and respite care providers have an opportunity to "feel each other out" as part of the training process. This reduces the need for trial-and-error learning that would otherwise have to take place during subsequent utilization of the respite care program.

Availability of Other Services   Another set of intervening variables that can influence the impact of a respite care program relates to the availability and utilization of support services other than respite by developmentally disabled persons and their families. Although respite services play a key role, they cannot substitute for other direct services needed by clients (e.g., skills training, occupational therapy, behavior management programs) or support services needed by their families (e.g., family training, family counseling, homemaker services). The relative degree to which these other service needs of clients and their families are being met may greatly influence the contribution that is felt when respite care is offered.

Ideally, there would be funding available to provide the entire panoply of needed services to all clients and their families. When funding constraints force choices between services, however, families themselves may judge that providing key resource therapies to their developmentally disabled son or daughter will be more effective in reducing their stress and anxiety than will the provision of respite care in the absence of these resource therapies. Although such trade-offs may be undesirable, they are almost inevitable with a publicly funded service system that is under the pressure of fiscal restraint.

Reasons for Requesting Respite Another set of intervening variables that influence the outcome of respite care relates to the reasons why families choose to request respite care. A study conducted by the Developmental Disabilities Council of Louisiana (1978) indicated that parents were nearly twice as likely to request and use respite services as a means for providing relief from a crisis situation as they were to use it for more routine needs, such as getting out of the house for an evening or taking a vacation. Aanes and Whitlock (1978) reported on an institution-based respite program that families used primarily for the purpose of taking vacations. Sometimes parents make a point to link up with a respite care program, but subsequently make little or no use of it because they view it primarily as an emergency back-up in case they ever *really* need help (Intagliata, Gibson, & Rinck, 1984).

Knowing the types of felt needs that trigger parents' requests for respite care services is important when evaluating the impact of a respite care program. For example, even if respite care services are made available in considerable amounts and in a responsive fashion, families are not likely to experience the potential impacts of respite—preventing stress and normalizing family life—if they wait until they are at or near the breaking point before requesting help.

As noted by a number of authors, families' guilt about using respite services for relief is often a barrier to their appropriate use of respite (Intagliata et al., 1984; Slater, Chapter 4). This guilt, in fact, probably needs to be addressed directly with parents as part of any training or orientation they might receive when becoming part of a respite care program. Conducting frank and open discussions about the reluctance that many parents feel about using respite may be a helpful way to encourage those families who are in dire need of support to ask for it before things begin to fall apart.

Use of Respite Time A final set of intervening variables that influence the impact of respite care services relates to how the family members who are relieved of their caring responsibilities make use of the respite time. Examples of how this time is used include rest and relaxation, going shopping, visiting friends, dealing with special needs of other siblings, and entertainment and recreation (Cohen & Warren, 1985). Knowing how parents and other family members use their respite time is important for understanding what sort of ultimate outcome or benefits can be expected from the respite care being provided. For example, if an intended outcome of a respite program is to have families reduce their social isolation and extend their social support networks, this is unlikely to happen if they spend their respite care time in solitary activities.

Respite care is a very generic type of intervention for families. What particular outcomes are realized by individual families will depend on the reasons for which they request it and the particular ways in which they make use of their relief time. It would be quite helpful, in fact, for parents participating in respite programs to be encouraged to think through the variety of ways that they can use their respite and to choose activities that are most effective in helping meet their most pressing needs.

Outcome Variables

There are a wide variety of outcomes that have come to be associated with the provision of respite care to developmentally disabled persons and their families. Although the weight and quality of evidence that exists to support the claims that respite care services produce these results are uneven at best, those advocating for the development and expansion of respite care services often promise that the following types of outcomes will be produced if their programs are funded:

1. Respite care services will be heavily utilized by the families to whom they are offered.
2. Levels of stress experienced by family members will be reduced, and their mental health and quality of life will improve.
3. Family dysfunctional patterns will diminish, and more healthy functioning will emerge.
4. The family will become less socially isolated and more socially active.
5. Parents will develop more positive attitudes toward their developmentally disabled son or daughter.
6. The behavior of the developmentally disabled person will improve.
7. The likelihood of out-of-home placement, especially institutionalization, will be reduced.

This section of the chapter assesses the extent to which there is evidence that respite care produces these outcomes and discusses how previously described independent and intervening variables are likely to influence whether such outcomes are actually realized.

Utilization of Services The degree to which respite services are utilized is a key variable that must be considered in any evaluation of a respite care program. Whether it is an independent, intervening, or outcome variable, however, depends somewhat on the design of the evaluation being conducted. In those cases where service utilization levels are fixed at a set number of hours that all families participating in the program must use, service use is an independent variable. The two studies described by Wikler and colleagues in Chapter 13 are examples of this type of evaluation. A slight variation on this model would be to elaborate the design somewhat and offer a different level of respite care to two different groups of parents (e.g., 50 hours versus 25 hours per month). Clearly, this approach is much more appropriate in a research context than in simply evaluating already established respite programs on their effectiveness.

The most common way in which service use has been treated as a variable in the respite evaluation literature to date, however, is as an outcome variable. As an outcome variable, the level of respite care use is a dependent measure that can vary from one family to another. Some evaluation reports seem to treat utilization level as an end in itself and interpret large numbers of respite hours requested and used as an index of program success. Although such use does provide evidence that helps substantiate claims that families are in need of respite, level of use is probably more appropriately viewed as an intermediate, rather than ultimate, program outcome. Utilization of respite care services is a meaningful index of program success only to the extent that this utilization can be linked to the range of beneficial impacts on clients and family members that are frequently promised by respite program providers and advocates.

Even when treated as an intermediate, rather than ultimate, outcome measure, however, level of respite utilization is a key variable that needs to be well understood when conducting evaluations of respite care programs. As described in earlier sections of this chapter, a variety of factors seem to influence the extent to which families utilize respite care services. These factors include such independent variables as the characteristics of the respite program itself, including where respite services are offered, the characteristics and qualifications of providers that are used, the availability and accessibility of the respite care, and the type of activities that take place with the client as part of the respite. Level of respite care use is also influenced by such intervening variables as the level of demand and stress that caring for a particular client has on his or her family, the family's attitudes regarding respite care use, the family's perception of the quality of respite care offered, and the degree to which the family's needs for support and relief are already being met by existing natural support networks.

In Chapter 4 Slater gives evidence of very uneven use of respite care by families, with nearly half of the families in one study (Apolloni & Triest, 1983) failing to use their full allocation and nearly half in another study (Halpern, 1982) using respite only once or twice. A great deal remains to be learned to ensure that respite is used in a fashion that makes it most effective.

As an intermediate outcome for respite programs, one natural question about utilization level is, "How does the amount of respite used relate to the degree of benefit experienced by families?" One hypothesis would be that those who use respite the most show the most positive outcomes. The evidence regarding this hypothesis is distinctly mixed. Cohen (1980) found that, when users of respite were contrasted with nonusers, the users were more likely to report improvement in family functioning, but were also more likely to be considering or planning out-of-home placement. In a study by Joyce, Singer, and Isralowitz (1983), positive impacts were noted for families receiving respite, but there was no significant relationship between number of hours received and overall ratings of improvement in life quality. Finally, Intagliata et al. (1984) reported that, although 25 families using a respite care program did not show significant improvements in levels of stress and mental well-being when considered as a single group, subdividing the sample by level of utilization revealed that those making greatest use of the program had shown improvement, whereas those using low/moderate levels of respite had not reduced their stress level or improved their mental well-being significantly.

The relationship between level of respite utilization and degree of beneficial impact realized is clearly complex. First, some families need greater amounts of respite than others, and all that may ultimately matter is that the amount received, regardless of its absolute level, matches the level of family need. Another factor confusing the issue at present is that most evaluation studies have not assessed the extent to which the families served in the programs evaluated are using other sources of respite and relief to meet their needs. Thus, high users of a program's respite service may have no additional respite available and show limited gains, whereas low users may have multiple alternative sources and show the most dramatic gains. It is unlikely that we will be able to understand the relationship between levels of respite care use and program outcomes without utilizing experimental designs that allow certain key variables (e.g., level of family need, extent of existing support networks) to be controlled systematically.

Levels of Stress One outcome that is typically associated with the provision of respite care and that is often explicitly highlighted by those developing respite programs is that the levels of stress in family members, especially that of the primary care provider, decrease as a result of respite care use. There are two important questions to ask regarding reduced stress as a respite care outcome: 1) What evidence is there that respite actually does reduce stress levels?, and 2) even if this outcome is achieved, what is its significance?

At this point in time, there is no solid or convincing empirical evidence that the provision of respite care reduces stress in family members. One of the most significant problems is the lack of sophistication with which stress has been measured. This problem has two aspects: 1) the choice of an appropriate stress measure, and 2) how and when the stress measures are employed. The most common approach to measuring stress has been to ask family members to rate how, if at all, their stress has changed as a result of receiving respite services. Generally, these ratings have been done at only one point in time, usually after respite has been used for a specified period. Although this approach (Halpern, 1982; Joyce et al., 1983) has resulted in families reporting stress reduction due to respite care, such evidence of positive program impact on stress levels is suggestive at best.

Two recent studies have either employed somewhat more sophisticated stress measures or have measured stress levels at more than one point in time. Wikler et al. (Study 2 cited in Chapter 13) had respite care providers rate the stress levels (a scale of 1 to 6) of the families they were serving after each of 10 respite care visits. Although such an approach has the built-in bias of the caregivers doing the ratings, at least the use of multiple ratings over time is a step in the right direction. If one uses a criterion of a change of at least 2 points on this 6-point scale as an indication of significant change, 5 of the 10 families assessed in the Wikler study showed noticeable stress reduction, whereas the others maintained the level of stress. In the same study, Wikler and her colleagues also used Holroyd's (1974) Questionnaire on Resources and Stress in a pre/post fashion. Results indicated significant positive changes on two subscales (less negative attitudes toward the child, less difficulty perceived in the child's characteristics) and significant negative changes on two others (felt lack of social support, felt lack of activities for the client). What the sum balance of these changes is on families' subjective experience of stress is difficult to determine.

Intagliata et al. (1984) used two measures of stress, both on a pre/post basis with a sample of 24 families using respite care over a period of 6 months. One was a simple rating scale, on which mothers rated their own level of stress on a scale of 1 to 5 before entering the respite program and then again after 6 months of participation. In addition, mothers completed (on a pre/post basis) the Bradburn Affect Balance Scale (1969), which assesses both positive and negative affects experienced by the respondents in the past 2 weeks. The report of negative affects on this scale has been strongly associated with individual's seeking supportive mental health services, whereas positive affects are treated as a measure of perceived quality of life. As discussed earlier, Intagliata and his colleagues found no significant changes in these measures over time for the sample as a whole. However, those families who used the greatest amounts of respite care were more likely to report reduced levels of subjectively rated stress, increased positive affect, and decreased negative affect when compared with low to moderate level users of respite.

Although the two more recent studies offer somewhat better methodologies for assessing changes in levels of stress, there is a need to conduct an experimental study with random assignment and a control group in order to develop more convincing evidence that respite services do reduce stress. In addition, results from both these studies suggest that even if respite can facilitate stress reduction it does not do so for all families. There is a need to explore which factors facilitate or inhibit respite from achieving its desired effect of stress reduction. As suggested in the earlier sections of this chapter, these factors may include initial levels of family stress, the sources of the stresses with which families are struggling, the availability of resources other than respite for families to reduce their stress, and the degree to which families make effective and health-enhancing use of their respite care time.

The other important question regarding stress reduction is why this change is a significant area to assess. In a very real sense, stress reduction can be viewed as more of an intermediate, rather than an ultimate, outcome with regard to respite care programs. Although reducing stress is an important objective to be met, the real significance of such an impact is that it leads to other key desired outcomes. Specifically, it is generally hoped that because of reduced levels of familial stress other more dramatic and important consequences follow. These include such benefits as improved physical and mental health and quality of life of family members, increased likelihood of families remaining intact, and decreased likelihood of families seeking out-of-home placement. If such changes do not follow from stress reductions, one could justifiably argue that the reduction in stress achieved has little practical significance. To date, the evaluation literature on respite care programs has had enough difficulty documenting stress reduction by itself and has had much less success evaluating these stricter, more dramatic outcome indices.

Family Functioning Another outcome often associated with the provision of respite care services is improved family functioning. Examples of ways in which this general notion of improved family functioning has been operationalized in evaluation studies of respite care programs include family members reporting: 1) getting along better with each other (Joyce et al., 1983), 2) being able to maintain their sanity (Halpern, 1982), 3) improved marital relations (Wikler et al., Chapter 13), 4) family regenerative power (Halpern, 1982) and 5) improved relationships with family members and more hope about the family's future (Cohen, 1980).

Just as with other respite evaluation studies already discussed, none of the above studies utilized a control group, and only the Halpern (1982) study employed its operationalized measure of improved family functioning in a pre/post fashion. Results from these studies are mixed, with significant positive results reported by three of the studies using retrospective, subjective measures of improved family functioning (Cohen, 1980; Halpern, 1982; Joyce et al., 1983). On the other hand, the Wikler et al. study (Chapter 13) found that 57% of subjects reported no change in marital relations, 9% reported negative changes, 20% reported mixed changes, and only 14% noted positive changes. Furthermore, the Halpern (1982) study found that, when users of respite services were contrasted with a comparison group of non-users, the users showed no significantly greater gains in regenerative power as a result of their receiving respite care.

Overall, improved family functioning is an outcome that has been imprecisely defined and inadequately operationalized. As with other outcomes discussed, it would be useful to assess the impact of respite care on family functioning using a truly experimental design. Further, even if those studies already conducted had indeed provided dramatic evidence of enhanced family functioning due to respite, it would remain the challenge of the authors to account for how providing respite care had produced such an outcome. This is where the importance of understanding intervening variables comes into play. Family dysfunction is a complex phenomenon that can be linked to established, if not entrenched, routines and patterns that may be largely intractable. It remains for us to learn what contribution respite services can make in enabling families to function in a more healthy fashion and to identify what other types of services or interventions are needed to help families make positive changes. At a minimum, respite care frees families and gives them time to do something other than child care. What they do with that time, however, may be the most crucial factor in determining the type and degree of benefits that are realized.

Social Isolation   Another outcome associated with providing respite care to families is that it may enable them to become more socially active and reduce their social isolation. Several studies have assessed social relations outcomes associated with respite care use. Wikler et al. (Study 2, Chapter 13) found that 53% of participants in a respite care program reported positive changes in social relations and 42% reported no change based on a retrospective self-report of participants. In Study 1 conducted by the same authors and also described in Chapter 13, the five participants receiving respite care reported ''going out'' one to two times more per month as a result of respite care. Finally, Joyce et al. (1983) found that participants in a respite program reported that their time for social activities and leisure had increased.

At best, the results of these studies are suggestive that respite care has the potential to improve the social activity level and social relations of families who receive it. If, indeed, reduced social isolation or enhanced social connectedness is the aim of respite care programs, these outcomes must be operationalized more specifically in future studies so that program success on this dimension can be better assessed. Further, as was just described with regard to the objective of enhancing families' healthy functioning, it is doubtful whether respite care as a solitary intervention is likely to produce significant positive changes in a family's social relationships. If changes of this type are desired, it may be wise to supplement respite care with other programmatic interventions that are designed specifically to help families build and enhance their natural support networks.

Attitudes toward Persons with Developmental Disabilities Another outcome sometimes associated with the provision of respite care services is that family members' attitudes toward the person with developmental disabilities become more positive. Several studies have included this outcome in their assessment efforts. Using retrospective subjective reports provided by program participants, Joyce et al. (1983) found that participants reported relating better to their disabled child, and Cohen (1980) found that users of respite care reported that their attitude toward the child had improved. Wikler et al. (Study 1, Chapter 13) used a pre/post test approach with the Itkin Scale to measure quantitative changes in parental feelings about their mentally retarded child and found no consistent changes, either in a positive or negative direction. Interestingly, parents in the same study had reported a significant *increase* in positive attitudes toward their child when it was assessed using an open-ended question. In Study 2, Wikler and her colleagues (Chapter 13) again assessed changes in parental attitude toward their handicapped child in a pre/post respite fashion using Holroyd's (1974) QRS scale. As described earlier in this chapter, there were significant decreases in parents' negative attitudes toward the child and in their perception of the difficulty of his or her personality characteristics.

As for many of the other outcome measures already discussed, findings related to changes in attitudes toward the developmentally disabled family member are generally positive. However, the methodology used to assess the changes is generally weak. Suggestions for strengthening the assessment of this important outcome area include routine use of pre/post measures; use of quantitative measures, such as the appropriate subscales of Holroyd's (1974) QRS; and the inclusion of family members other than mothers (e.g., father, siblings) when assessing family attitude changes. Furthermore, it would be helpful for program providers and evaluators to delineate better why improved attitudes toward the child is a meaningful objective. If the reason is that such improved attitudes will result in other key consequences, such as higher expectations for the child, more parental energy devoted to skill development, decreased likelihood of seeking out-of-home placement, and so forth, then these hoped-for consequences should be made explicit and measured along with the attitudinal changes.

Improved Client Behavior This is an outcome that is discussed somewhat less frequently than the others, but is still relevant in assessing the variety of possible outcomes associated with respite care. The only study reviewed that specifically assessed behavioral changes in the client was conducted by Wikler et al. (Study 1, Chapter 13). In this study respite services were provided to families whose developmentally disabled child had significant behavioral problems. Results indicated that all children either improved or maintained their initial level of problem behavior. Although it is interesting to consider the possible behavorial impacts that providing respite care can have on the client, the degree to which significant change is a realistic expectation would depend greatly on: 1) the amount of respite being provided (it must be considerable) and 2) the systematic nature with which respite care time is used by the provider to work with the child on specific skill areas. Perhaps it is somewhat more realistic to approach respite care time as an opportunity for the provider to build on or be consistent with the skill-building behaviors already being focused on by parents and other family members, rather than viewing it as a separate training-focused intervention in and of itself.

Decreased Likelihood of Out-of-Home Placement Of all the outcomes associated with respite care programs, the promise that respite care will help prevent institutionalization is perhaps the most dramatic. As such, it is one that is frequently mentioned when supporters of respite programs are trying to persuade legislators and other funding sources to support respite care. Funding respite care is presented as a way not only to support families but also to save money. There is no question that this is a very attractive promise to make for any program. What evidence do we have that this promise is warranted? Unfortunately, very little.

On a case-by-case basis, the existing evidence consists of the following:

1. *Pagel and Whitling (1978)* reported in a study of 22 cases in which clients from natural homes were readmitted to an institution that the most frequently given reason was lack of respite care.
2. *Joyce et al. (1983)* reported that, of a sample of 32 families actively using respite over a 4-month period, 30% reported that they would not be able to care for their son or daughter at home without respite care.
3. *California Institute on Human Services (1982)* reported that, of a sample of 98 parents using respite care services in California, 47% said they would have to consider out-of-home placement if respite were unavailable.
4. *Cohen (1980)* reported that, of 107 respite care users surveyed, 29% felt

that they "would not have been able to cope" without respite. However, when the user group was compared with a control group of 35 nonuser families, a significantly higher proportion of user families indicated that out-of-home placement (not necessarily to an institution) was likely.

In summary, the positive evidence that respite care reduces the likelihood of out-of-home placement is generally weak and based on either indirect evidence (Pagel & Whitling, 1978) or on parents' hypothetical speculation of the probable consequences of discontinuing the respite care services they were receiving when surveyed. In the only study in which a group using respite services was contrasted with a nonuser comparison group (Cohen, 1980), users were actually more likely to indicate out-of-home placement as a high probability. Although Cohen and Warren (1985) attribute this finding to the larger proportion of older (over age 18) clients in the user group, the users were *not* any less likely than the nonusers to consider out-of-home placement when the sample was restricted to only those families with clients under 18 years of age.

Clearly, if those promising that respite care reduces institutionalization and out-of-home placement were challenged to provide solid supporting evidence for their assertion, they would be hard pressed to do so. Until we are able to conduct a longitudinal study involving an experimental and control group (one receiving respite, the other not), it will be difficult to support this assertion empirically. In the meantime, advocates of respite care services should be cautious about attempting to develop support for their programs by highlighting the promise of reduced placement pressure, an outcome that, although the most dramatic of those benefits associated with respite care programs, may also be the one with the least empirical evidence to support it.

CONCLUSIONS AND RECOMMENDATIONS

Evaluation studies have an important role to play in the continued development and refinement of respite care services in this country. There is no question that respite care is a valuable support service needed by many families with developmentally disabled members. However, a great deal remains to be learned about the kinds of benefits that respite care can realistically be expected to produce, as well as which contextual factors facilitate or inhibit these benefits from being realized.

We cannot afford to ignore the call for not only more respite care evaluation studies but also for a higher level of quality in such studies. There has been and will continue to be a great deal of competition for the shrinking amounts of public dollars available to fund a wide array of important human services. As a result, those advocating for respite care services may not only be pressed to provide better evidence of how effective and important those services are but also to convince funding agencies that respite care represents a more effective investment of dollars than other, perhaps equally needed, service programs.

As was made clear in this chapter, the existing literature of outcome studies of respite care services is generally weak and fails to address a number of important issues adequately. If the quality of future evaluation efforts in the respite care area is to be significantly enhanced, those conducting such evaluations will need to address the following points:

1. The design of respite care evaluations ought to be guided by broader conceptual frameworks that not only take client, family, and programmatic factors into consideration but that also identify the particular outcomes that respite care is intended to produce. The framework offered in this chapter is an effort in this direction.

2. Respite care evaluations should be influenced by and be consistent with current relevant psychosocial theories, especially those relating to family structure and functioning, stress at both an individual and familial level, and the role of social support and other constructive mechanisms for coping with stress. Greater attention to these theories and to their supporting research literatures can aid respite care providers and evaluators in identifying program outcomes that are more realistically achievable and explainable.

3. Far greater sophistication must be demonstrated in selecting and designing the measures to be used in respite care evaluation. It simply is not sufficient to measure levels of stress by asking individuals to rate how much stress they are experiencing on a scale from 1-to-7. Similarly, how well a family is functioning as a whole must be assessed in a more sophisticated fashion than merely asking a family member to rate his or her perception of family functioning on a scale ranging from very poor to excellent. There are many excellent measures of stress, mental well-being, anxiety, and family function/dysfunction. Respite care evaluators, however, must be willing to search beyond the relatively limited developmental disabilities literature to find these measures.

4. Evaluators must work with respite care program designers and providers in order to have the opportunity to control key program variables when conducting an evaluation study. Efforts must be made to conduct studies with true control (no respite) groups to determine program impacts more powerfully and reliably. When this is not possible, the use of comparison groups that differ on key program dimensions (e.g., number of hours of respite received) can be an attractive alternative. Further, evaluation designs must begin to administer measures at multiple, rather than single,

points in time in order to do a better job of assessing change. At the very least, measures should be administered on a pre/post basis as an alternative to relying on program participants' retrospective judgments of how respite care has affected them.

5. Evaluators must do a more thorough job of assessing the broader context within which a respite care program is operating. It is essential, for example, to be mindful of such variables as: 1) the degree to which a family is meeting its needs for respite through natural support networks independent of a specific respite program in which they participate, and 2) the degree to which the developmentally disabled client is engaged in needed programs and services outside the home. Such factors as these can greatly influence the magnitude and types of impacts that a respite care program has on participating families.

6. Much more attention needs to be given to assessing the impact of providing respite care on the individual with developmental disabilities. The majority of evaluations conducted to date have focused on the effects on parents or the family as a whole (as perceived by parents). What type of impact respite care makes on the individual client will, of course vary greatly depending on how often respite is provided and what occurs during respite times. The collection of data regarding the impact of respite care on developmentally disabled persons may be particularly crucial to programs whose funding agencies see their primary role as serving these individuals, rather than their family members (see Chapter 15 by Castellani).

7. Evaluators must wrestle with the difficult issue of the time frame over which certain intended respite care outcomes can be achieved or demonstrated. For example, if the outcome being assessed is a significant change in family functioning patterns that have developed over many years, how much sense does it make to look for substantive change after 6 months of participation in a respite care program? Similarly, how does one demonstrate that respite care programs reduce rates of institutionalization or out-of-home placement without doing a longitudinal study? Clearly, if we hope to assess whether respite care programs produce some of their most potential dramatic benefits, the time frame over which the respite must be provided and the evaluation conducted must be considerably longer than is currently the norm in the respite evaluation literature.

There are two final issues that deserve consideration not only from those evaluating respite care but perhaps even more so from those designing and providing respite care programs. The first issue relates to the variability in the degree to which families are ready not only to request respite care but also to use their respite care time in ways that help them achieve desired program outcomes. If respite care program providers intend to achieve certain objectives, such as stress prevention or reduced social isolation for participating families, they may need to do more than simply make respite care available. They may, for example, have to work actively with families to help overcome psychological barriers (e.g., guilt) that may deter them from using respite care in situations that are not clearly crises or emergencies. If reducing families' social isolation is an intended outcome, program providers may have to assist parents in learning how to use their respite time in ways that will increase their likelihood of expanding their social networks and perhaps even provide some training in social interaction skills. In order for respite care to produce some of the outcomes that many program providers expect or promise, respite care may itself need to be supplemented by additional supportive services in order to maximize its potential benefits for participants.

The second issue is that respite care must be viewed as only one of a wide range of supportive services that families with a developmentally disabled member may need. Chapter 4 by Slater makes this point quite effectively. There are a variety of other family support services (e.g., homemaker services, financial assistance, family training) that can assist families in experiencing the same outcomes that are associated with respite care—reduced levels of stress and enhanced quality of life. Although respite may make an important contribution regarding these outcomes, its benefit may be enhanced greatly if families are also receiving the supplemental forms of assistance and support that they need.

In conclusion, respite care program administrators and evaluators must address a number of significant issues if respite care programs are not only to continue to expand but also to demonstrate their effectiveness and value more clearly. This chapter has attempted to describe these issues and to offer some suggestions and recommendations regarding how they can be addressed. Respite care has an important role to play in assisting persons with developmental disabilities and their families. If respite program administrators and evaluators take the steps needed to meet the challenges they are facing, it is these individuals and families who will reap the benefits.

REFERENCES

Aanes, D., & Whitlock, A. (1978). A parental relief program for the mentally retarded. *Mental Retardation, 13*(3), 36–38.

Apolloni, A. H., & Triest, G. (1983). Respite services in California: Status and recommendations for improvement. *Mental Retardation, 21,* 240–243.

Association for Retarded Citizens (1982). *Characteristics of respite care programs.* Arlington, TX: Author.

Bradburn, N. M. (1969). *The structure of psychological well-being.* Chicago: Aldine Publishing Co.

Brickey, M. (1982). *Preliminary report on respite care needs in four Appalachian counties.* Athens: Ohio University.

California Institute on Human Services. (1982). *Respite services for Californians with special developmental needs.* Sacramento: California State Council on Developmental Disabilities.

Cohen, S. (1980). *Final report: Demonstrating model continua of respite care and parent training services for families of persons with developmental disabilities.* New York: City University of New York, Graduate School, Center for Advanced Study in Education, Education Development Center.

Cohen, S. & Warren, R. (1985). *Respite care: Principles, programs and policies.* Austin, TX: Pro-Ed Publishers.

Hagen, J., Reasnor, R., & Jensen, S. (1980). *Report on respite care services in Indiana.* South Bend: Northern Indiana Health Systems Agency.

Halpern, P. L. (1982). *Home-based respite care and family regenerative power in families with a retarded child.* Ann Arbor, MI: University Microfilms International.

Holroyd, J. (1974). The Questionnaire on Resources and Stress: An instrument to measure family response to a handicapped member. *Journal of Community Psychology, 2*(1), 92–94.

Home aid resources program (1978). Olympia, WA; Washington Division of Developmental Disabilities.

Intagliata, J., Gibson, B., & Rinck, R. (1984, May). Evaluating the impact of respite care on respite utilization and family well-being. Paper presented at the Annual Conference of the Association on Mental Deficiency. Minneapolis, MN.

Joyce, K., Singer, M., & Isralowitz, R. (1983). Impact of respite care on parents' perception of quality of life. *Mental Retardation, 21,* 153–156.

Knutson, A. A. (1969). Evaluation for what? In H. C. Schulberg, A. Sheldon, & F. Baker (Eds.), *Program evaluation in the health fields.* New York: Behavioral Publications.

Louisiana Developmental Disabilities Council. (1978). *Agency and parent needs assessments (respite care).* Baton Rouge: Louisiana State Planning Council on Developmental Disabilities.

Moos, R. H., Insel, P. M., & Humphrey, B. (1974). *Family environment scale.* Palo Alto, CA: Consulting Psychologist Press.

Pagel, S. E., & Whitling, B. (1978). Readmissions to a state hospital for mentally retarded persons: Reasons for community placement and failure. *Mental Retardation, 16*(2), 164–166.

Upshur, C. C. (1982). An evaluation of home-based respite care. *Mental Retardation, 20,* 58–62.

Chapter 15

DEVELOPMENT OF RESPITE SERVICES
POLICY ISSUES AND OPTIONS

Paul J. Castellani

Respite is clearly the most salient among the family support services that have attracted attention in the field of services to people with developmental disabilities. Advocacy for these services has increased among parents, and both parents and professionals have worked to develop a variety of programs to provide respite services. Often these programs have been responses to local needs and manifestations of local resources and service patterns. Increasingly, policymakers have been establishing and implementing policies and programs that deal with statewide and service-system-wide issues and problems in this area.

The purpose of this chapter is to discuss some of the central issues that must be addressed in developing policies and programs to enhance the availability and accessibility of respite services. Following a brief review of some recent history that is instructive for the future direction of policy, the chapter examines the many emerging approaches and problems from the perspectives from which policymakers most often deal with these issues. Specifically, this chapter considers the development of statewide respite policy and programs in terms of these questions:

What policy objectives are expected to be achieved?
What specific services will be provided?
Who will receive respite services?
How will they be delivered?
How will respite services be financed?

RECENT HISTORY OF RESPITE SERVICES

An appreciation of the development of respite care programs can be gained by considering them in the context of the development of general family support services. A number of services in addition to respite care typically comprise the family support services framework. These services include transportation, recreation, information and referral and parent training. The development and provision of these services have helped facilitate the large-scale deinstitutionalization of developmentally disabled people in the past 10 to 15 years (Scheerenberger, 1975).

The manner in which family support services became the focus of attention in the field of services to developmentally disabled people is particularly significant for the consideration of respite services. Initially, the question of the availability and accessibility of important community-based support services for people with developmental disabilities was not raised nor addressed very effectively by those administering the large-scale movement of these people from large institutions to community-based residences. Several studies of deinstitutionalized individuals subsequently pointed out that those so-called generic services were not generally available or, if available, were not accessible to people with developmental disabilities or their families. The absence of those support services was shown to be related to reinstitutionalization and lack of success in community living (Bachrach, 1981; Braddock, 1981; Bruininks, 1979; Gollay, Friedman, Wyngaarden, & Kurtz, 1978; Intagliata, Krauss, & Willer, 1980).

The support services that were available and accessible to developmentally disabled people, such as diagnosis and evaluation, speech therapy, or physical therapy, were often provided as an adjunct to their day programs, such as sheltered workshops or clinic services (New York State OMRDD, 1983). Indeed, these day services were largely developed to accommodate those individuals who had been deinstitutionalized. Many of these services, such as transportation and recreation, were provided directly to individuals who had been placed in community residences and were more accurately "placement support services." Overall, the need for family support services first became apparent to policymakers when their absence was shown to be related to reinstitutionalization, although the overwhelming majority of people with developmental disabilities live at home with their families and often need the same services. To a large degree, support services to those living at home have been developed subsequent to and with less resources than services for deinstitutionalized individuals. Therefore, services that have become widely known as family support services were initially and largely developed as placement support services. This historical perspective continues to be important for the future development of these services because it affects such policy concerns as who is to receive family support services and what objectives are expected to be achieved through their delivery. These concerns are especially important with respect to respite services because they are largely oriented toward families with a developmentally disabled family member living at home.

POLICY OBJECTIVES

When the family becomes the primary focus of services, as in such family support services as respite, an important policy shift is involved. The objectives policymakers are asked and seek to achieve with the provision of respite programs change in important ways. Salisbury and Griggs (1983) define respite care as "planned or emergency care provided to the disabled individual in or out of the home, for the purpose of providing relief to the family from the daily responsibilities of caring for a developmentally disabled family member" (p. 51). Although this definition raises the question of who is the recipient of respite services, a more overarching issue of policy objectives must first be addressed.

Respite services represent a departure from the primary and fundamental thrust of developmental services; namely, the welfare of the developmentally disabled person. A service that is aimed primarily at the welfare of the family of the disabled person creates an important new set of complexities and ambiguities that permeate the policy response to demands for respite care. Others have addressed this problem by linking respite and other family support services more closely to the welfare of the disabled family member. For example, Agosta, Bradley, Jennings, Feinberg, and Gettings (1984) propose that the goals of these services are: 1) to strengthen the family structure to enhance the quality of care families provide to a developmentally disabled member, and 2) to prevent undue out-of-home placement. This formulation seems to narrow the policy objectives somewhat, although there is little evidence that clearly and directly links the provision of respite services to either the strengthening of family structure, quality of care, or prevention of out-of-home placements. As more attention is directed at respite services, the assumptions that those linkages exist will be increasingly challenged as policymakers consider whether respite services represent an expansion in policy focus from developmental services to family policy in general.

Policymakers have been attuned to programs that have been designed to address the individual developmental needs of disabled people. Despite some ambiguities about clientele, those individuals are relatively identifiable, the interventions and resources required to address their needs are understood, and the expected developmental outcomes are reasonably well articulated. The goal of ''strengthening the family structure'' involves major uncertainties for policymakers, at least those in this particular policy arena. The needs of parents, siblings, and other family members must be taken into account, and doing so obviously increases the number of people to be served. Moreover, the resources required to serve them are uncertain, and the desired policy outcome, ''strengthened families,'' is an ambiguous one with which policymakers in the field of developmental disabilities have little experience or expertise. Even legislators who have been responsive to demands for respite programs have informally expressed concern for the implications for ''family'' policy. Ultimately accountability will be required for resources expended, and those operating these programs are likely to find it extremely difficult to provide reliable information to demonstrate that families have been strengthened.

WHAT SPECIFIC SERVICES CONSTITUTE RESPITE?

The questions—what specific services constitute respite and where they are delivered—involve several policy problems that must be addressed in enhancing the availability and accessibility of respite. One of the primary issues is the locus of service; the distinction between in-home and out-of-home respite is a major one that is usually made in examining these services. Whether respite services are delivered day/evening or overnight and whether they are specifically developed or a secondary outcome of other programs are other major sets of policy considerations.

Although parents generally prefer that overnight (as well as other types) of respite services be provided in their home, the bulk of capacity for overnight respite is in institutional settings (OMRDD, 1984). Developmental centers, community residences, and community-based Intermediate Care Facilities (ICFs) are more restrictive than home settings (Salisbury & Griggs, 1983), but other natural family homes or free-standing respite centers are relatively scarce sources of overnight respite and tend to be in great demand on weekends and underutilized on weekdays. More restrictive rate-setting methodologies, regulations on use of these facilities, and concerns that use of temporarily vacant beds in group homes is not appropriate, further limit capacity for out-of-home respite. Moreover, those congregate care facilities do not typically serve young children or adolescents for whom services are very much in demand (OMRDD, 1983). Overall, overnight respite is a very costly option.

The development of respite services in the day and evening hours involves other policy problems. One of the most salient issues is the trade-off between service to single or multiple families. For example, homemaker and chore services are typical of single family service and have been the primary type of in-home services in New York State. In order to meet the increase in demand for sitter/companion-type respite services, a family's need for a one-to-one service will have to be more carefully evaluated and probably limited to cases where few alternatives exist. A more cost-effective way to increase services to meet the larger demand, especially for families without special problems in mobility, will undoubtedly involve greater use of group respite settings and services.

Weekend and early evening drop-in and recreation programs are examples of this mode, but their development encompasses other problems. Schools, churches, neighborhood centers, and other locations that would seem to be likely sites for group respite are often not readily available. The cost of utilities and after-hours maintenance staff, as well as liability insurance concerns, has hampered the development of group respite services in those places even when staff and other program resources have been available. Public policy initiatives in the form of revised guidelines on the use of public facilities, pool liability insurance, and logistical support are required to foster enhancement of this mode of respite services.

In summary, the diversity of services encompassed within the respite framework presents a variety of policy problems. It is becoming clearer that, as the demand for respite services increases and more specific programs are designed and implemented, a number of important policy choices will have to be made concerning what services are to be delivered in what settings.

WHO WILL RECEIVE RESPITE SERVICES?

The issue of eligibility for respite services is one of the most crucial and troublesome policy issues in this area. The resolution of this issue requires that strategic and operational problems be first addressed.

At the strategic level, the goal articulated for respite—that is, ". . . providing relief to the family from the daily responsibilities of caring for a developmentally disabled family member." (Salisbury & Griggs, 1983, p. 51) represents a substantial departure from the primary focus of the developmental services system, the disabled individual. As the demand for and delivery of respite services becomes more prominent, the anomaly inherent in this policy goal is likely to become more problematic. When the needs of the family become a policy objective, policymakers must deal with a possible exponential increase in those served and a clientele whose needs for respite are related to but must be determined independently of the needs of the disabled individual.

The criteria for services have, to this point, been almost exclusively based on the disabled person's needs. A wide variety of assessment tools are available to ascertain a disabled person's developmental deficits and service requirements. However, the goals of enhancing a family's capacity to provide quality of care at home and prevention of out-of-home placement require that we be able to identify and measure the familial and situational characteristics that affect those outcomes.

Several of these familial and situational characteristics have been suggested in the growing body of literature in this area. In addition to the level of disability experienced by the disabled person, these characteristics fall into three main categories: age, family structure, and limitations on access to services (Tausig & Epple, 1982). Age encompasses a variety of concerns. It is becoming apparent that families experience crises that affect their ability to cope with a developmentally disabled member at a number of stages in the life cycle, including: 1) the period around the birth of a developmentally disabled child with the problems involved in identifying needs and obtaining early intervention services, 2) the period when a disabled child enters school, 3) adolescence, and 4) when a child "ages out" of school programs. Another important stress occurs when the increasing age of the parent(s) of a developmentally disabled person brings diminished physical or economic capacity to care for that individual at home. Family structure involves such factors as single-parent families, excessive stress caused by the presence of a disabled member, and the number and characteristics of other siblings or family members either requiring care or able to provide care. Access issues involve persons not currently enrolled in mentally retarded/developmentally disabled (MRDD) programs, and ethnic, racial, and language minorities who tend to be unserved and underserved by MRDD programs. Similarly unserved and underserved are persons with low-incidence developmental disabilities, such as autism and Prader-Willi syndrome, and families with low incomes or who are geographically and socially isolated from MRDD services (Downey, 1984). Although these familial and situational characteristics have been suggested as factors affecting a family's ability to care for a developmentally disabled member at home, it is extremely difficult to measure their impact and use them to establish priorities for respite services.

Bird's survey of family support services, including respite, in 17 states indicates that relatively few of these eligibility criteria have been employed in state programs (1984). Eight of the 17 states surveyed required that risk of out-of-home placement be established as a condition of service. Family income, used by 9 of the 17 states as a criterion, can be a surrogate measure for several of the other factors suggested in the literature. Otherwise, there was no direct inclusion of criteria that are linked to such needs of other family members as number of siblings, other members' need for care, capacities of parents or other family members to give care, or housing problems.

It is clear that, as states develop and implement respite programs, the issues of who is to be provided service will be central strategic and operational concerns. Substantially greater attention will have to be paid to devising explicit and equitable mechanisms for making choices among those demanding what are likely to be limited respite services.

DELIVERING RESPITE SERVICES

The question of how respite services are to be delivered is one of the most important emerging policy problems in this area. As indicated above, the bulk of respite services has been delivered as out-of-home short-term care in congregate care facilities and as homemaker-type in-home services. Overall, there have been few options, and families have had limited choice in the amount, type, source, and use of respite services.

An emerging issue concerns the structures of services and the mechanisms families can use to gain access to respite services. The degree to which families are empowered to exercise choice in the amount, type, source, and use of respite is another important policy issue.

As was pointed out earlier, many states began support services programs when it became apparent that people who had been placed out of institutions were returning or having problems because the so-called generic services that were expected to be available were not. States provided support services to families only as spin-offs of placement support services or in belated recognition of the needs of families caring for a developmentally disabled member at home. Thus, the progression has been to ensure first that those services that had been available in institutions were provided to individuals placed in the community and then attempt to make those services available to people living at home with their families. In many instances, these family support services are provided as direct service adjuncts to core residential and day programs (OMRDD, 1983).

The increasing demand for and use of respite and other family support services have raised several problems and concerns with the direct provision of services model. As experience grows, it is becomingly increasingly apparent that families are radically different from public residential care facilities, even those that are community-based. The structure of service delivery to all residential care facilities is primarily institutional, and the problems and opportunities families present seem to confound or be confounded by that structure.

The family is often the setting where family support services are provided. In many instances, the family is the provider of services. The family is also the consumer of services, and these roles often occur at the same time. Government regulations, policies, guidelines, and funding formulas do not typically or easily deal with the somewhat simultaneous overlap of roles that occurs in providing family support services, including respite.

One response to these problems has been to increase the array of respite services available in family support programs. However, this still results in a product-driven system. That is, families' choices are limited to the respite services made available by the state or agencies contracted to provide services.

Another response to these concerns is an increasing number of family support services programs employing cash subsidies and/or vouchers (Bird, 1984). Cash subsidies and vouchers, although limited in amount and occasionally to specific types of services, represent a substantial alternative to direct provision of services. They increase the discretion of the family and in light of the complexity of dealing with the family as provider and consumer, the simplicity of cash subsidy approaches may become more attractive to governments. It does seem, nevertheless, that the same political energy that is demanding more respite services is also resulting in greater demands for approaches and mechanisms that empower the family.

The answer to the question of how should we deliver respite services is obviously complex. These issues, perhaps more than any of the others involved in the entire area of family support services, are highly conditioned by each state's experience in delivering services to people with developmental disabilities and the political-economic environment in each state. New York State for example, has a large state-operated system of services, as well as a major voluntary agency role in the full range of services for people with developmental disabilities and their families. Local governments play a very limited role in the direct provision of developmental services, and there has been virtually no experience with vouchers or cash subsidies and little apparent movement in that direction. In contrast, Pennsylvania has had a very large family support services program for a number of years that operates largely through direct provision of services through county government. Other states are similarly conditioned by their history in this area.

Nevertheless, there are factors that seem either inherent to the nature of respite and other family support services or at work in the political-economic environment that will shape the direction of delivery of these services. These services are closely linked to the communities in which the needs arise, and it would appear that local governments will have to play an important role in managing and/or delivering them. The continuing pressure to contain government spending on social programs seems likely to create more pressure to increase the role of the private vis-a-vis the public sector in the area of family support services. Those cost pressures, as well as the generic character of many family support services, will also encourage greater integration of service delivery and less separate and parallel services specific to people with developmental disabilities.

The generally increasing role of proprietary for-profit providers in virtually all areas of human service delivery will undoubtedly be seen in family support services as well. Entrepreneurial opportunities are certain to increase to the degree that cash subsidies and consumer sovereignty in their use increase. As suggested earlier, the demand for cash subsidies, vouchers, and other mechanisms that tend to empower families seems to be emerging as a companion to the demand for these services in general. None of these observations should be especially surprising. However, taken together, they indicate that respite services represent an increasingly significant departure in the way in which services are provided to people with developmental disabilities and their families, and they may ultimately have a reciprocal effect on the entire system of services for disabled people.

FINANCING RESPITE SERVICES

The financing of respite services is obviously a central concern in this area. Moreover, it has been particularly important in the recent discussion and debate surrounding the Home and Community Care Waiver (Sec. 2716, PL 97-35) and the Community and Family Living Amendments of 1983 (S.2053), the Chafee bill.

Current Sources

Much of the discussion about respite services concerns strategies for increasing their funding levels. To some extent it ignores the current bases of funding, which are usually the best predictors of the future (Wildavsky, 1964). Moreover, this discussion also ignores some problems that threaten the current bases of funding respite services.

State tax levy dollars constitute the largest source of funding for respite and other family support services (Braddock, 1984). Despite the importance of the issues raised in the debates on S.2053 and the Home and Community Care Waiver, arguments for increasing the amounts of funding for these services should take into account the fiscal commitment made in each state to these services. Another important aspect of the issue that was pointed out by a study of family support services in New York State was that funds for these respite services were often not specifically identified or budgeted (OMRDD, 1983), although homemaker funds used for in-home day respite services were separately identified. That is, respite services were often provided as adjuncts to routine day and residential programs. In addition, many of these programs, including ICFs/MR, community residences, and day treatment programs, are supported in part with federal funds. Thus, at least some federal funds are used indirectly in respite services. Nonetheless, as rate-setting methodologies established tighter controls on the use of funds or as funding was constrained, the respite services that lacked an explicit fiscal rationale became increasingly vulnerable to cutbacks (Castellani & Puccio, 1984). It is very likely that the large number of states without explicit family support services programs may indeed fund respite services in similar ways, and they may be similarly vulnerable. Overall, the available information on the funding of respite services indicates that states themselves provide the bulk of funds for their support. Although there are some federal funds used at least indirectly to support respites, these programs are small and/or not explicitly identified in funding bases.

Sources for Additional Funds

As suggested above, there has been an extraordinary amount of discussion and debate around proposals that affect the sources of funding for additional respite family support services. Federal funds are seen by many as a primary source of support for these services. Since the mid-1960s when the federal government expended almost no funds on state developmental services, the fiscal participation of the federal government in this area has increased enormously (Gettings, 1980). Moreover, the overwhelming proportion of federal funds is devoted to ICFs/MR, and the majority of those funds to larger facilities of over 15 beds (Braddock, 1984). Overall, the federal government has assumed almost one-half of the cost of operating public facilities for the developmentally disabled, and that program is the fastest growing component of the entire Medicaid program (Fernald, 1984). Clearly, the enormous role of federal funds in this area has also focused attention there on sources of additional funds for respite and other family support services. Two proposals have been at the center of the discussion; specifically, the Home and Community Care Waiver and the Community and Family Living Amendments of 1983.

The Home and Community Care Waiver would allow a state to finance a community-based system of care by eliminating ICF/MR beds and reinvesting those funds in home and community-based services. The waiver has obviously been suggested as a vehicle to increase the availability of respite services. However, it is widely recognized that the waiver is intended to be a mechanism for cost containment (Fernald, 1984). The waiver formula requires that the number of Medicaid beneficiaries after the waiver be less than or equal to the number of beneficiaries before the waiver. Thus, there is a fiscal disincentive for states to use the waiver to expand and extend services to new recipients, particularly the large number of families caring for a disabled member at home and currently not receiving any services. Despite some initial enthusiasm about the prospects for expanding respite services through the Home and Community Care Waiver mechanism, state developmental disabilities agencies seem to be experiencing problems in designing, implementing, and continuing waiver programs.

The Community and Family Living Amendments of 1983 (Senate 2053), introduced by Senator Chafee, are intended to bring about a radical change in the states' fiscal incentives to use Medicaid funds for community vis-a-vis institutional services. In summary, the intent of the Chafee Bill would be to remove and/or create substantial fiscal penalties over time in the federal financial support for residential facilities serving over 15 persons. Since the initial introduction of the legislation there have been a variety of modifications and counterproposals that would generally soften its immediate impact on states with substantial institutional populations. Nonetheless, the intent of the proposal remains substantially the same. Supporters of the proposal argue that the impact of this legislation would be to force states to accelerate rapidly the phase-out of large institutions; conversely it would provide a large financial incentive for states to develop community and family support services programs, including respite. Opponents of the proposal have argued that size alone is not an adequate measure of quality of care and that the provisions for implementation create a differential and inequitable impact on states. Most opponents of the specific proposal, S.2053, do, nonetheless, tend to acknowledge the desirability of a community-based rather than institutional system of care.

Major public policy changes, such as those involved in the Community and Family Living Amendments, typically take place over a period of time, often a number of years. Nonetheless, there seems to be considerable energy within the MRDD field for changes in the general direction of the Chafee Bill. Moreover, there is substantial pressure being exerted by the federal government to contain Medicaid costs, and such proposals as S.2053 tend to complement those efforts in some important respects. Community and family support services are perceived to be less costly than institution-based services. Thus, there is a good possibility that a variation of S.2053 will ultimately be enacted, resulting in an increase of federally funded community-based and family support services.

States, as pointed out earlier, are currently the primary source of funding for family support services (Braddock, 1984). Thus, it would also seem likely that they will be a major source of additional funds. Indeed, the expansion of state-funded respite services programs indicates that these programs are one important area of new program development in the states (Agosta et al., 1984; Bird, 1984). The attention devoted to respite services suggests that programs in this area are likely to increase in number and size.

The role of local government in this area is uncertain. On the one hand, it is generally assumed that governments at this level that depend in large measure on property and sales taxes for revenues have neither the capacity nor willingness to fund respite and other family support services programs. However, some core family support services, such as transportation and recreation, are usually provided by local governments. Transportation is often crucial to the provision of respite services, and recreation is often an important source of secondary respite. Voluntary agencies that provide substantial amounts of these services also rely in part on funding from local government sources. Moreover, school districts, either as independent local entities or as components of municipal governments, are being pressed to provide more family support services, such as afterschool programs, as adjuncts to special education services mandated by PL 94-142. Thus, the role of local government in funding respite and other family support services has not been particularly prominent in discussions on this topic, but it seems that closer attention must be paid to the problems and opportunities of financing at this level of government.

Some attention has been paid to private sources of funding for respite services (Agosta et al., 1984), particularly the possibilities for inclusion of family support services in either privately purchased or employer-provided health insurance programs. The potentially large and usually long-term costs associated with services (including family support services) for persons with developmental disabilities tend to either confound basic insurance principle or prove to be prohibitively expensive (Kane & Kane, 1978). Proposals for publicly financed national childhood disability insurance (Gliedman & Roth, 1980) have not generated as much interest as direct government provided or funded services programs. Generally, the focus of attention for funding family support services has been on public rather than private sources.

Summary of Funding Issues

Discussions concerning the funding of services are typically complex. The specific issues and various mechanisms are indeed very often difficult for lay people and professionals to understand. These discussions often obscure the fundamental and relatively straightforward issues at stake: the connected questions of whether to fund an expansion of respite services and who will pay for these services.

Clearly, families caring for a developmentally disabled member at home have borne virtually the entire burden of cost, as well as care. The advocacy for increased public funding for these services is a political demand for socialization of the costs and risks (Lowi, 1979). Typically, the first priority in this process is to generate the political energy necessary to place the issue on the policy agenda. This seems to have been achieved to a considerable degree at the federal and state level. Next steps include the identification of funding opportunities. State funds themselves have been an initial and major source of funds for the development of respite services programs, and the energy and diversity associated with those programs are likely to result in an increase in their number and size.

The opportunity for using Medicaid funds for community and family support services, including respite, has become an overriding issue in the developmental disabilities field. Although advocacy for overall expansion of these programs continues, it seems that a major portion of the political energy is devoted to efforts to reallocate the institutional and community services shares of the Medicaid "pie." In light of the possibility that Medicaid funding will contract, the energy devoted to reallocating what is now available for developmental services may dissipate the political energy needed to increase funds available for all services, including respite services.

One final overarching concern in the area of funding respite services is the extent to which these services are items on the agenda for long-term care reform. Gettings (1980) and others have pointed to the need to broaden the base of funding services beyond a health base. Boggs (1981) points toward that direction in observing

> . . . a newly emerging constituency for long-term care, as earlier defined, appears to be making headway toward legislative reform, what is sought is an alternative funding stream for noninstitutional support services in which it will not be necessary to differentiate between homemakers or personal care givers by whether they earn "health" dollars or "social service" dollars. (p. 76)

It is apparent that most of the core family support services identified earlier, such as respite, transportation, recreation, counseling, homemaker services, and information and referral, are not especially MRDD-specific. It is likely, therefore, that funding for respite services may indeed be an important part of reform of long-term care.

CONCLUSION

When dealing with the often desperate needs of families caring for a member with a developmental disability, it is difficult to recognize that addressing those needs is the outcome of political processes. "Politics" is a term that occasionally has a pejorative connotation, and seems out of place in a field dominated by clinical practice and somewhat objective professional standards. Nonetheless, the answers to the questions *What policy objectives should be pursued?*, *What kinds of respite services should we provide?*, *Who will receive them?*, *How are they to be delivered?*, and *How should respite services be funded?* are fundamentally political questions. They involve choices that must be made in the policy process.

In many respects, the most crucial stage in the policy process has been reached. Respite and other family support services are on the policy agenda of the federal, state, and local level. Although important, it is not sufficient merely to be on the policy agenda, and a variety of difficult policy choices remain to be addressed. The degree to which broad or narrow ranges of respite services are identified will depend largely on the tactical opportunities available to advocates. The determination of who will be served is potentially one of the most divisive within the MRDD community as cleavages surface and become resolved among advocates for the previously and never institutionalized persons, individuals with various developmental disabilities, and groups that have been traditionally unserved and underserved by formal developmental services. The issue of how respite services are to be delivered may result in basic restructuring of the provision and use of social services and relationships between government and its clientele as families seek greater empowerment. Finally, the question of how respite services are to be funded will likely be part of a major reform of federal, state, and local fiscal responsibilities for long-term care. It is likely that the political energy that has put respite services on the policy agenda will also force the resolution of these issues in the near future.

REFERENCES

Agosta, J. M., Bradley, V. J., Jennings, D. M., Feinberg, B., & Gettings, R. (1984). *Family support programs for families with members who are developmentally disabled: Review of the literature with an emphasis on financial assistance strategies.* Boston: Human Services Research Institute.

Bachrach, L. L. (1981). A conceptual approach to deinstitutionalization of the mentally retarded: A perspective from the experience of the mentally ill. In R. Bruininks, C. Meyers, B. Sigford, & C. Lakin (Eds.) *Deinstitutionalization and community adjustment of mentally retarded people,* Washington, DC: American Association on Mental Deficiency.

Bird, W. A. (1984). *A survey of family support programs in seventeen states.* Albany: New York State Office of Mental Retardation and Developmental Disabilities.

Boggs, E. M. (1981). Behavioral Fisics. In J. J. Bevilacqua (Ed.), *Changing government policies for the mentally disabled,* Cambridge, MA: Ballinger Publishing Co.

Braddock, D. (1981). Deinstitutionalization of the retarded: Trends in public policy. *Hospital and Community Psychiatry, 32,* 607–615.

Braddock, D. (1984, February). *Statement on S.2053, The Community and Family Living Amendments of 1983.* U.S. Senate Finance Committee, Subcommittee on Health, Washington, D.C.

Bruininks, R. H. (1979). The needs of families. In R. H. Bruininks & G. C. Krantz (Eds.), *Family care of developmentally disabled members: Conference proceedings,* Minneapolis: University of Minnesota.

Castellani, P. J., & Puccio, P. S. (1984). *The development of family support services for the developmentally disabled: An administrative and political perspective.* Paper presented at the American Society for Public Administration National Conference, Denver, CO.

Downey, N. A. (1984). *Eligibility for family support services.* Albany: New York State Office of Mental Retardation and Developmental disabilities.

Fernald, C. D. (1984). *Too little too late: Deinstitutionalization and the development of community services for mentally retarded people.* Bush Institute for Child and Family Policy, University of North Carolina.

Gettings, R. M. (1980). *Federal financing of services to mentally retarded persons: Current issues and policy options.* Paper prepared for U. S. Office of Human Development Services.

Gliedman, J., & Roth, W. (1980). *The unexpected minority: Handicapped children in America.* New York: Harcourt Brace Jovanovich.

Gollay, E., Freedman, R., Wyngaarden, M., & Kurtz, N. R. (1978). *Coming back.* Cambridge, MA: Abt Books.

Intagliata, J., Kraus, S., & Willer, B. (1980). The impact of deinstitutionalization on a community-based service system, *Mental Retardation,* 305–307.

Kane, R. L., & Kane, R. A. (1978). Care of aged: Old problems in need of new solutions. *Science* 20, 913–919.

Lowi, T. (1979). *The end of liberalism* (2nd ed.). New York: W. W. Norton.

New York State Office of Mental Retardation and Developmental Disabilities (OMRDD). (1983). *Local services project: The provision of planning of support services Phase I report.* Albany, NY: Author.

New York State Office of Mental Retardation and Developmental Disabilities (OMRDD). (1984). *Respite services for developmentally disabled individuals in New York State.* Albany, NY: Author.

Salisbury, C., & Griggs, P. A. (1983). Developing respite care services for families of handicapped persons. *The Journal for The Association for Persons with Severe Handicaps, 8,* 50–57.

Scheerenberger, R. (1975). *Current trends and status of public residential services for the mentally retarded.* Madison, WI: National Association of Superintendents of Public Residential Facilities for the Mentally Retarded.

Tausig, M., & Epple, W. (1982). *Placement decision-making: A study of factors that lead to out-of-home placement.* Study Report 82-01. Albany: New York State Office of Mental Retardation and Developmental Disabilities.

Wildavsky, A. (1964). *The politics of the budgetary process.* Boston: Little, Brown & Co.

Chapter 16

PARENTS' PERSPECTIVES
FOCUS ON IMPACT

Noreen Quinn Curran

Each individual family member experiences personal issues regarding respite care, particularly regarding the access and implementation of respite services (e.g., issues of sibling rivalry, issues of care and personal responsibility, and issues of support, especially for the primary provider of care, but actually for all family members).

Our son, when young, loved the attention of the respite worker. This charming, engaging sibling, however, had to have some limits set or Christine's needs would have been eclipsed. Eventually, in Sean's preadolescence, the respite worker came to be perceived by him as a special person for Christine, whom he was graciously able to accept. There have been times in mid-adolescence, however, when he objects to a respite worker and feels he can and should take care of Christine himself. This feeling, I believe, should be encouraged in moderation, for we hope as he grows older that he develops a healthy attitude toward his involvement in her care.

Christine's father was somewhat resistant to respite care and uncomfortable with having strangers in our home. As I became more comfortable with utilizing respite services and the respite workers proved to be responsible, he began to accept respite as part of the family experience of raising a child with developmental disabilities.

Each family member's attention to working through these issues prepares them for more productive and fulfilling care of the family member with a disability.

IMPACT

Respite care provided me a chance for personal renewal and a renewed sense of family cohesiveness. The most important single impact of respite care was that the time away rejuvenated my marital relationship, my most important support system. I had renewed energy to deal with my children, particularly the child with special needs, in more loving and creative ways. Having new energy to invest in the various "systems" involved in my child's life as well as accomplishing some neglected household chores, was a side benefit. I gained a better perspective on all family members' needs, rather than having the handicapped child's needs overwhelm all others. The family's needs as a well-functioning unit were in sharper focus for me.

ADJUSTMENT PERIOD

When our children were younger, our return home after a break was followed by a short period of upset (1 to 2 days). Our children typically showed some anger because we parents were away. I often felt overwhelmed, adjusting to the everyday realities of living with a child with special needs. The transition became easier with more experience, with good respite services, and with more independence on my child's part.

SOME SUGGESTIONS FOR PARENTS

1. Use respite services. In Massachusetts, families are given an allotment by a legislative act. If families do not use respite services, the legislature or other governing body will most likely substantially decrease respite services.
2. Design your respite services so that they fit your needs, your family's needs and the needs of the child/adult with handicaps.
3. Use good babysitters for respite workers. They are a terrific resource, if they are age-eligible to serve. It would be well worth the effort to encourage your babysitter to apply to the agency and receive the necessary training as a respite worker. We parents are more likely to take advantage of respite if we feel very comfortable with the worker.
4. Listen to the sensitivities of your children. They will give you clues about the design the respite service must take to be as successful as possible for the whole family. For example, our teenage son does not feel comfortable with a respite worker in his home. His sister loves having a respite worker. We parents need it! So we ask him to try to arrange an overnight that night with friends.
5. Evaluate the experience informally after each respite so that you have information to use for the next planned respite. As in any good service or project, we design, implement, and evaluate for maximum benefit.
6. Plan your respite times. Know your needs for a break and plan them into

the family calendar. I have seen far too many middle-aged and older parents who have "burnt out" without respite as they cared for a young adult with moderate retardation. Nobody benefits in this situation. I've also seen a parent of a profoundly retarded child who, after finally taking advantage of respite and vacations, returned to her youthful, energetic, rational, and attractive self. Everybody benefits from that!

7. Do not wait for or expect your extended family to offer assistance so that you can take a break. If it is offered, it is a bonus, and enjoy it. For our needs, the nonemotional nature of the respite worker's relationship has made it easier for us to take a break than when we leave our children with family members. It is on our schedule at our request and is a more business-like arrangement than family dealings, which can get a little too emotionally tangled. The major caregiver needs a rest, not a relapse!

Harriet Horowitz Bongiorno

As I am writing this I am looking out the back window and gazing at a child's swing set, a swing set that was never used by Alan. My heart is aching. The question of "What might have been?" haunts me now as it has haunted me for the past 15 years. Would Alan be living away from home today had respite care been available? I love my son with all my heart and I wish that we had had more time together. Had some person, some organization or group come forth to offer us a helping hand we might have been able to postpone our decision to institutionalize our son for a few more years. Perhaps our families' ties would have been strengthened by the outreaching hands of others, and through the love and sharing of others perhaps our burden could have been shared. Allowing others to share in Alan's day-to-day care might have caused us to become more open with our friends and family, and instead of feeling totally isolated in our grief, perhaps we might have been able to share our experiences with other parents many years sooner.

To you, a parent of a handicapped child who might be reading this book, I can only offer this advice: Please try to understand that you are not alone in your grief, even though it may seem so at times. Many parents have walked the path that you are walking today. Do not be afraid or embarrassed to seek any type of help for yourself or your child or both. Respite care might literally be only a phone call away. It may not be a total solution to the problem, but perhaps by reaching out and seeking help you might be giving yourself and your child a few more years to grow together in love.

INDEX

Numbers in *italic* indicate illustrations or tables.